Intervention
Pulmonary Medicine

LUNG BIOLOGY IN HEALTH AND DISEASE

Executive Editor

Claude Lenfant

Former Director, National Heart, Lung, and Blood Institute
National Institutes of Health
Bethesda, Maryland

1. Immunologic and Infectious Reactions in the Lung, *edited by C. H. Kirkpatrick and H. Y. Reynolds*
2. The Biochemical Basis of Pulmonary Function, *edited by R. G. Crystal*
3. Bioengineering Aspects of the Lung, *edited by J. B. West*
4. Metabolic Functions of the Lung, *edited by Y. S. Bakhle and J. R. Vane*
5. Respiratory Defense Mechanisms (in two parts), *edited by J. D. Brain, D. F. Proctor, and L. M. Reid*
6. Development of the Lung, *edited by W. A. Hodson*
7. Lung Water and Solute Exchange, *edited by N. C. Staub*
8. Extrapulmonary Manifestations of Respiratory Disease, *edited by E. D. Robin*
9. Chronic Obstructive Pulmonary Disease, *edited by T. L. Petty*
10. Pathogenesis and Therapy of Lung Cancer, *edited by C. C. Harris*
11. Genetic Determinants of Pulmonary Disease, *edited by S. D. Litwin*
12. The Lung in the Transition Between Health and Disease, *edited by P. T. Macklem and S. Permutt*
13. Evolution of Respiratory Processes: A Comparative Approach, *edited by S. C. Wood and C. Lenfant*
14. Pulmonary Vascular Diseases, *edited by K. M. Moser*
15. Physiology and Pharmacology of the Airways, *edited by J. A. Nadel*
16. Diagnostic Techniques in Pulmonary Disease (in two parts), *edited by M. A. Sackner*
17. Regulation of Breathing (in two parts), *edited by T. F. Hornbein*
18. Occupational Lung Diseases: Research Approaches and Methods, *edited by H. Weill and M. Turner-Warwick*
19. Immunopharmacology of the Lung, *edited by H. H. Newball*
20. Sarcoidosis and Other Granulomatous Diseases of the Lung, *edited by B. L. Fanburg*
21. Sleep and Breathing, *edited by N. A. Saunders and C. E. Sullivan*
22. *Pneumocystis carinii* Pneumonia: Pathogenesis, Diagnosis, and Treatment, *edited by L. S. Young*
23. Pulmonary Nuclear Medicine: Techniques in Diagnosis of Lung Disease, *edited by H. L. Atkins*
24. Acute Respiratory Failure, *edited by W. M. Zapol and K. J. Falke*

For information on volumes 25–182 in the *Lung Biology in Health and Disease* series, please visit www.informahealthcare.com

183. Acute Exacerbations of Chronic Obstructive Pulmonary Disease, *edited by N. M. Siafakas, N. R. Anthonisen, and D. Georgopoulos*
184. Lung Volume Reduction Surgery for Emphysema, *edited by H. E. Fessler, J. J. Reilly, Jr., and D. J. Sugarbaker*
185. Idiopathic Pulmonary Fibrosis, *edited by J. P. Lynch III*
186. Pleural Disease, *edited by D. Bouros*
187. Oxygen/Nitrogen Radicals: Lung Injury and Disease, *edited by V. Vallyathan, V. Castranova, and X. Shi*
188. Therapy for Mucus-Clearance Disorders, *edited by B. K. Rubin and C. P. van der Schans*
189. Interventional Pulmonary Medicine, *edited by J. F. Beamis, Jr., P. N. Mathur, and A. C. Mehta*
190. Lung Development and Regeneration, *edited by D. J. Massaro, G. Massaro, and P. Chambon*
191. Long-Term Intervention in Chronic Obstructive Pulmonary Disease, *edited by R. Pauwels, D. S. Postma, and S. T. Weiss*
192. Sleep Deprivation: Basic Science, Physiology, and Behavior, *edited by Clete A. Kushida*
193. Sleep Deprivation: Clinical Issues, Pharmacology, and Sleep Loss Effects, *edited by Clete A. Kushida*
194. Pneumocystis Pneumonia: Third Edition, Revised and Expanded, *edited by P. D. Walzer and M. Cushion*
195. Asthma Prevention, *edited by William W. Busse and Robert F. Lemanske, Jr.*
196. Lung Injury: Mechanisms, Pathophysiology, and Therapy, *edited by Robert H. Notter, Jacob Finkelstein, and Bruce Holm*
197. Ion Channels in the Pulmonary Vasculature, *edited by Jason X.-J. Yuan*
198. Chronic Obstructive Pulmonary Disease: Cellular and Molecular Mechanisms, *edited by Peter J. Barnes*
199. Pediatric Nasal and Sinus Disorders, *edited by Tania Sih and Peter A. R. Clement*
200. Functional Lung Imaging, *edited by David Lipson and Edwin van Beek*
201. Lung Surfactant Function and Disorder, *edited by Kaushik Nag*
202. Pharmacology and Pathophysiology of the Control of Breathing, *edited by Denham S. Ward, Albert Dahan, and Luc J. Teppema*
203. Molecular Imaging of the Lungs, *edited by Daniel Schuster and Timothy Blackwell*
204. Air Pollutants and the Respiratory Tract: Second Edition, *edited by W. Michael Foster and Daniel L. Costa*
205. Acute and Chronic Cough, *edited by Anthony E. Redington and Alyn H. Morice*
206. Severe Pneumonia, *edited by Michael S. Niederman*
207. Monitoring Asthma, *edited by Peter G. Gibson*
208. Dyspnea: Mechanisms, Measurement, and Management, Second Edition, *edited by Donald A. Mahler and Denis E. O'Donnell*
209. Childhood Asthma, *edited by Stanley J. Szefler and Søren Pedersen*
210. Sarcoidosis, *edited by Robert Baughman*
211. Tropical Lung Disease, Second Edition, *edited by Om Sharma*
212. Pharmacotherapy of Asthma, *edited by James T. Li*

213. Practical Pulmonary and Critical Care Medicine: Respiratory Failure, *edited by Zab Mosenifar and Guy W. Soo Hoo*

214. Practical Pulmonary and Critical Care Medicine: Disease Management, *edited by Zab Mosenifar and Guy W. Soo Hoo*

215. Ventilator-Induced Lung Injury, *edited by Didier Dreyfuss, Georges Saumon, and Rolf D. Hubmayr*

216. Bronchial Vascular Remodeling in Asthma and COPD, *edited by Aili Lazaar*

217. Lung and Heart–Lung Transplantation, *edited by Joseph P. Lynch III and David J. Ross*

218. Genetics of Asthma and Chronic Obstructive Pulmonary Disease, *edited by Dirkje S. Postma and Scott T. Weiss*

219. *Reichman and Hershfield's* Tuberculosis: A Comprehensive, International Approach, Third Edition (in two parts), *edited by Mario C. Raviglione*

220. Narcolepsy and Hypersomnia, *edited by Claudio Bassetti, Michel Billiard, and Emmanuel Mignot*

221. Inhalation Aerosols: Physical and Biological Basis for Therapy, Second Edition, *edited by Anthony J. Hickey*

222. Clinical Management of Chronic Obstructive Pulmonary Disease, Second Edition, *edited by Stephen I. Rennard, Roberto Rodriguez-Roisin, Gérard Huchon, and Nicolas Roche*

223. Sleep in Children, Second Edition: Developmental Changes in Sleep Patterns, *edited by Carole L. Marcus, John L. Carroll, David F. Donnelly, and Gerald M. Loughlin*

224. Sleep and Breathing in Children, Second Edition: Developmental Changes in Breathing During Sleep, *edited by Carole L. Marcus, John L. Carroll, David F. Donnelly, and Gerald M. Loughlin*

225. Ventilatory Support for Chronic Respiratory Failure, *edited by Nicolino Ambrosino and Roger S. Goldstein*

226. Diagnostic Pulmonary Pathology, Second Edition, *edited by Philip T. Cagle, Timothy C. Allen, and Mary Beth Beasley*

227. Interstitial Pulmonary and Bronchiolar Disorders, *edited by Joseph P. Lynch III*

228. Chronic Obstructive Pulmonary Disease Exacerbations, *edited by Jadwiga A. Wedzicha and Fernando J. Martinez*

229. Pleural Disease, Second Edition, *edited by Demosthenes Bouros*

230. Interventional Pulmonary Medicine, Second Edition, *edited by John F. Beamis, Jr., Praveen Mathur, and Atul C. Mehta*

Interventional Pulmonary Medicine
Second Edition

Edited by

John F. Beamis, Jr.
Lahey Clinic Medical Center
Burlington, Massachusetts, USA

Praveen Mathur
Indiana University School of Medicine
Indianapolis, Indiana, USA

Atul C. Mehta
Sheikh Khalifa Medical City managed by the Cleveland Clinic
Abu Dhabi, UAE

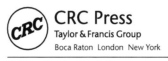
CRC Press
Taylor & Francis Group
Boca Raton London New York

CRC Press is an imprint of the
Taylor & Francis Group, an **informa** business

CRC Press
Taylor & Francis Group
6000 Broken Sound Parkway NW, Suite 300
Boca Raton, FL 33487-2742

First issued in paperback 2019

ISBN-13: 978-1-4200-8184-8 (hbk)
ISBN-13: 978-0-367-38482-1 (pbk)

This book contains information obtained from authentic and highly regarded sources. While all reasonable efforts have been made to publish reliable data and information, neither the author[s] nor the publisher can accept any legal responsibility or liability for any errors or omissions that may be made. The publishers wish to make clear that any views or opinions expressed in this book by individual editors, authors or contributors are personal to them and do not necessarily reflect the views/opinions of the publishers. The information or guidance contained in this book is intended for use by medical, scientific or healthcare professionals and is provided strictly as a supplement to the medical or other professional's own judgement, their knowledge of the patient's medical history, relevant manufacturer's instructions and the appropriate best practice guidelines. Because of the rapid advances in medical science, any information or advice on dosages, procedures or diagnoses should be independently verified. The reader is strongly urged to consult the relevant national drug formulary and the drug companies' and device or material manufacturers' printed instructions, and their websites, before administering or utilizing any of the drugs, devices or materials mentioned in this book. This book does not indicate whether a particular treatment is appropriate or suitable for a particular individual. Ultimately it is the sole responsibility of the medical professional to make his or her own professional judgements, so as to advise and treat patients appropriately. The authors and publishers have also attempted to trace the copyright holders of all material reproduced in this publication and apologize to copyright holders if permission to publish in this form has not been obtained. If any copyright material has not been acknowledged please write and let us know so we may rectify in any future reprint.

Library of Congress Cataloging-in-Publication Data

Interventional pulmonary medicine / edited by John F. Beamis, Praveen Mathur, Atul C. Mehta.—2nd ed.
    p. ; cm.—(Lung biology in health and disease ; 230)
  Includes bibliographical references and index.
  ISBN-13: 978-1-4200-8184-8 (hardcover : alk. paper)
  ISBN-10: 1-4200-8184-5 (hardcover : alk. paper) 1. Bronchoscopy. I. Beamis, John F. II. Mathur, Praveen N. III. Mehta, Atul C. IV. Series: Lung biology in health and disease ; v. 230.
  [DNLM: 1. Lung Diseases—therapy. 2. Bronchoscopy. 3. Thoracoscopy. W1 LU62 v.230 2009 / WF 600 I6178 2009]
  RC734.B7I588 2009
  616.2'307545—dc22

                                            2009036250

Visit the Taylor & Francis Web site at
http://www.taylorandfrancis.com

and the CRC Press Web site at
http://www.crcpress.com

*Dedicated to interventional pulmonologists throughout the world—
past, present, and future*

Introduction

There is no question that in 1816 when Rene-Theophile-Hyacinth Laennec reported his invention of the stethoscope, chest diseases began to be viewed in an entirely different way. It is interesting that Laennec first called his new medical instrument the "cylinder," and it is only later that it was named the "stethoscope," derived from two Greek words, one meaning "breast" and the other "to view."

Was the stethoscope the first step toward "interventional pulmonary medicine?" Probably, yes! Indeed, before Laennec, Aristotle and Galen among others had given us insights on pulmonary diseases, but their main tool was observations of postmortem tissue. The publication of *De humani corporis fabrica* by Andreas Verslicus in 1543 had a remarkable impact on medicine in general, and lung disease in particular. Then, the invention of chest percussion by Leopold Auenbrugger in 1764 became an important landmark and tool for physical examination of chest disease patients.

During the last century, lung surgery was developed, which led not only to remarkable advances in treatment but also to the understanding of lung disease. Microscopy had also found its way in the armamentarium of what has been used to diagnose respiratory disease, and bronchoscopy, invented in 1887, had also become the preferred instrument for diagnosis and treatment of some specific lung conditions.

Despite all these advances, and what each in their own way contributed to research, in clinical chest medicine and treatment, the field of respiratory disease gained a new momentum with the development of a new discipline, interventional pulmonary medicine.

In 2004, the series of monographs Lung Biology in Health and Disease introduced the first edition of *Interventional Pulmonary Medicine*, edited by John F. Beamis, Jr., Praveen Mathur, and Atul C. Mehta. At that time, we of course knew of the success of this new discipline, but we were hoping that this particular volume would stimulate the relevant research and clinical communities. Today, five years later, we are pleased to introduce this new edition that reports on new advanced diagnostic procedures and new therapeutic options from which patients can benefit.

In their preface, the editors of this new volume (and of the previous edition) underscore that interventional pulmonary medicine has enormous potential, but for it to be realized requires a workforce trained and proficient in this discipline.

For more than 31 years, the series Lung Biology in Health and Disease has aimed to bring to its readership the latest information available on specific research and clinical areas; our goal has always been to do the best we can for the patients. It is hoped that this new edition of *Interventional Pulmonary Medicine* will stimulate students of medicine and clinicians to take advantage of this emerging and critically important discipline.

As the executive editor of this series of monographs, I am grateful to the editors and authors for giving us the opportunity to introduce this new volume and to present to our readership the most recent approaches and therapies from which patients are certain to benefit.

Claude Lenfant, MD
Vancouver, Washington, U.S.A.

Preface

We are very pleased to organize the second edition of *Interventional Pulmonary Medicine*. Interventional pulmonology continues to grow as a specialty within the broader field of pulmonary/critical care medicine. IP, as it is often referred to, has become the mainstream, and an increasing number of pulmonary groups, both academic and private practice, are employing dedicated interventional pulmonologists. The demand for expertise in interventional pulmonary procedures continues to increase. The web site of the American Association for Bronchology and Interventional Pulmonology now lists 12 North American fellowships in interventional pulmonology. There are multiple courses dedicated to various interventional pulmonary procedures in the United States and Canada and throughout the world, including France, China and Lebanon, Spain, India, Germany, and Singapore among others.

The initial development of interventional pulmonology was spurred on by the epidemic of lung cancer, which resulted in many patients presenting with severe central airway obstruction, requiring endobronchial therapy such as laser and stenting. Interventional pulmonology has now branched out into other areas including advanced diagnostic procedures such as endobronchial ultrasound, navigational bronchoscopy, and autoflorescence bronchial imaging. There is an increasing interest in the use of newer interventional pulmonology procedures to treat nonmalignant pulmonary diseases such as asthma and chronic obstructive pulmonary disease.

The purpose of this volume is to update recent advances in several of the classic interventional pulmonology procedures such as endobronchial therapy and medical thoracoscopy. More importantly, this volume addresses in detail some of the advanced diagnostic procedures that have recently been validated or are currently being studied. These include navigational bronchoscopy for the diagnosis of peripheral lesions and use of endobronchial ultrasound for staging of lung cancer. Newer therapeutic procedures such as the use of tunnel pleural catheters for the management of pleural effusion, endobronchial treatment for asthma, and chronic obstructive pulmonary disease and bronchoscopic therapy for peripheral lesions will be addressed.

As in the first edition, the last chapter is dedicated to training in interventional pulmonology. This area continues to be problematic in the United States. Although up to 12 interventional pulmonology fellows will now be graduated each year, this number is insufficient to meet the current demands, especially if high-quality interventional pulmonologists are to be provided to outside of known centers of excellence.

We have dedicated this book to interventional pulmonologists throughout the world. As the three of us have traveled internationally for various meetings and courses, we have found that pulmonologists in every country face similar clinical problems whether related to thoracic malignancy or benign conditions such as tracheal stenosis and foreign body aspiration. We hope that this book will serve as a summary of recent advances in interventional pulmonology and that it will improve the competence and performance of interventional pulmonologists and contribute to improved outcomes for their patients.

As in the past, we wish to acknowledge and thank the many experts who contributed to this endeavor. All are busy practicing physicians who are committed to sharing their expertise with others. We particularly thank Sandra Beberman and her team at Informa Healthcare for encouraging us to take on this project and for her gentle prodding of us and the contributors to bring it to fruition. We also thank our families and local colleagues for their love and support to our many projects.

John F. Beamis, Jr.
Praveen Mathur
Atul C. Mehta

Contributors

C. T. Bolliger   Division of Pulmonology, Faculty of Health Sciences, University of Stellenbosch, Cape Town, South Africa

Mario Castro   Washington University School of Medicine, St. Louis, Missouri, U.S.A.

Prashant Chhajed   Department of Pulmonology and Centre for Sleep Studies, Fortis Hiranandani Hospital, Vashi, Navi Mumbai, India

Enrique Diaz-Guzman   University of Kentucky, Lexington, Kentucky, U.S.A.

Anne Gonzalez   McGill University Health Centre, Montreal, Quebec, Canada

David Feller Kopman   The Johns Hopkins Hospital, Baltimore, Maryland, U.S.A.

Elif Kupeli   Mesa Hospital, Ankara, Turkey

Tim Lahm   Indiana University School of Medicine, Indianapolis, Indiana, U.S.A.

Carla Lamb   Lahey Clinic Medical Center, Burlington, Massachusetts, U.S.A.

Pyng Lee   Singapore General Hospital, Singapore

Robert Lee   Lahey Clinic Medical Center, Burlington, Massachusetts, U.S.A.

Paul MacEachern   University of Calgary, Calgary, Alberta, Canada

Praveen Mathur   Indiana University School of Medicine, Indianapolis, Indiana, U.S.A.

Martin L. Mayse   Washington University School of Medicine, St. Louis, Missouri, U.S.A.

Atul C. Mehta   Sheikh Khalifa Medical City, managed by Cleveland Clinic, Abu Dhabi, UAE

Perry Nystrom   Indiana University School of Medicine, Indianapolis, Indiana, U.S.A.

David Ost   The University of Texas M.D. Anderson Cancer Center, Houston, Texas, U.S.A.

Jonathan Puchalski   Yale University School of Medicine, New Haven, Connecticut, U.S.A.

David Riker   Department of Pulmonary and Critical Care Medicine, University of California, San Diego, San Diego, California, U.S.A.

Francis D. Sheski   Indiana University School of Medicine, Indianapolis, Indiana, U.S.A.

Gerard A. Silvestri   Medical University of South Carolina, Charleston, South Carolina, U.S.A.

David Stather   University of Calgary, Calgary, Alberta, Canada

Daniel Sterman   University of Pennsylvania Medical Center, Philadelphia, Pennsylvania, U.S.A.

Alain Tremblay   University of Calgary, Calgary, Alberta, Canada

Andrew G. Villanueva   Lahey Clinic Medical Center, Burlington, Massachusetts, U.S.A.

Christophe von Garnier   Bern University Hospital, Bern, Switzerland

Jessica S. Wang   Medical University of South Carolina, Charleston, South Carolina, U.S.A.

Lonny Yarmus   The Johns Hopkins Hospital, Baltimore, Maryland, U.S.A.

Kazuhiro Yasufuku   Toronto General Hospital, University Health Network, Toronto, Ontario, Canada

Contents

Introduction   Claude Lenfant   . . . .   *ix*
Preface   . . . .   *xi*
Contributors   . . . .   *xiii*

1. **New Bronchoscopic Instrumentation: A Review and Update in Rigid Bronchoscopy** *1*
   Lonny Yarmus and David Feller Kopman

2. **Laser Bronchoscopy, Electrosurgery, APC, and Microdebrider** *9*
   C. T. Bolliger

3. **Update on Cryotherapy, Brachytherapy, and Photodynamic Therapy** *25*
   Tim Lahm and Francis D. Sheski

4. **Airway Stents** *45*
   Pyng Lee, Elif Kupeli, and Atul C. Mehta

5. **High-Resolution Bronchoscopy: Bringing These Modalities into Focus** *61*
   David Riker

6. **Endoscopic Staging of Lung Cancer** *84*
   Kazuhiro Yasufuku

7. **Medical Thoracoscopy** *98*
   Andrew G. Villanueva and Anne Gonzalez

8. **Tunneled Pleural Catheters** *122*
   Paul MacEachern, David Stather, and Alain Tremblay

9. **Bronchoscopic Lung Volume Reduction in COPD** *141*
   Enrique Diaz-Guzman and Atul C. Mehta

10. **Bronchial Thermoplasty** *152*
    Martin L. Mayse and Mario Castro

11. **Sedation, Analgesia, and Anesthesia
    for Airway Procedures** *168*
    Perry Nystrom and Praveen Mathur

12. **Advanced Bronchoscopic Techniques for Diagnosis of
    Peripheral Pulmonary Lesions** *186*
    Robert Lee and David Ost

13. **Bronchoscopic Treatment of Peripheral Lung Nodules** *200*
    Jonathan Puchalski and Daniel Sterman

14. **Percutaneous Dilational Tracheostomy** *209*
    Carla Lamb

15. **Training in Interventional Pulmonology** *224*
    Jessica S. Wang and Gerard A. Silvestri

16. **Role of Bronchoscopy in Transplant Patients** *235*
    Christophe von Garnier and Prashant Chhajed

Index *247*

1

New Bronchoscopic Instrumentation: A Review and Update in Rigid Bronchoscopy

LONNY YARMUS and DAVID FELLER KOPMAN
The Johns Hopkins Hospital, Baltimore, Maryland, U.S.A.

I. Introduction

For over 100 years, rigid bronchoscopy has been an invaluable resource for the pulmonologist and surgeon. The first rigid bronchoscopy performed by Dr Gustav Killian in the late 1800s offered physicians a new glimpse into human anatomy and sparked the growth of pulmonary medicine. Throughout its history, the use of the rigid bronchoscope has waxed and waned as the approaches to intrapulmonary processes have shifted. The procedure has proven itself to stand the test of time and remains an integral tool in the diagnosis and treatment of airway pathology. This chapter focuses on the history of the rigid bronchoscope, reviews new technological updates in rigid bronchoscopy, and discusses current ventilatory strategies utilized during rigid bronchoscopy.

II. History

In 1887, Gustav Killian, of Freiburg, Germany, removed a pork bone from the right main stem bronchus of a farmer who had aspirated while eating soup. Dr Killian used a head mirror as an external light source and a 33.5-cm esophagoscope to remove the 11×3–mm bone fragment while performing the first documented foreign body retrieval utilizing bronchoscopy. The procedure was reported by his assistant, Kollorath, who stated that, "On March 30th of this year I had the honor to assist my admired principal, Herrn Prof. Killian in extraction of a piece of bone from the right bronchus. This case is of such peculiarity with respect to its diagnostic and therapeutic importance that a more extensive description seemed justified" (1). One of Dr Killian's early observations regarding the anatomy of the bronchial tree helped pave the way for advances in bronchoscopic technology (2) (Picture 1):

> The bronchial tubes are elastic, mildly flexible and can be dilated. But most importantly, they can be displaced. One should not imagine the bronchial tree to be stiff as if it were made of wrought iron. On the contrary, both the entire structure and the different branches show pulsating and respiratory movement. It is therefore obvious that the bronchi do not resist the movement of the instruments. It is hence possible under local anesthesia to carefully insert the instrument into the branches of different sizes and to view the small branches. Bearing this in mind, I do not think it would be too risky to try a direct bronchoscopy approach.

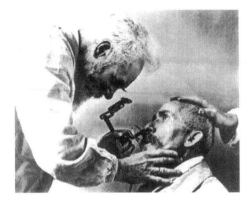

Picture 1 "Dr. Killian performing an early rigid bronchoscopic examination."

In 1904, Chevalier Jackson, the "father of American bronchoesophagology" further advanced the field of rigid bronchoscopy by equipping his bronchoscope with a suction channel and a small light bulb at the distal tip to provide illumination. By 1922, Dr Albricht, a pupil of Dr Killian, reported on 703 patients undergoing rigid bronchoscopy for foreign body aspiration between 1911 and 1921. He reported successful removal in 691 (98.3%) of the cases (3).

The rigid bronchoscope quickly became an indispensable piece of equipment for otolaryngologists across the world and remained the only medical instrument to access the airways until 1963 when Shigeto Ikeda from the National Cancer Center Hospital in Tokyo, Japan, introduced the flexible fiberoptic bronchoscope (4,5) (Picture 2).

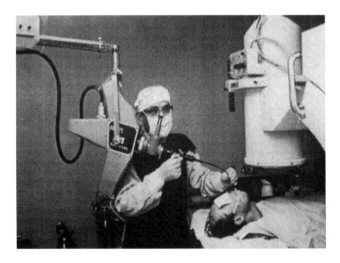

Picture 2 "Dr. Shigeto Ikeda performing an early fiberoptic bronchoscopic examination."

For the next 30 years, the use of rigid bronchoscopy declined as flexible bronchoscopy quickly gained worldwide acceptance and almost completely replaced the rigid bronchoscope as the diagnostic instrument of choice for pulmonary disease. In a survey performed in 1989, 8% of responders were performing rigid bronchoscopy (6). In a repeat survey in 1999, this number had declined to only 4% (7).

It was not until the lung cancer epidemic of the 1980s and the associated increase in central airway obstruction that the utility of the rigid bronchoscope reemerged (8). In addition, recognition of certain advantages that rigid bronchoscopy has over flexible bronchoscopy, such as airway control and ventilation during intervention as well as the ability to simultaneously use larger forceps and suction catheters, has also led to the increase in rigid bronchoscopies being performed today (9).

III. New Innovations in Rigid Bronchoscopy

The design of the rigid bronchoscope has not significantly changed since first used by Jackson in 1897 (Picture 3). It is a stainless steel, hollow cylindrical tube with a lumen, which is equal along its length. The external diameter of the adult rigid bronchoscope ranges from 9 to 14 mm and is usually 40 cm long. There is a distal beveled end to allow for lifting of the epiglottis and safer insertion through the vocal cords. The beveled end also facilitates dilation of a stenotic lesion and allows one to "core" through the tumor, achieving rapid airway patency. Fenestrations are present at the distal one-third of the bronchoscope to allow for contralateral lung ventilation when the bronchoscope is inserted into a main stem bronchus. Of note, the 30 cm length of the rigid tracheoscope is shorter than the bronchoscope to allow more maneuverability within the trachea to relieve proximal central airway obstructions. Since single-lung ventilation cannot be achieved while operating within the central airway, the tracheoscope does not have the distal fenestrations seen on the bronchoscope. The proximal end of the tracheoscope/ bronchoscope varies by manufacturer, as discussed further in the text. Most systems have several ports to allow passage of the telescope, suction catheters, as well as a variety of instruments used for tumor destruction, tumor excision, dilation, and foreign body removal (Picture 4).

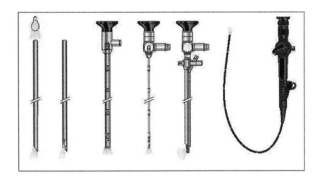

Picture 3 "Basic design of the rigid and flexible bronchoscope."

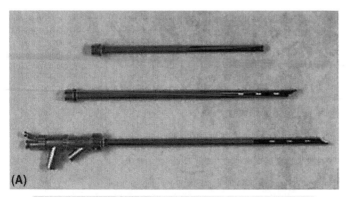

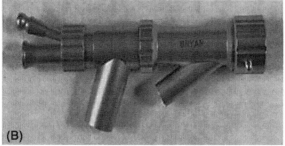

Picture 4 "(**A**) Examples of a rigid tracheoscope (top), a rigid bronchoscope (middle) and a rigid bronchoscope with a ventilating adaptor attached to the proximal end (bottom). (**B**) A close up view of a ventilating adaptor and 'universal instrumentation barrell'."

Over the past several years, several new designs and modifications of the standard rigid bronchoscope have given the interventional pulmonologist new tools to advance the field.

The Bryan-Dumon Series II rigid bronchoscope (Bryan Corp., Woburn, Massachusetts, U.S.) was the first major modification to the rigid bronchoscope since the time of Gustav Killian. It features an operator head with a universal instrumentation barrel. This is an interchangeable piece that can be placed on the proximal end of any of the color-coded bronchial and tracheal tubes. The universal instrumentation barrel is also equipped with three side ports for instruments, ventilation, and anesthesia. This unique design permits the physician to utilize various endoscopic tools, suction catheters, and laser fibers simultaneously, maintaining the visualization capabilities of the rigid telescope. The Bryan-Dumon line also offers a stent placement kit for the placement of silicone tracheobronchial stents. This system corresponds to the color-coded bronchial and tracheal tubes of the Series II rigid bronchoscope. The steel stent introducers and pushers allow for loading of the Y-stent in a musket barrel–type fashion. The deployment of the stent can be achieved through the barrel of the rigid bronchoscope (Picture 5).

There are several ventilatory strategies that can be used during rigid bronchoscopy. In the 1990s, the most common technique was to use spontaneous assisted

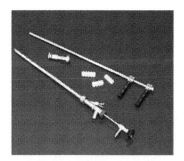

Picture 5 "The Bryan-Dumon rigid bronchoscope and stent-introducer system with a variety of silicone stents."

ventilation with intravenous anesthesia. During this ventilatory strategy, recurrent episodes of hypoxemia in a high-risk patient population, with many patients suffering from central airway obstruction, led to a paradigm shift from this mode over the past several years (10).

A desire for a ventilatory approach by interventional pulmonologists, which provided continuous oxygenation and ventilation with optimal airway control, led to the reemergence of jet Venturi ventilation. Originally described in 1967 by Sanders (11), this method of low-frequency jet ventilation has been shown to effectively ventilate and oxygenate the patient while keeping the proximal end of the bronchoscope free to allow passage of instruments.

Jet ventilation is achieved through an open system where 100% oxygen is injected at 50 psi though one of the operator ports at the proximal end of the bronchoscope. This is achieved manually, usually at a rate of 8 to 15 breaths per minute, by the anesthesiologists who observe chest rise to ensure adequate ventilation. Given that the system is open to atmosphere, room air is also entrained into the bronchoscope, and as a result there is a variable FiO_2 that is transmitted to the distal airways (12). Although a safe oxyhemoglobin saturation is usually easily obtained, potential downsides to this system are a limited ability to monitor minute ventilation as well as airway pressures. As such, there is a potential increased risk of iatrogenic pneumothorax because of dynamic hyperinflation distal to a stenotic airway (13).

The Wolf Company (Richard Wolf Medical Instruments, Vernon Hills, Illinois, U.S.) recently produced the Hemer bronchoscope that introduces a measuring port that can allow levels of carbon dioxide and oxygen as well as pressure fluctuations during the procedure. The pressure on inspiration resulting from the jet nozzle and room air entrainment reaches a plateau in the working channel at a distance of approximately 10 cm from the proximal end of the bronchoscope. As a result, the inspiratory pressure distal to this point can be taken as being representative of the mean inspiratory pressure. The Hemer bronchoscope has an internal port at 14 cm from the proximal end of the bronchoscope and can be connected to pressure transducers and gas sensors to monitor end-tidal CO_2 (Picture 6).

When used with the Monsoon high-frequency jet ventilator (Acutronic Medical Systems, Hirzel, Switzerland), ventilation will be discontinued if a set pressure limit is

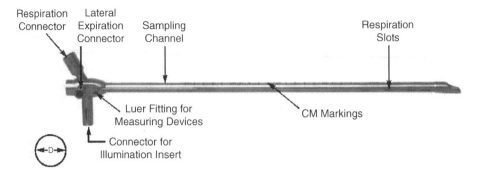

Respiration Connector · Lateral Expiration Connector · Sampling Channel · Respiration Slots · Luer Fitting for Measuring Devices · CM Markings · Connector for Illumination Insert

Picture 6 "The Hemer bronchoscope. *Source*: Courtesy of Richard Wolf Medical Instruments, Vernon Hills, Illinois, U.S.A."

exceeded (14). The measuring devices for pressure and breath gas and the jet pressure control are connected via a three-way stopcock and connecting tubes to the Luer connector of the measuring tube.

Another rigid bronchoscope recently produced by Wolf is the Texas R.I.B (Rigid Integrated Bronchoscope). The bronchoscope was designed by Dr Garrett Walsh at the MD Anderson Hospital in Houston, Texas, and features separate channels for optics and instruments to allow for a larger working area with continuous visualization. The innovative design combines the operator head with the camera, which limits the loss of working space within the bronchoscope channel taken up by larger optics. This may also allow increased efficiency during the procedure, as the telescope does not need to be removed prior to the insertion of accessory devices. There is also an irrigation port at the proximal operator end to allow washing of the distal lens for optimal visualization. At the distal tip of the bronchoscope, there are additional fenestrations to provide a 360° viewing. The bronchoscope is also compatible with all stent systems (Picture 7).

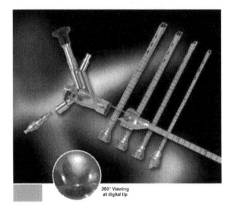

360° Viewing at digital tip

Picture 7 "The Texas R.I.B. bronchoscope. *Source*: Courtesy of Richard Wolf Medical Instruments, Vernon Hills, Illinois, U.S.A."

A. Optical Forceps

Rigid forceps are perhaps the most useful accessory to the rigid bronchoscope. They are used for multiple modalities of bronchoscopic interventions including stent placement, repositioning, and removal, as well as foreign body extraction and tumor excision. The first major new design in optical forceps is now being offered by Wolf. The new Optical Holding Forceps 3XL "Cyclops Forceps" has a centrally positioned 5.5-mm telescope that ensures optimum visualization in combination with mechanical stability (Picture 8).

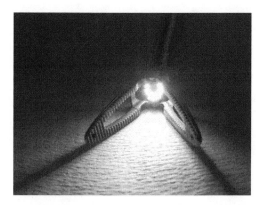

Picture 8 "The Cyclops forceps. *Source*: Courtesy of Richard Wolf Medical Instruments, Vernon Hills, Illinois, U.S.A."

IV. Conclusion

As Chevalier Jackson said, "In the future, as at present, the internist will tap and look and listen on the outside of the chest; the roentgenologist will continue to look through the patient; but in continually increasing proportions of cases, the surgeon, the internist and the roentgenologist will ask the bronchoscopist to look inside the patient." Rigid bronchoscopy has stood the test of time and remains the single most important instrument for the interventional pulmonologist for the diagnosis and treatment of airway pathology.

References

1. Kollorath O. Entfernung eines Knochenstücks aus dem rechten Bronchus auf natürlichem Wege und unter Anwendung der directen Laryngoskopie. München Med Wochen 1897; 38: 38–43.
2. Killian G. Ueber direkte Bronchoskopie. München Med Wochen 1898; 27:844–847.
3. Alberti PW. The history of laryngology: a centennial celebration. Otolaryngol Head Neck Surg 1996; 114(3):345–354.
4. Ikeda S, Yanai N, Ishikawa S. Flexible bronchofiberscope. Keio J Med 1968; 17(1):1–16.
5. Ohata M. History and progress of bronchology in Japan. JJSB 1998; 20:539–546.
6. Prakash UB, Offord KP, Stubbs SE. Bronchoscopy in North America: the ACCP survey. Chest 1991; 100(6):1668–1675.

7. Colt HG, Prakash UBS, Offord KP. Bronchoscopy in North America: survey by the American Association for bronchology, 1999. J Bronchol 2000; 7:8–25.
8. Ayers ML, Beamis JF Jr. Rigid bronchoscopy in the twenty-first century. Clin Chest Med 2001; 22(2):355–364.
9. Wahidi MM, Herth FJF, Ernst A. State of the art: interventional pulmonology. Chest 2007; 131(1):261–274.
10. Perrin G, Colt HG, Martin C, et al. Safety of interventional rigid bronchoscopy using intravenous anesthesia and spontaneous assisted ventilation. A prospective study. Chest 1992; 102(5):1526–1530.
11. Sanders RD. Two ventilating attachments for bronchoscopes. Del Med J 1967; 39:170–192.
12. Godden DJ, Willey RF, Fergusson RJ, et al. Rigid bronchoscopy under intravenous general anaesthesia with oxygen Venturi ventilation. Thorax 1982; 37(7):532–534.
13. Fernandez-Bustamante A, Ibanez V, Alfaro JJ, et al. High-frequency jet ventilation in interventional bronchoscopy: factors with predictive value on high-frequency jet ventilation complications. J Clin Anesth 2006; 18(5):349–356.
14. Pobloth A, Reichle G, Deimel G, et al. A new rigid bronchoscope with a measuring tube for pressure and capnometry. Pneumologie 2001; 55(3):120–125.

2
Laser Bronchoscopy, Electrosurgery, APC, and Microdebrider

C. T. BOLLIGER
Division of Pulmonology, Faculty of Health Sciences, University of Stellenbosch, Cape Town, South Africa

I. Clinical Background

At the time of diagnosis, a good 80% of all lung cancers are inoperable and their treatment is mainly palliative. Obstruction of the major airways is one of the most serious complications of advanced stage tumors and can vary from asymptomatic airway narrowing to life-threatening dyspnea caused by airway occlusion. Significant central airway obstruction (CAO) with imminent suffocation requires immediate action to promptly regain airway passage (1,2). Airway obstruction is caused by intraluminal tumor growth, extraluminal tumor compression, or their combination of both (Fig. 1). Depending on staffing and equipment of the local health care facilities, patients with or without previous treatment are referred to the interventional pulmonologist. In developing countries—usually with limited access to health care—such patients often seek medical aid at an advanced stage of disease, sometimes exhibiting severe CAO, whereas in first world setups they usually present with recurrences after previous surgical treatment or failed chemoradiotherapy. In addition, imminent suffocation and poor physical condition may provide little room for timely and safe intervention, thus immediate action is warranted. Therefore, treatment plans must be diligently considered and executed to obtain an optimal benefit. Tumor coagulation to reduce profuse bleeding followed by debulking, with additional stenting in case of significant residual extraluminal stenosis, is the time-honored accepted strategy (1,2).

For patients with resectable cancers, radical surgical resection with systemic nodal dissection is the standard approach (3), while lesser resection in the absence of nodal disease is now being increasingly explored, primarily in Japan (4). Especially for tumors up to 2 cm in diameter—stage T1a in the newly proposed 7th edition of the TNM classification system for NSCLC (5)—sublobar resections hold promise. Should sublobar resections become the new standard of care for small peripheral tumors, the importance of nonsurgical curative attempts of such lesions by techniques such as brachytherapy (6) or radiofrequency ablation (7) might increase as well, as they would not be restricted to patients unfit or unwilling to undergo surgery. Within the central airways, advancements of bronchoscopic techniques allow diligent observation of the target tissues, that is, in the preneoplastic and carcinoma in situ stage. Increasing experience with endobronchial ultrasound (EBUS) seems to indicate that, in the absence of nodal disease, early lung cancer in the central airways, defined as tumor not extending

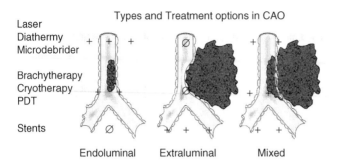

Figure 1 Types and treatment options in CAO. Schematic illustration of three basic types of CAO. A 50% narrowing of the lumen at the distal trachea is chosen for each type. The value of various treatment modalities for each type is indicated: from Ø = N/A to +++ = excellent.

beyond the cartilagenous layer of the airway wall, can be cured by endoscopic techniques (8). Medically unfit patients with early stage cancer have been treated successfully with intraluminal bronchoscopic treatment for some time (9). Similarly to peripheral lesions, the advent of newly available imaging techniques such as EBUS, autofluorescence bronchoscopy, and narrow band imaging (10) might also lead to increased use of endoscopic treatment with curative intent in surgically fit patients with early stage lung cancer of the central airways. However, before such minimal resections/ablations both for peripheral and for central airway lesions become the standard of care, carefully planned prospective comparative trials will have to be conducted. This chapter will discuss the role and limitations of electrocautery, argon plasma coagulation (APC), and laser resection in the palliative and curative endoscopic setting, and also describe the newly available modality of the microdebrider.

II. Indications
A. Palliative Treatment

As many as 30% of all lung cancer patients may present with central airway involvement already at the time of diagnosis. Most of these situations present locally advanced tumor stages, which irrespective of their cell type are not amenable to surgical resection. Depending on the degree of obstruction, but also on the availability on oncological services, these tumors are treated with chemoradiotherapy with palliative intent. The initial treatment often leads to excellent local tumor control and symptom relief. The duration of this effect, however, is often short-lived and rarely exceeds months or at best a few years. In many such situations, the oncologist's armamentarium is then severely limited. Often the total dose of external beam irradiation has been exhausted or first-line chemotherapy is not effective any more, or too toxic. If such patients present with endobronchial tumor obstruction of the central airways with a significant amount of normal lung parenchyma distal to the obstruction, reopening of the affected airway by endoscopic means can provide palliation with excellent symptom relief and limited local tumor control.

The large majority of patients with even marked CAO should first undergo an orientating flexible bronchoscopy, lung function measurements, and a CT scan of the chest to help planning of the therapeutic endoscopic procedure. Imminent respiratory failure, however, accompanied by symptoms such as stridor and severe dyspnea requires immediate action precluding the above-mentioned investigations (2). The immediate action taken is similar to tracheal intubation for lifesaving resuscitation. It has been a consensus that individuals presenting with imminent suffocation usually present with ≥50%, often even subtotal obstruction of their central airways (3). With such a clinical presentation, the interventional pulmonologist has to anticipate intra- and extraluminal airways' stenoses (Fig. 1). For extraluminal CAO ≥50% of the normal lumen, airway dilation, often followed by stent implantation, is the only choice. In case expertise is lacking, immediate intubation using the fiberoptic bronchoscope, passing distal of the stenosis and cleaning the distal airways of pus and mucus prior to referral, can be lifesaving. Inflation of the tracheal cuff helps compress the tumorous section. Thereafter, the patient can be transported safely to a referral center for further treatment.

In the setting of such a center, the interventional pulmonologist can perform tumor coagulation and debulking in the same session by either using the rigid scope or working through the endotracheal (ET) tube with the flexible scope. The rigid scope with the whole barrel lumen available as a large working channel provides better access, allowing safer manipulation as ventilation is better preserved, and hemorrhage can be controlled by direct compression of bleeding tissue by the instrument itself (1). Despite increasing availability of devices suited for the flexible bronchoscope, its blocking effect within the ET tube often limits adequate ventilation, and the smaller working channel may jeopardize safety, especially when dealing with emergency situations, and prolongs treatment time. From the clinical perspective, immediate symptomatic relief by tumor coagulation using laser resection or electrocautery followed by mechanical debulking is straightforward and has been the accepted consensus strategy (1,2,11–14). The effectiveness of stent placement for significant extraluminal disease has also been established.

B. Treatment with Curative Intent
Benign Conditions
Benign conditions amenable to curative endoscopic treatment are usually benign tumors, originating from central airway walls, as well as circumscribed scar tissue, leading to severely narrowed airway lumen. Frequent benign tumors are lipomas, hamartomas, chondromas, papillomatosis, but also inflammatory granulation tissue from foreign bodies or suture materiel. The most frequent scar situations are postintubation tracheal stenoses, which range from simple weblike stenoses with an intact airway wall to complex stenoses with varying degrees of wall destruction and remodeling, often exhibiting some degree of tracheomalacia as well. The interventional pulmonologist is ideally suited to deal with all tumors described above as well as with the management of weblike stenoses. For all more complex situations involving airway wall destruction, the best curative treatment should be sought with an interdisciplinary approach involving the interventional pulmonologist, the ENT, and/or thoracic surgeon.

Malignant Tumors in the Central Airways
Arguments have been raised that the limited number of patients with occult cancer treated with various intraluminal bronchoscopic techniques does not justify their role. However, less extensive surgical resection, for example, segmentectomy and surgical bronchoplasty, has been accepted as a legitimate approach for patients considered to be

high-risk surgical candidates because of limited pulmonary function (15). This concept is based on the recognition that minute early stage lesions within the bronchoscopically visible range, according to strict criteria as proposed by S. Ikeda in 1976, never have nodal disease (16). Meticulous histopathological studies from various Japanese centers and from the Mayo screening study confirmed the superficial nature of these lesions and the absence of lymph nodes' metastasis (17–20), while it is long known that these lesions are only several millimeters thick. All these data have raised increased interest to apply photodynamic therapy (PDT) for treatment with curative intent and to move to early detection and localization, and apply methods for accurate staging prior to any treatment decision.

A vast array of early detection and staging methods are increasingly being investigated: sputum cytometry, autofluorescence bronchoscopy, local staging with EBUS, high-resolution computed tomography, virtual bronchoscopy, and fluoro-deoxy-glucose positron emission tomography (FDG-PET) scan. These investigational techniques combined with minimally invasive intralesional treatment can therefore provide a cost-effective early interventional management in the current screening area (8,9,21–23). This has driven a paradigm shift toward early intervention, recognition of the individuals at highest risk, biomolecular research, predictive algorithms for those at risk, and early interventional strategy such as chemoprevention at the preneoplastic stage of early detected potentially malignant lesions. As far as endoscopic treatment of early lung cancer is concerned, most reports mention the use of either PDT or electrocautery (24,25).

A detailed description of this topic is, however, beyond the scope this chapter, which emphasizes the role of endoscopic tools used for the resection of endobronchial tumors or mixed airway obstructions with an important endobronchial component (Fig. 1). These tools can be divided further by their onset of action: immediate versus delayed. This chapter exclusively discusses three modalities: laser resection, electrocautery, including APC, and the microdebrider, all with immediate effect. Modalities with delayed effect, such as PDT and brachytherapy, but also cryotherapy—which is increasingly used with immediate effect as well—are dealt with elsewhere in this book. Further, the treatment of extrinsic airway compression by stents is discussed in chapter 4.

It is clear from the outset that treatment modalities used with the same indications and outcomes are largely competitive in nature, and the practicing interventional pulmonologist often has to decide which one he wants to use (Fig. 1). Even in very specialized centers with high patient loads, one uses either laser or electrocautery. Although both laser and electrocautery will be described individually later, the technical approach is virtually identical, both modalities provide excellent results, and the choice of the one or the other technique often depends on the physician preference, the local setup, and financial considerations. The microdebrider, on the other hand, is a very recent addition to the pulmonary endoscopist's toolbox and can be considered a complementary modality for the rapid removal of bulky tissue. The individual techniques are discussed later.

III. Laser Resection

The word "laser" is an acronym for *L*ight *A*mplification of *S*timulated *E*mission of *R*adiation. Laser resection is the application of laser energy delivered via rigid and/or flexible bronchoscopes to manage (palliate or cure) different endobronchial lesions.

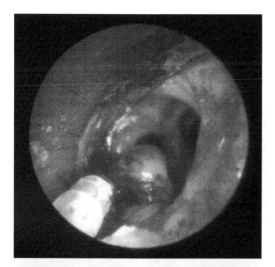

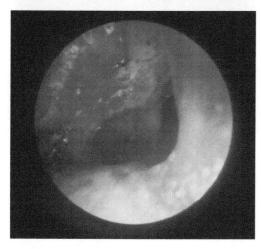

Figure 2 Laser resection. Laser resection of recurrent endoluminal growth of thymoma needing repetitive laser resection after exhaustion of chemo- and radiotherapy options. (Top) Before resection, the rigid bronchoscope is in place with tip of Nd:YAG laser probe left and suction catheter right at distal end of barrel, approximately 1.0 to 1.5 cm from tumor. (Bottom) View five minutes later with tumor resected. Note significant residual narrowing of tracheal lumen because of extraluminal component of tumor, in this case, not necessitating stent placement.

The use of laser resection in the tracheobronchial tree has been firmly established for decades (26–30). The following description of the equipment and technical background is therefore an update and not a repetition of a detailed discussion of laser physics (Fig. 2).

A. Equipment and Technical Background

Most laser lights can be delivered through optical fibers and are suitable for bronchoscopic applications. Three main characteristics determine the suitability of a particular laser for therapeutic bronchoscopy, which are (*i*) power density rating, (*ii*) ratio of absorption and scattering coefficients in soft tissue, and (*iii*) the delivery system. Power density depends on laser technology and on factors such as target tissue and exposure time. By determining the volume of tissue that is heated, absorption and scattering make the difference between cutting and hemostasis. Lasers with high absorption coefficients and high scattering coefficients are good coagulators. The different types of laser and their characteristics are listed in Table 1. The Nd-YAG (neodynium:yttrium aluminium garnet) equipment is the most widely used type of laser for bronchoscopic interventions because it has sufficient power to vaporize tissues and produces an excellent coagulation effect. With its wavelength of 1064 nm, which is in the invisible range, it needs a pilot light usually in the red color range. Both contact and noncontact probes are available. In the noncontact mode, the tip of the probe is held at about 1 cm proximal to the target. An initial power setting of 20 to 40 W with a pulse duration of 0.5 to 1 second represents a safe initial setting to obtain devascularization. To carbonize tissue one either moves the tip of the probe closer to the target at about 3 mm or applies several pulses at the same location. When treating obstructing lesions of the central airways, the aim is to devascularize the tumor and subsequently core out the tumor bulk with the tip of the rigid bronchoscope. When working with a flexible bronchoscope, the lesion is either devascularized or carbonized and the remaining tissue removed by forceps, or the whole lesion is vaporized. Both rigid and flexible techniques are used successfully (29,32,33). Protective eyewear is mandatory when the laser beam is activated.

The CO_2 laser with a wavelength of 10.600 nm is an excellent cutting tool with an almost scalpel-like precision. Its application in the tracheobronchial tree has, however, been limited by its poor coagulating properties and more importantly by the need of a cumbersome articulated arm delivery system, which precludes its use distal to the main carina. The CO_2 laser is quite popular with ENT surgeons for the upper respiratory tract.

Laser resection delivered via a rigid or flexible bronchoscope requires anesthesia (topical anesthesia with or without conscious sedation, or general anesthesia). Procedures done with the rigid scope always require general anesthesia.

Table 1 Laser Equipment for Bronchoscopic Applications

Type of laser	Wavelength (nm)	Biological effects	
		Vaporization	Coagulation
Nd-YAG	1064	+++	+++
CO_2	10,600	+[a]	−
Argon	488–514	−	++
Dye	360–700	Activate photochemicals	
Diode	810	+	++
Excimer	193–351	Tissue destruction by mechanical effect	
YAP-Nd	1340	?	++

[a]Precise cutting effect. Note: ? indicates unknown result.
Source: Reproduced from Ref. (31).

B. Clinical Experience and Results

For nearly 80 years in the history of bronchology, therapeutic interventions were limited to foreign body removal and suctioning of airway secretions. In 1976, Laforet et al. (34) reported the first applications of laser for the management of airway tumors. Toty et al. (35), Dumon et al. (26), and Cavaliere et al. (27) published their experiences with the application of Nd-YAG laser in endoscopic tracheobronchial surgery, which became the most frequently used nonsurgical technique in the management of malignant as well as benign endobronchial disorders.

The main indication for laser bronchoscopy comprises obstructive lesions of the trachea, the left and right main bronchi, the bronchus intermedius, and the lobar orifices that compromise ventilation and produce severe symptoms (including dyspnea, stridor, intractable cough, and hemoptysis) (Table 2) (Fig. 3). Laser treatment of obstructions of a single segmental bronchus does not improve ventilation significantly but is worth trying from two segments (i.e., middle lobe) upward. The most frequent indication is inoperable lung cancer with endobronchial manifestations. The main goal of the intervention is palliation. In many cases, laser bronchoscopy is combined with other treatment modalities, that is, stenting, external beam irradiation, and brachytherapy.

The only absolute contraindication is external compression. There are relative contraindications such as intractable hypoxemia, bronchoesophageal fistula, and coagulopathy. Complications of laser bronchoscopy include hypoxemia, bleeding, perforation, fistula formation, and fire. The risk of fire necessitates a limitation of the inspired

Table 2 Indications for Laser Resection and Electrocautery

Malignant disorders	Primary lung cancer
	Endobronchial metastasis (from breast, colon, kidney, thyroid gland, esophagus)
	In situ carcinoma[a]
	Typical carcinoid[a]
Benign tumors[a]	Papilloma, fibroma, lipoma, hamarthochondroma, leiomyoma
Stenoses	As a result of the following:
	Anastomosis (lung transplantation, surgical resection)
	Intubation
	Tracheotomy, tracheostomy
	Tuberculosis
	Sarcoidosis
	Wegener's granulomatosis
	Trauma
	Inhalation injury
	Radiation therapy
	Granulation tissue
Miscellaneous	Reduction of bleeding
	Amyloidosis
	Endometriosis
	Closure of esophagobronchial fistulas
	Foreign body removal (lithotripsy)

Endobronchial obstruction in the central airways.
[a]Intended to be curative.
Source: From Ref. 31.

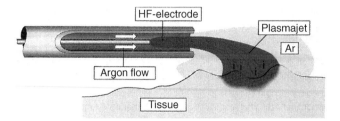

Figure 3 Argon plasma coagulation. Schematic illustration of the flexible catheter tip for delivery of argon into the tracheobronchial tree. The argon gas (Ar) flows around a high-frequency electrode and spreads out into the airway lumen. When the gas is activated and ionized it is called plasma. A spark through the plasma jet dessicates tissue (depicted by the brown area) to a specific depth.

oxygen concentration (FiO$_2$) to $\leq$40% (but strictly $\leq$ 50%) (36). In patients requiring higher FiO$_2$ values a safe alternative is the use of cryotherapy.

The channel of the rigid bronchoscope is large enough to simultaneously allow ventilation, passage of different laser fibers, and a suction tube. In addition to photo-coagulation, mechanical dilation with rigid tubes of increasing diameter can also be performed. For resection of bulky lesions, the rigid technique is clearly favored for speed and safety by bronchoscopists skilled in both techniques (26,29,37).

In the treatment of early-stage lung cancer with curative intent, however, the flexible bronchoscope is comparable to the rigid method.

IV. Electrocautery and Argon Plasma Coagulation

The use of electrical current for tissue destruction by heat is called electrocautery or diathermy. Because of voltage difference between probe and target tissue, electrons will flow and current density can be controlled using probes that conduct the electrons toward the target (38). Electrons will generate heat for tissue coagulation because of the higher resistance of the target tissue. APC uses ionized argon gas jet flow (=plasma) to conduct electrons allowing a noncontact mode of treatment (lightning effect) (39).

A. Equipment and Technical Background

The high frequency electrical generator is a standard instrument in every hospital to generate alternating current that prevents neural and muscular response. A plate is attached to the patient to ground electrons. APC has been popular in gastrointestinal endoscopy for superficial coagulation of large mucosal surfaces. The argon gas quite flexibly flows around bends and corners (Fig. 3). Coagulated tissue has a higher resistance, which automatically drives the argon gas flow away to nearby untreated tissue. APC is therefore suited to treat bronchial segments, which take off at an acute angle from the major airways, such as apical and posterior segments of the upper lobes or the apical lower lobe segments. This is an advantage over laser bundles, which always leave the probe in a straightforward fashion.

Various probes are available to perform controlled conductance of electrons: biopsy forceps, knives, blunt probes, suction rods, cutting loops, and snares. Each can be chosen to match personal expertise and need. Current density is the issue to be remembered as the size of the probe functions as the focusing point for electrons. Ultimate tissue effect therefore depends on voltage difference between probe and tissue (i.e., the wattage setting), the surface area of contact (e.g., smaller probe will increase current density), the duration of energy application (i.e., the time duration electrons are allowed to pass) in the absence of leak (mucus, blood, and conductance of metal part of the bronchoscope or other instruments). More importantly, one sees the immediate effect during electrocautery treatment, which corresponds well with the histological effect of coagulative necrosis (40).

The vast array of instruments (rigid or flexible), both for contact or for noncontact mode, is appealing for every purpose to match personal expertise and need (Fig. 4). Purchase price and maintenance cost of equipment are low, reusable applicators are cheap, while the principle is straightforward and easy to comprehend especially in comparison to Nd-YAG laser, which is the most popular technique in larger institutions (11,42,43) The contact mode, that is, palpation to coagulate tumor is similar to Nd-YAG laser by way of the sapphire probe, while the noncontact mode of APC is similar to the noncontact mode of the Nd-YAG laser for achieving superficial coagulation. One may perform coagulation, cutting, fulgurate, vaporize, and all combinations with mechanical debulking for quick airway recanalization. Significant residual extraluminal stenosis or airway wall collapse can be managed by stent placement (see chap. 4).

Arguments have been raised that compared to Nd-YAG laser, the effect of electrocautery and APC are superficial. Nd-YAG laser is the most popular technique for coagulation because of its enormous heat sink effect, as photons of 1064 nm deeply scatter causing profound tissue necrosis. In contrast, electrons do not scatter and dissipate in the deeper layers beneath the point of impact, leading to superficial necrosis, similar to CO_2 laser for treating watery tissue. Deep tissue coagulation, however, may not always be preferable because of the vicinity of major vessels in the central airways, especially in the changed anatomy following previous treatments (surgical resection, chemoradiotherapy). The importance of coagulation to minimize

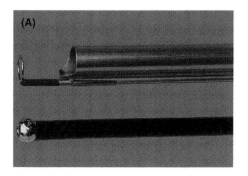
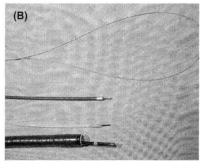

Figure 4 Electorcautery probes (A rigid, B flexible). (**A**) Rigid electrocautery tools. (Above) Combined hollow electrocautery/suction probe as used at Tygerberg Academic Hospital. (Below) Rigid bronchoscope with distal electrocautery loop. (**B**) The various flexible tools from top to bottom: snare, hook, knife, blunt probe. Note the green ring on certain probes, this should be visible during electrocautery to guarantee safety distance between cauterizing tip of probe and distal end of flexible bronchoscope. *Source*: For part (A): From Ref. 41.

profuse bleeding prior to debulking is the accepted strategy in restoring airway passage (1,2,29).

Logistics for applying electrocautery and APC are simple (no goggles and coverage of reflecting surfaces), and the system runs on much less electrical energy. The ease of using the instrument and flexible applicators as additions to standard flexible bronchoscopes is a great advantage (similar to the flexibility of a brachytherapy catheter vs. the rigidity of microlens and cylindrical diffuser for PDT).

APC as a noncontact mode using argon plasma jet also clears the pool of mucus and blood and conducts electrons around the corner. It allows spraying larger surface areas to obtain homogeneous and superficial necrosis. Electrocautery and APC are therefore elegant tools for treating early-stage superficial squamous cell cancer known to be only several cell layers' thick similar to using CO_2 laser or ultraviolet light illumination for PDT using Photofrin II$^{\circledR}$ sensitizers (12).

B. Clinical Experience and Results

Various authors such as Hooper (42,43) and Sutedja et al. (11) reported the use of electrocautery through the fiberoptic bronchoscope and its economic potential, but the initial popularity of Nd-YAG laser was overwhelming. The obvious advantages of electrocautery were not fully appreciated until cost-effectiveness became increasingly important (11,12). In palliative interventional pulmonology, various available methods can currently be applied. Hot techniques achieve rapid hemostasis enabling mechanical debulking of obstructing tumors. This combination of techniques has become the cornerstone approach for immediate recanalization (1,2,29). Brachytherapy and PDT with their delayed effects are therefore less appropriate. Electrocautery and APC are straightforward techniques, enabling simpler clinical application than Nd-YAG laser (11,13,44,45).

V. Microdebrider

In contrast to the well-established modalities of laser resection and electrocautery, the microdebrider (Xomed, Jacksonville, Florida, U.S.) is a new addition to the armamentarium of the interventional pulmonologist, used to cut and simultaneously remove obstructing endoluminal tissue from the airway with immediate effect.

A. Equipment and Technical Background

The microdebrider is a powered rotary dissection instrument with incorporated suction, previously used in orthopedics and sinus surgery and newly adapted for CAO (46–48). It consists of the blade (Fig. 5), the hand piece (Fig. 5), and the control console (Fig. 6). The blade is disposable and is composed of a hollow metal tube inside another hollow tube. The blade can be smooth or serrated. It can rotate in the forward and reverse direction or can oscillate between the two. The hand piece allows the user to control its movement. It holds the motor that moves the blade up to 10,000 rpm, though working speeds are in the 1000 to 2000 rpm range. It also contains the suction port through which debris and blood may be removed. The control console operates the hand piece through a foot pedal and allows for changes in speed and direction. The microdebrider blade comes in two lengths: 37 cm, allowing access to lesions of the trachea and at the most of the proximal main bronchi, and 45 cm, for more distal lesions (49).

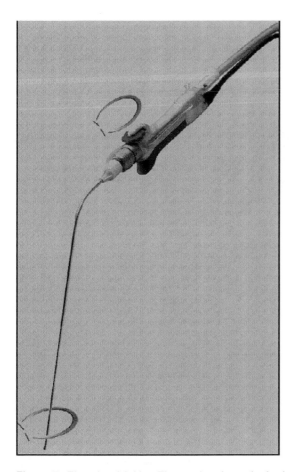

Figure 5 The microdebrider. The rotating tip tracheal microdebrider with the hand piece and suction tube in top right hand corner. *Source*: From Ref. 49.

The microdebrider has several advantages over the thermal modalities of desobstruction. Because of the combination of dissection and suction, there is immediate removal of debris and blood, maintaining a clear operating field. This can make for shorter operating times. There is no need to limit inspired oxygen concentration as airway fires are a nonissue. Patients with high oxygen requirements may be accommodated. For the operators, eye protection is not necessary.

On the other hand, hemostasis is a potential problem, as a separate instrument to control bleeding (a separate thermal modality or tamponade using the rigid bronchoscope) is necessary. In rounded cyst-like lesions, a laser or other modality has to be used to cut into the lesion before the microdebrider can bite into the edges. An important limitation of microdebrider use is its rigidity and diameter of 5 to 7 mm, which limit its use to rigid bronchoscopy or suspension laryngoscopy.

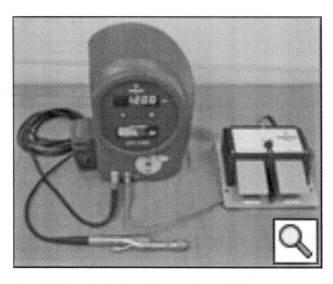

Figure 6   The microdebrider. The control console for selection of blade speed and direction with use of foot switches. *Source*: From Ref. 50.

B.   Clinical Experience and Results

The microdebrider has been in use for sinus surgery since its introduction in 1985 by Kennedy and Kennedy (46). The success of this modality prompted further experimentation. The first use of the tool for airway desobstruction was by Simoni et al. in 2003 (48). In 2005, Lunn et al. (50) reported on the utility of the microdebrider in CAO. Twenty-three cases of postintubation granulation tissue, tracheal stenosis, and malignant obstructions underwent treatment. Lesions were at the trachea or main-stem bronchi. Rigid bronchoscopy and, in four cases, suspension laryngoscopy were employed for the procedure. In 2008, Lunn et al. (51) expanded on their previous work. Using the longer, 45 cm instrument instead of the previous 37 cm, they were able to reach lesions more distal to the mainstem bronchi. While various airway blades are available, Lunn and Ernst (52) favor an angled tip tracheal blade with a serrated edge, as the slight angle to the tip of the blade allows for excellent maneuverability in the airway with the ability to reach most lesions in the trachea and proximal portions of the mainstem bronchi. They prefer the serrated blades to smooth blades, as they found them superior for cutting redundant tissue and pulling it into the orifice of the blade. Further, they prefer an oscillating mode rather than a forward or reverse mode, as they found the oscillating blade to clog up less with tissue. In terms of blade speed, they use slower speeds in the range of 1000 to 2000 rpm, as they allow more time for tissue to be drawn up into the aperture of the blade and result in rapid debridement.

Whether the microdebrider enjoys vast use will depend on the cost of the blades, but also on whether it proves superior both in terms of speed and safety in comparison to simple coring out with the barrel of the rigid bronchoscope of tissue previously devascularized by thermal ablation methods.

VI. How I Do It
A. Equipment

At our institution, a large teaching hospital in the greater Cape Town area, more than 90% of all therapeutic bronchoscopies involving resection of endobronchial tissue are performed with the rigid bronchoscope under general anesthesia. An important consideration is cost-effectiveness due to significant financial constraints. In many instances, the flexible instrument is used through the barrel of the rigid scope, and tissue resection is performed in a combined fashion; more proximal and bulky lesions being treated with rigid applicators, smaller and more distal lesions situated at angles not easily accessible with the rigid tube being treated with the flexible instrument and its tools.

The exclusive use of the flexible bronchoscope is limited to procedures that generally are expected to last a maximum of 30 to 40 minutes and are done under local anesthesia. Such procedures require removal of little tissue such as pure weblike post-intubation stenoses of the trachea or treatment of early lung cancer.

As all our interventional pulmonologists involved in therapeutic bronchoscopies are versed in both the rigid and flexible techniques, the reasons to generally prefer the rigid instrument are (*i*) safety and (*ii*) speed. The better airway control in terms of ventilation and hemostasis is achieved with the rigid tube as mentioned earlier. The major concern even in experienced hands is the occurrence of significant hemorrhage. In such a situation, the combined use of the rigid barrel tip to compress the bleeding site and the ability to use one or more large caliber suction tubes to clear the blood, and simultaneously being able to apply thermal energy to achieve lasting hemostasis present the safest approach. As for speed, the much larger applicators used during rigid bronchoscopy allow much shorter intervention times for the resection of a given amount of tissue. Further, since the defining contributions made by Dumon (26,29), it has become standard practice to remove bulky tissue masses by only devascularizing them with thermal energy and subsequently resecting the tissue mechanically by coring it out with the bevel of the rigid bronchoscope and removing it by forceps (2,14,30,31,53). With the advent of the microdebrider, tissue resection and removal can be achieved in one go, thermal applicators being used to achieve hemostasis where necessary.

B. Thermal Energy

By and large laser resection or electrocautery are competitive techniques (Fig. 1), both being used successfully. At our institution we have opted for electrocautery for financial reasons. We use both flexible and rigid probes. When using the rigid probe, the time-honored combined suction/cautery probe by Storz was found to be extremely safe and fast. Firstly, the probe can be used to palpate tissue; secondly, the continuous suction combined with simultaneous application of electrocautery provides two tools in one, and finally, because of the large suction tube, removal of tissue is often possible by the probe without the need for a forceps.

C. Anesthesia

The most important part is the careful planning and discussion of the procedure with the anesthetist well ahead (36). Potential complications such as bleeding, hypoxia, barotrauma often depend on the nature of the lesion and/or the overall condition of the patient. In case of doubt, a bed in high or intensive care should be reserved for the immediate postoperative period.

Procedures exclusively performed with the flexible bronchoscope are usually done under local anesthesia, with or without transtracheal application of 1% lidocaine. All patients get additional intravenous conscious sedation with midazolam and/or propofol. If a patient is unable to maintain proper airway control, we use mostly a laryngeal mask or an ET tube, both with spontaneous ventilation.

Most procedures are, however, performed under general anesthesia. When using the Dumon bronchoscope, ventilation is assisted-controlled through a large side-port of the scope. When using Storz equipment, jet ventilation is used (36). Most of our procedures are performed with the Dumon scope, as this allows the use of different diameter tubes within a large tracheostomy tube without the need for repetitive extubation/ reintubation maneuvers. This saves time and protects the larynx. Tubes of varying diameters are used for dilatation of airways, exhibiting mixed stenoses with an endoluminal component to be resected and an extraluminal component to be dilated, often combined with stent placement to obtain a durable effect.

Summary

Tracheobronchial therapeutic approaches form a well-established part of the practice of interventional pulmonology both for palliative and for curative intent.

In the palliative setting, the techniques of laser resection, electrocautery, argon plasma coagulation, and microdebrider resection aim at alleviating central airway obstruction. In contrast to brachytherapy and photodynamic therapy with delayed clinical effects they can provide immediate relief. For early stage lung cancer and benign lesions of the central airways, various intraluminal techniques can also be used with curative intent.

References

1. Dumon JF, Shapshay S, Bourcereau J, et al. Principles for safety in application of neodymium-YAG laser in bronchology. Chest 1984; 86:163–168.
2. Bolliger CT, Mathur PN, Beamis JF, et al. European Respiratory Society/American Thoracic Society. ERS/ATS statement on interventional pulmonology. European Respiratory Society/ American Thoracic Society. Eur Respir J 2002; 19:356–373.
3. Ginsberg RJ, Rubinstein LV. Randomized trial of lobectomy versus limited resection for T1 N0 non-small cell lung cancer. Lung Cancer Study Group. Ann Thorac Surg 1995; 60:615–622.
4. Okada M, Nishio W, Sakamoto T. Effect of Tumor size on prognosis in patients with non-small cell lung cancer: the role of segmentectomy as a type of lesser resection. J Thorac Cardiovasc Surg 2005; 129:87–93.
5. Goldstraw P. Lung cancer staging: the sixth and latest revision. Oral Presentation at ATS Congress, Toronto, May 20, 2008.
6. Harms W, Krempien R, Grehn C, et al. Electromagnetically navigated brachytherapy as a new treatment option for peripheral pulmonary tumors. Strahlenther Onkol 2006; 182(2):108–111.
7. Zhu JC, Yan TD, Morris DL. A systematic review of radiofrequency ablation for lung tumors. Ann Surg Oncol 2008; 15(6):1765–1774 [Epub March 2, 2008].
8. Miyazu Y, Miyazawa T, Kurimoto N, et al. Endobronchial ultrasonography in the assessment of centrally located early-stage lung cancer before photodynamic therapy. Am J Respir Crit Care Med 2002; 165(6):832–837.

9. Sutedja TG, van Boxem AJ, Postmus PE. The curative potential of intraluminal bronchoscopic treatment for early-stage non-small-cell lung cancer. Clin Lung Cancer 2001; 2:264–270.

10. Herth FJ, Eberhardt R, Ernst A. The future of bronchoscopy in diagnosing, staging and treatment of lung cancer (Review). Respiration 2006; 73(4):399–409.

11. Sutedja G, van Kralingen K, Schramel FM, et al. Fibreoptic bronchoscopic electrosurgery under local anaesthesia for rapid palliation in patients with central airway malignancies: a preliminary report. Thorax 1994; 49:1243–1246.

12. van Boxem T, Muller M, Venmans B, et al. Nd-YAG laser vs bronchoscopic electrocautery for palliation of symptomatic airway obstruction: a cost-effectiveness study. Chest 1999; 116:1108–1112.

13. Coulter TD, Mehta AC. The heat is on: impact of endobronchial electrosurgery on the need for Nd-YAG laser photoresection. Chest 2000; 118:516–521.

14. Ernst A, Feller-Kopman D, Becker HD, et al. Central airway obstruction. Am J Respir Crit Care Med 2004; 169:1278–1297.

15. Endo C, Sagawa M, Sato M, et al. What kind of hilar lung cancer can be a candidate for segmentectomy with curative intent? Retrospective clinicopathological study of completely resected roentgenographically occult bronchogenic squamous cell carcinoma. Lung Cancer 1998; 21:93–99.

16. Ikeda S. Atlas of Early Cancer of Major Bronchi. Igakushoin Publisher, 1976.

17. Woolner LB, Fontana RS, Cortese DA, et al. Roentgenographically occult lung cancer: pathologic findings and frequency of multicentricity during a 10-year period. Mayo Clin Proc 1984; 59:453–466.

18. Usuda K, Saito Y, Nagamoto N, et al. Relation between bronchoscopic findings and tumor size of roentgenographically occult bronchogenic squamous cell carcinoma. J Thorac Cardiovasc Surg 1993; 106:1098–1103.

19. Konaka C, Hirano T, Kato H, et al. Comparison of endoscopic features of early-stage squamous cell lung cancer and histological findings. Br J Cancer 1999; 80:1435–1439.

20. Nagamoto N, Saito Y, Ohta S, et al. Relationship of lymph node metastasis to primary tumor size and microscopic appearance of roentgenographically occult lung cancer. Am J Surg Pathol 1989; 13:1009–1013.

21. McWilliams A, MacAulay C, Gazdar AF, et al. Innovative molecular and imaging approaches for the detection of lung cancer and its precursor lesions. Oncogene 2002; 21:6949–6959.

22. Sutedja G. New techniques for early detection of lung cancer. Eur Respir J Suppl 2003; 39:57s–66s.

23. Sutedja G, Venmans BJ, Smit EF, et al. Fluorescence bronchoscopy for early detection of lung cancer: a clinical perspective. Lung Cancer 2001; 34:157–168.

24. van Boxem AJ, Westerga J, Venmans BJ, et al. Photodynamic therapy, Nd-YAG laser and electrocautery for treating early-stage intraluminal cancer: which to choose? Lung Cancer 2001; 31:31–36.

25. Mathur PN, Edell E, Sutedja G, et al. Treatment of early stage non-small cell lung cancer. American College of Chest Physicians. Chest 2003; 123(1 suppl):176S–180S.

26. Dumon JF, Rebound E, Garbe L, et al. Treatment of tracheobronchial lesions by laser photoresection. Chest 1982; 81:278–284.

27. Cavaliere S, Foccoli P, Farina P. Nd:YAG laser bronchoscopy: a 5-years experience with 1,396 applications in 1,000 patients. Chest 1988; 94:15–21.

28. Cavaliere S, Foccoli P, Toninelli C. Endobronchial laser treatment. In: Strausz J, ed. Pulmonary Endoscopy and Biopsy Techniques. European Respiratory Monograph, Vol 3. 1998:49–64.

29. Cavaliere S, Dumon JF. Laser bronchoscopy. In: Bolliger CT, Mathur PN, eds. Interventional Bronchoscopy. Prog Respir Res. Basel: Karger, 2000; 30:108–119.

30. Ernst A, Gerard A, Silvestri GA, et al. Interventional pulmonary procedures guidelines from the American College of Chest Physicians. Chest 2003; 123:1693–1717.

31. Bolliger CT, Sutedja TG, Strausz J, et al. Therapeutic bronchoscopy with immediate effect: laser, electrocautery, argon plasma coagulation and stents. Eur Respir J 2006; 27:1258–1271.
32. Mehta AC, Lee FY, Cordasco EM, et al. Concentric tracheal and subglottic stenosis. Management using the Nd:YAG laser for mucosal sparing followed by gentle balloon dilatation. Chest 1993; 104:673–677.
33. Lee P, Kupeli E, Mehta AC. Therapeutic bronchoscopy in lung cancer. Laser therapy, electrocautery, brachytherapy, stents, and photodynamic therapy. Clin Chest Med 2002; 23: 241–256.
34. Laforet EG, Berger RL, Vaughan CW: carcinoma obstructing the trachea. Treatment by laser resection. N Engl J Med 1976; 294:941.
35. Toty L, Personne C, Colchen A, et al. Bronchoscopic management of tracheal lesions using Nd:YAG laser. Thorax 1981; 36:175–178.
36. Studer W, Bolliger CT, Biro P. Anesthesia for interventional bronchoscopy. In: Bolliger CT, Mathur PN, eds. Interventional Bronchoscopy. Prog Respir Res. Basel: Karger, 2000; 30:44–54.
37. Cortese DA. Rigid versus flexible bronchoscope in laser bronchoscopy. J Bronchol 1994; 1:72–75.
38. Barlow DE. Endoscopic applications of electrosurgery: a review of basic principles. Gastrointest Endosc 1982; 14:61–63.
39. Grund KE, Storek D, Farin G. Endoscopic argon plasma coagulation (APC) first clinical experiences in flexible endoscopy. Endosc Surg Allied Technol 1994; 2:42–46.
40. van Boxem TJ, Westerga J, Venmans BJ, et al. Tissue effects of bronchoscopic electrocautery: bronchoscopic appearance and histologic changes of bronchial wall after electrocautery. Chest 2000; 117:887–891.
41. Fenton JL, Beamis JF. Laser bronchoscopy. In: Beamis JF, Mathur PN, eds. Interventional Pulmonology. New York: McGrwa-Hill, 1999:43–67.
42. Hooper RG, Jackson FN. Endobronchial electrocautery. Chest 1985; 87:712–714.
43. Hooper RG. Electrocautery in endobronchial therapy. A letter to the editor. Chest 2000; 117:1820.
44. Reichle G, Freitag L, Kullmann HJ, et al. Argon plasma coagulation in bronchology: a new method—alternative or complementary? Pneumologie 2000; 54:508–516.
45. Morice RC, Ece T, Ece F, et al. Endobronchial argon plasma coagulation for treatment of hemoptysis and neoplastic airway obstruction. Chest 2001; 119:781–787.
46. Kennedy DW, Kennedy EM. Endoscopic sinus surgery. AORN J 1985; 42(6):932–936.
47. Reed AL, Flint R. Emerging role of powered instrumentation in airway surgery. Curr Opin Otolaryngol Head Neck Surg 2001; 9:387–392.
48. Simoni P, Peters GE, Magnuson JS, et al. Use of the endoscopic microdebrider in the management of airway obstruction from laryngotracheal carcinoma. Ann Otol Rhinol Laryngol 2003; 112:11–13.
49. Kennedy MP, Morice RC, Jimenez CA, et al. Treatment of bronchial airway obstruction using a rotating tip microdebrider: a case report. J Cardiothorac Surg 2007; 2:16.
50. Lunn W, Garland R, Ashiku S, et al. Microdebrider bronchoscopy: a new tool for the interventional bronchoscopist. Ann Thorac Surg 2005; 80:1485–1488.
51. Lunn W, Bagherzadegan N, Munjampalli S, et al. Initial experience with a rotating airway microdebrider. J Bronch 2008; 15(2):91–94.
52. Lunn W, Ernst A. The microdebrider allows for rapid removal of obstructing airway lesions. Available at: http://www.CTSNet.org.
53. Wahidi MM, Herth FJF, Ernst A. State of the art. Interventional pulmonology. Chest 2007; 131:261–274.

3

Update on Cryotherapy, Brachytherapy, and Photodynamic Therapy

TIM LAHM and FRANCIS D. SHESKI
Indiana University School of Medicine, Indianapolis, Indiana, U.S.A.

I. Introduction

While the use of laser therapy, electrocautery, or argon plasma coagulation in patients with endobronchial lesions leads to immediate tissue destruction, cryotherapy, photodynamic therapy (PDT), and brachytherapy often demonstrate a delayed onset. Therefore, the latter techniques are generally limited to situations in which rapid tissue destruction and rapid symptom relief are not crucial. Each modality has unique characteristics, indications, and clinical advantages, as reflected in recent evidence-based clinical practice guidelines of the American College of Chest Physicians, which support cryotherapy, brachytherapy, and PDT as treatment options for patients with superficial non–small cell lung cancer (NSCLC), who are not surgical candidates (1). In many situations, these methods are complementary. A common requirement is that the pathology be endobronchial. It is the purpose of this chapter to discuss the history, scientific background, practical and technical aspects, indications, and potential complications of each of these three modalities.

II. Cryotherapy

Endobronchial cryotherapy (ECT) refers to the application of cold to destroy tissue via repetitive freeze-thaw cycles.

A. History

In 1845, James Arnott published the first report of "cold" for the treatment of malignancy, using it to treat uterine cancer (2). Gage was the first to report the use of cryotherapy for endobronchial lesions, applying this in 1968 via rigid bronchoscopy (3). Initially, the technique received little attention, but over the next 25 years, several studies were published on ECT for either malignant or benign conditions, and cryotherapy through a rigid bronchoscope became widespread in Europe (4–8). The development of a flexible cryoprobe in 1994 (ERBE-USA, Inc., Marietta, Georgia, U.S.) allowed for the use of ECT via a flexible bronchoscope, making the technique popular in North America. In 1996, Mathur et al. published the initial report in the United States, detailing the use of the technique via flexible bronchoscopy mainly for palliative treatment in patients with malignancy (9). Today, ECT via a flexible bronchoscope is commonly used in a variety of settings. Current studies investigate the potential for synergistic effects between ECT and chemotherapy in the treatment of NSCLC (10,11).

B. Scientific Basis

Cryotherapy damages and destroys cells through multiple mechanisms (12). Contact between the cryoprobe and tissue leads to an immediate adherence between the surfaces. This phenomenon allows removal of blood clots, mucous plugs, or foreign bodies, as described later in this chapter. When the temperature drops further, molecular processes in the cell slow and ultimately stop. At tissue temperatures of $-15°C$ to $-40°C$ or colder, intracellular dehydration occurs, intracellular and extracellular ice crystals form, intracellular pH and tonicity change, and venous and capillary blood flow cease. In addition, vasoconstriction of arterioles and venules as well as increases in capillary permeability and formation of platelet aggregates are observed. These processes result in thrombosis, ischemia, and cell death. The vascular effects explain the hemostatic effects of cryotherapy. The effects of cryotherapy on cell death are dependent on freezing time, thawing time, lowest temperature achieved, and number of freeze-thaw cycles (13–15). Freezing and thawing times play a central role in this process. When tissue is cooled, extracellular ice crystals form, while the intracellular matrix remains liquid (16). When tissue is cooled slowly, the dehydration results in an intracellular increase in solute concentration that prevents intracellular freezing. However, with rapid cooling, water does not have time to pass the membrane and intracellular ice crystals form. Because of the extremely destructive nature of this process, damage of mitochondria, endoplasmatic reticulum, and other intracellular structures occurs, eventually resulting in complete crystallization of the cell. Slow thawing, in contrast to rapid thawing, fosters intracellular crystallization (17). Therefore, cryotherapy is most destructive to tissue when cells are frozen rapidly and thawed slowly. The vascular effects occur 6 to 12 hours after the physical insult, thereby completing cell destruction via local infarction. Around the area of the cryoprobe, cell death occurs through necrosis (18). Tissue destruction more peripherally is heterogeneous and occurs mainly through apoptosis (18). In a study by Homasson et al. (18), necrosis was found near the cryoprobe impact site and was maximal two hours after treatment, with a second peak being observed after four days. Around this central necrosis, apoptotic cells were found and apoptosis was maximal after eight hours. In contrast to ECT, chemotherapy induced apoptosis in a fewer number of cells, and this effect was time independent.

The above-mentioned processes result in an area of tissue destruction with a diameter of approximately 1 cm when a 3-mm-diameter probe is used (18). Cytotoxicity occurs to a depth of 3 to 5 mm. One to two weeks after the procedure, nonhemorrhagic tissue necrosis will occur. Poorly vascularized tissues, such as cartilage or fat, are cryoresistant. This minimizes the risk of bronchial perforation or scarring with fibrosis and stenosis, contributing to procedure safety (5,12). In contrast, highly vascularized tissues, such as malignant tumors or granulation tissue, are particularly susceptible to cryotherapy (19,20). The cytotoxic effects are most pronounced in proximity to the cryoprobe, and they are characterized by a delayed onset that is completed by a late hemostatic effect.

C. Technical Aspects

Two types of cryogens exist: liquid nitrogen and nitrous oxide. While the former is very potent, its use is limited by inconvenience in handling and by unavailability in the United States. With both agents, cooling occurs by the sudden expansion of a gas from a high to a low pressure (Joule–Thomson principle). As mentioned previously, both rigid and flexible cryoprobes are available, and choice depends on personal preference and

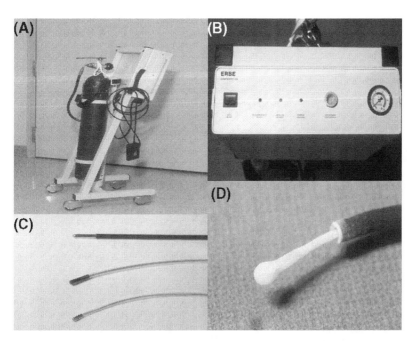

Figure 1 Equipment used at our institution for endobronchial therapy. (**A**) ERBOCRYO®CA cryotherapy unit (ERBE-USA, Inc., Marietta, Georgia, U.S.). Only nitrous oxide–driven cryoprobes are available in the United States. The unit uses the Joule–Thomson principle where pressurized gas expands through a fine orifice producing a rapid drop in temperature, thereby freezing the probe tip and the surrounding tissue. (**B**) Control unit, which can be combined with either rigid or flexible cryoprobes (**C, D**). The rigid probe requires rigid bronchoscopy.

institutional infrastructure. Rigid cryoprobes have a 3-mm contact area and the advantage of a footpad or a trigger on the handle that allows for immediate and active thawing after cooling. These probes require rigid bronchoscopy. In contrast, with the flexible cryoprobe, thawing is a passive process, resulting in a longer freezing and thawing cycle as compared to the rigid probe. However, with a diameter of <3 mm, flexible probes can be used through a flexible bronchoscope, eliminating the need for rigid bronchoscopy and general anesthesia (9). Recently, reinforced cryoprobes were developed that allow for the removal of tumor pieces after the adherence phase (21). Only the tip of the probe causes freezing, the rest of the device is insulated. In contrast to laser with its associated risk of airway fire, high oxygen concentrations can be used during ECT (Fig. 1).

With both rigid and flexible probes, the cryoprobe is advanced through the working channel of the bronchoscope and then either pushed into protruding tissue or applied laterally onto more infiltrative or superficial tissue. In general, three cycles of freezing and thawing are performed at each location. Each freezing period lasts about 30 to 60 seconds. Thawing occurs through body heat and takes 30 to 60 seconds. After three cycles, the tip of the cryoprobe is advanced to an adjacent part of the tumor or granulation tissue. While a treated area is about 10 mm in size, the adjacent impact of the

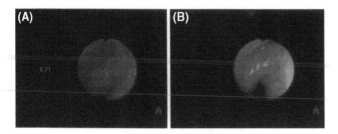

Figure 2 Autofluorescence (**A**) and white light images (**B**) of lung cancer occurrence at the site of a previous right upper lobe resection. The autofluorescence images demonstrate marked hetero-geneity and discoloration indicating atypical tissue, while the white light images only reveal non-specific inflammatory changes. This is also an example of a tumor possibly suitable for cryotherapy, brachytherapy, or photodynamic therapy in case the patient is a poor surgical candidate.

probe should be made about 5 mm from the first impact so that the frozen areas overlap. In case of malignancy, it is crucial to cover the entire surface of the tumor. Often, 30 or more cycles are required. If early stages of lung cancer are treated, autofluorescence bronchoscopy may provide important information regarding the borders of the lesion (22) (Fig. 2). If autofluorescence is unavailable, a margin of 5 mm around the visible borders of the lesion should be treated. Interestingly, immediately after treatment is complete, the tissue usually appears undamaged. For the reasons outlined above, the occurrence of tissue death is delayed. Approximately one week after the ECT session, necrotic sloughed tissue either is spontaneously removed by expectoration or needs to be removed by bronchoscopy. In general, when ECT alone is used for lung cancer, a second session is needed to treat residual tumor.

D. Indications

Because of the delayed onset of effects, ECT is only indicated for situations where immediate relief of airway obstruction is not required. However, the cryoadherence that is generated when the probe comes in contact with biologic tissue can be used to facilitate removal of clots, mucus plugs, or foreign bodies such as food, pills, or peanuts. This is of particular importance when other devices (like forceps) are not capable of grasping extremely soft and pliable tissues such as clots, mucus plugs, or food. Recently, the successful removal of a broncholith using ECT during flexible bronchoscopy has been reported (23). On the other hand, the method is less efficient for teeth, bone, or metallic foreign bodies (12). In addition, after rapid tumor debulking has been achieved by using the tip of a rigid bronchoscope, electrocautery, or laser, ECT can be used in the same session in order to treat any remaining or infiltrating tumor. Cryotherapy is highly effective for cellular and well-vascularized tissues, such as bronchial carcinomas, car-cinoids, adenoid cystic carcinomas, or granulation tissue (Fig. 3) (24). The technique has also been successfully used for endobronchial metastases (25). In lung cancers ECT is successful in approximately 75%, regardless of the cell type or the endoluminal aspect (6,7,12,19). Furthermore, the vascular effects of the method make it effective for tumor-related hemoptysis. The characteristics of ECT also make it a safe and effective tech-nique for the treatment of carcinomas in situ or microinvasive tumors. In a French study of 35 patients with early superficial bronchogenic carcinoma treated with this method,

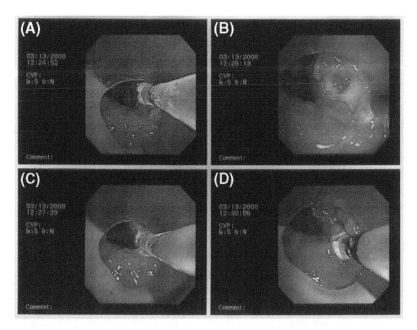

Figure 3 Endobronchial cryotherapy for removal of granulation tissue at the distal end of a Y-stent. In a step-wise fashion using several freeze-thaw cycles (**A–D**), the obstructing granulation tissue is removed, allowing for significant improvement in dyspnea and respiratory mechanics.

the complete response rate after one year was 91% (26). Fifty percent of patients were long-term survivors (follow-up >4 years) (26). A recurrence rate of 28% within four years was reported, and a long-term response of 63% was achieved. Some authors also use the technique for the removal of residual stalks of resected tumors (12,27). Since collagen-rich tissue, scar tissue, and poorly cellular tumors are not cryosensitive, ECT alone is not indicated for benign tracheobronchial strictures, fibromas, lipomas, or postintubation stenoses (12,28). In addition, this method is not indicated in situations with extrinsic compression of the airways. Recent data suggest a synergistic effect when ECT is combined with other treatment modalities such as chemotherapy or radiation therapy. While promising results have been reported in both animals and humans (7,11,29,30), large randomized trials are needed to confirm these data.

E. Complications
As compared to other methods, ECT is a safe and predictable method that is not associated with the risk of airway perforation, tracheobronchomalacia, or residual stenosis. The most commonly observed side effects are fever and sloughing of necrotic tissue. The fever is usually self-limiting and because of an inflammatory response induced by cell death and subsequent cytokine release. If bothersome, the fever can be treated with antipyretics. Sloughing of necrotic airway tissue can be excessive and result in cough, dyspnea, and even airway obstruction. To prevent this complication, flexible bronchoscopy for pulmonary toilet is recommended 8 to 10 days after the procedure.

Rare complications include fatal hemoptysis, tracheoesophageal fistulas, cardiopulmonary arrest, pneumothorax, bronchospasm, cardiac arrhythmias, and exacerbation of
cold-agglutinin anemia (7,9,30).

III. Brachytherapy

Endobronchial brachytherapy (EBT) describes the process of local irradiation via
placement of radioactive material within or close to an endoluminal or peribronchial
tumor. The radioactive source usually is iridium-192 (Ir-192). The technique is usually
applied as high dose rate (HDR) brachytherapy.

A. History

After having gained experience with radioactive implants in gynecologic oncology,
radium capsules were used endobronchially in 1922 by Yankauer (31). Initially, the
radioactive source was instilled directly into the tumor, but this was associated with high
irradiation exposure to medical personnel. In the 1950s and 1960s, Henschke introduced
modern afterloading techniques (32,33), thereby allowing for the widespread use of the
technique. The procedure was initially performed using rigid bronchoscopy and general
anesthesia. The use of a plastic catheter with the flexible bronchoscope was reported two
decades later (34,35). The use of Ir-192 evolved around the same time (34). The small
size of the iridium source and its high activity allowed for fast, highly active treatment
via a hollow guidance catheter and the flexible bronchoscope. As a result, low and
intermediate dose rate brachytherapy, which were used initially, were soon replaced by
HDR brachytherapy in the 1980s (36,37). The introduction of automated and computer-
controlled steering devices has further advanced the field. Brachytherapy has mainly
been used for palliative purposes in cases of hemoptysis, cough, or dyspnea caused by
malignancy. In the case of NSCLC, the method is usually employed in patients who
have failed or are not candidates for other forms of therapy, such as surgery or external
beam irradiation. However, in recent years, the use of EBT alone or in combination with
other modalities has emerged as a treatment option for early stage lung cancer.

B. Scientific Basis

The basic principle of EBT is the delivery of therapeutic irradiation to malignant tissue,
while minimizing injury to the normal airway. The irradiation effect decreases from the
source inversely proportional to the radius of the airway lumen. As a result, a high
irradiation dose can be achieved at the center of the irradiation source, with a rapid
decrease towards the periphery (Fig. 4). While this aspect limits the area that can be
treated, it also limits toxicity. The effects of irradiation are single-chain breaks in the
DNA of irradiated cells, resulting in apoptosis and decreased cell proliferation. As a
consequence, the effects of EBT are delayed, and the maximum histological and visible
changes are usually present after three weeks. This explains why EBT is often used as a
stabilizing measure in conjunction with fast-acting debulking techniques such as Nd:
YAG laser therapy. Malignant tissue is clearly more susceptible to the effects of irradiation than nonmalignant tissue (38,39).

C. Technical Aspects

To perform EBT, a flexible polyethylene catheter (usually 2–3 mm in diameter) is
placed adjacent to and beyond the malignancy using flexible bronchoscopy so that the

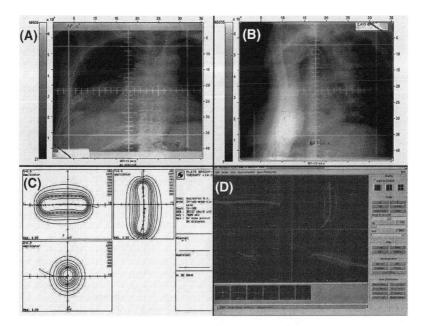

Figure 4 Brachytherapy planning and treatment. A set of radiographs is obtained to verify correct placement of the afterloading catheter within the tumor and determine the required irradiation length (**A, B**). The dose distribution is generated by specifying the dwell positions to be used along the catheter and importing this information into the brachytherapy planning software. The dwell time of the HDR source at each position is optimized to create a uniform dose distribution (**C**). The treatment dose is usually described as 1 cm from the middle of the source axis. The plan is then transferred to the Nucletron HDR unit and the patient's catheter is connected to the unit (**D**). *Source*: Images courtesy of Achilles J. Fakiris, MD.

irradiation can be delivered close to the tumor. Thus, complete airway obstruction must not be present. However, initial debulking with other bronchoscopic methods may allow for the subsequent application of EBT. If laser is used for debulking, a three-day interval is recommended before EBT is initiated, even though this recommendation has been questioned (12,40,41). Under bronchoscopic and fluoroscopic guidance, the catheter is advanced over a guidewire. Both the bronchoscope and guidewire are then removed, leaving the catheter in place. A radiopaque "dummy" insert with marker pellets is then placed into the catheter to simulate the pathway of the radiation source. After proper placement is confirmed fluoroscopically, the system is fastened externally to the patient. The radiation oncologist determines the irradiation dosing using radiographic and bronchoscopic visualization of tumor load and location (Fig. 4). As mentioned previously, HDR using Ir-192 is the usual delivery mode. The dose is described as 1 cm from the source (42). Centering devices such as balloons, cages, or sheaths can be used to keep the irradiation source in the center of the airway lumen and avoid dose inhomogeneity (43). Total dose and fractionation vary from institution to institution. The procedure is performed in a shielded room, and the irradiation is delivered automatically by an afterloader, thereby limiting exposure to medical personnel. The irradiation source is advanced to the desired position and is then drawn backward at 5-mm intervals. It remains in each position as long as needed to deliver the computed dose. Source position and dwelling time can thus be varied, achieving individual computer-assisted dose distribution. A 1-cm safety margin should be applied at each end of the tumor. Irradiation length is defined as the length between the first and the last dwell point of the Ir-192 (in case of HDR brachytherapy). HDR brachytherapy with Ir-192 employs delivering a 3- to 10-Gy fraction over several minutes. This fraction is repeated every one to two weeks for a total of two to four sessions. Only one controlled, randomized study evaluated dose rate, overall irradiation dose, fractionation, and localization of the afterloading catheter (44). Two regimens with a similar total irradiation dose of 15 Gy but different doses per fraction (four fractions of 3.8 Gy per week vs. two fractions of 7.2 Gy three weeks apart) did not find any differences in survival time (19 weeks), local control time, or complication rates. Fatal hemorrhage occurred in 21% of patients. The procedure is usually performed on an outpatient basis. Since the maximal effect is appreciated after about three weeks, a repeat bronchoscopy three to six weeks after completion of treatment is usually performed.

D. Indications

The major advantage of EBT is its longer lasting effect and greater tissue penetration as compared to other endobronchial antineoplastic therapies. Brachytherapy also destroys tissue outside the bronchial wall and behind cartilage tissue. With HDR brachytherapy, a high irradiation dose can be applied over a short period, while minimizing damage to the surrounding airway and lung parenchyma. As a consequence, EBT is an elegant method for long-lasting destruction of tumor tissue inside and outside the bronchial wall. However, imminent and significant endotracheal or endobronchial obstruction must not be present. Initial debulking with faster acting methods is indicated in these cases. In addition, the presence of fistulas between bronchi and surrounding structures represent contraindications as well.

Similar to cryotherapy and PDT, EBT can be used with curative or palliative intent. In most cases, EBT is performed for palliation of dyspnea, hemoptysis, or cough in patients with malignancy and poor performance status. The technique can also be used in patients who have received their maximal dose of external beam radiation therapy (EBRT). Success rates vary between 53% and 95% (12,45,46). Hemoptysis and endobronchial obstruction seem to be most responsive, while dyspnea, cough, and pain are less so. In most patients, the palliative effects seem to be sustained (41,47–52), and limited data suggest a survival benefit in selected cases (53,54). In the curative setting, EBT is indicated for microscopically positive resection margins after surgery, as an adjunct to EBRT, and for early lung cancer. Brachytherapy has been used in conjunction with EBRT to reduce the volume of irradiated lung parenchyma and improve local control (48,49,54–57). EBT can reduce the irradiation of normal tissues by 32% (58), thereby attenuating the amount of radiation fibrosis. While a survival benefit of combination therapy with EBT and EBRT has not been clearly demonstrated, evidence exists that local control can be improved when the two methods are combined (57). Recently, the successful use of navigated brachytherapy with an electromagnetic navigation system was reported in a patient with medically inoperable NSCLC of the peripheral right upper lobe that was not amenable to conventional bronchoscopy (59).

Brachytherapy in early lung cancer has been used for patients who were not surgical candidates, had recurrence after surgery or EBRT, or were in conjunction with other treatment modalities such as chemotherapy, laser, or cryotherapy. Radiosensitization may occur when used in conjunction with systemic chemotherapy (60). Unfortunately, a clear definition of "early stage" lung cancer (dysplasia vs. carcinoma in situ vs. microinvasive carcinoma) is lacking in most publications, and no randomized, controlled comparison studies exist to date. The current literature suggests that HDR, either alone or in combination with EBRT, seems to be a treatment option with good results and low morbidity (51,55,61–68). The deeper tissue penetration makes this method an attractive modality, but further investigation in form of randomized, prospective trials is needed before definitive recommendations can be made.

HDR-EBT in nonmalignant cases has mainly been used for the treatment of granulation tissue around stents or airway anastomoses after lung transplantation (69–73). Tendulkar et al. (71) recently reported eight patients with refractory benign airway obstruction that were treated with HDR-EBT. Six patients had a good or excellent subjective early response, but only one patient maintained this response beyond six months. HDR-EBT increased mean FEV_1 and allowed for a decrease in the mean number of bronchoscopic interventions. Five patients died from causes related to their chronic pulmonary disease, including one death from hemoptysis resulting from a bronchoarterial fistula. The authors suggested that performing HDR-EBT within 24 to 48 hours after excision of obstructive granulation tissue might further improve outcomes. In a series of five refractory patients with significant airway compromise from recurrent granulation tissue treated with HDR-EBT, all patients experienced a reduction in the number of therapeutic bronchoscopic procedures after HDR brachytherapy compared with the pretreatment period (72). With the exception of possible radiation-induced bronchitis in one patient, no other treatment-related complications were reported. Optimal timing, dose fractionation, and candidate selection have not yet been defined.

E. Complications

Two serious complications of EBT are massive hemoptysis and fistula formation. Fatal hemoptysis rates of 0% to 42% have been reported, with an overall incidence of 10% (4,12,46,52,57,74). However, most studies were neither prospective nor randomized, and different selection criteria have been applied. It is also unclear what percentage of hemoptysis is because of tumor infiltration of blood vessels versus direct irradiation effects. It has been postulated that the increase in bleeding correlates with a longer survival time as a result of EBT rather than with the treatment itself (12). Squamous cell carcinoma and tumor localization in the main stem or upper lobe represent risk factors for hemoptysis (66,75,76). Whether prior EBRT or the combination of EBT and EBRT are risk factors has not been clearly defined. In contrast, irradiation in vicinity of major blood vessels and an increase in the dose per fraction over 10 Gy clearly increase the bleeding risk (77,78). The incidence of fistula formation is comparable to that of hemoptysis, and the same concerns with regard to study quality and selection criteria hold true.

Similar to EBRT, radiation bronchitis and stenosis may occur weeks to months after treatment. The usual symptoms are cough and wheezing. Concurrent EBRT, radiation with curative intent, large cell lung cancer, and prior laser resection represent risk factors (47). Bronchial stenosis has been reported to occur in 10% of patients (79).

Treatment of radiation bronchitis consists of inhaled corticosteroids, while radiation stenosis is treated with balloon dilatation, laser resection, and/or stenting.

Acute complications at the time of the procedure include cough, bronchospasm, bronchorrhea, and pneumothorax or pleuritic chest pain because of catheter placement. However, the incidence of these complications is similar to that of regular bronchoscopy (12). Patients with poor performance status and preexisting respiratory compromise are at higher risk for periprocedural complications.

IV. Photodynamic Therapy

Photodynamic therapy (PDT) refers to tissue destruction that relies on the excitation of a chemical photosensitizer by an appropriate light, whose wavelength matches the absorption band of this substance. In the presence of oxygen, this process results in a photodynamic reaction that leads to cell necrosis via the generation of reactive oxygen species.

A. History

The therapeutic effects of sunlight and light-activated chemical substances have been recognized for several centuries (12). The scientific basis of modern phototherapy stems from the work of Finsen in the early 20th century (80). The first case of clinical PDT was published by Lipson et al. in 1966 (81), reporting a patient with a recurrent ulcerating breast tumor that was treated by injection of a hematoporphyrin derivate followed by exposure to a filtered xenon arc lamp. In the 1970s, several investigators studied the photodynamic effects of various chemicals and their corresponding activating light. Hematoporphyrin derivative and light in the red spectrum evolved as the most suitable combination (82,83). Dougherty et al. (84) advanced the field by demonstrating that systemic administration of hematoporphyrin derivate followed by exposure to red light from a xenon arc lamp can eradicate transplanted murine mammary tumor material without causing significant damage to the surrounding healthy tissue. This group also demonstrated the effectiveness of PDT in a variety of malignancies in clinical trials (82,84,85). The era of bronchoscopic PDT began in 1982 in Tokyo, where Hayata et al. applied this technique to treat a patient with early lung cancer that refused surgical treatment (86). PDT resulted in complete eradication of the tumor. Interestingly, the patient died four years later from non-cancer-related causes (87). Because of its high incidence, advanced stage at the time of diagnosis, and high rate of unresectable tumors, lung cancer was one of the first cancers addressed in clinical PDT trials (88–91).

B. Scientific Basis

The basis of PDT rests in the preferential retention of a photosensitizing agent by malignant or premalignant tissue. As mentioned above, PDT destroys tissue through excitation of this photosensitizer by an appropriate light. The resulting photodynamic reaction is dependent on the presence of oxygen, leading to the generation of reactive oxygen species and subsequent cytotoxicity and cell death. In addition, vascular and ischemic effects seem to play a role as well. The photodynamic process also leads to an inflammatory response with complement activation and red cell extravasation, thereby promoting further tissue damage (92–94). In addition to direct effects on cellular mechanisms, cytotoxicity is also mediated by effects on the extracellular milieu. Similar to cryotherapy, cell death results from necrosis as well as apoptosis.

C. Technical Aspects

The process of bronchoscopic PDT consists of two stages: photosensitization and illumination. The photosensitization stage is achieved by the intravenous administration of a photosensitizer to the patient. Hematoporphyrin derivative, which was used initially, was later replaced by purified and manipulated derivates. At the present time, porfimer sodium (Photofrin®, Axcan Pharma, Birmingham, Alabama, U.S.) is the most commonly used photosensitizer. The agent has a long-standing safety record (91,95–97). The recommended dose is 2 mg/kg body weight. However, the drug is not entirely selective, and indiscriminate illumination can potentially lead to collateral damage to adjacent areas with edema or inflammation. Other photosensitizers (such as chlorin-based agents) have been developed in the interim. Recent literature suggests excellent antitumor effects and safety of the second-generation photosensitizer mono-L-aspartyl chlorin e6 (NPe6) (98,99). Inhaled photosensitizers such as 5-aminolevulinic acid (5-ALA) have been studied as well, but their use is limited by a high false-positive rate (100).

During illumination, the presensitized tumor is exposed to a light of a specific matching wavelength. This exposure results in necrosis of tumor tissue. Two different illumination techniques exist: in interstitial illumination, light exposure is from within the tumor, while in surface illumination, exposure is over the surface of the tumor. The actual depth of light penetration is rather unpredictable, but is thought to be <1 cm (101). As a consequence, PDT is most effective for local and superficial disease.

The light that activates porphyrin-based sensitizers such as porfimer sodium has a wavelength of 630 nm (red region of the spectrum). Several sources are available to deliver the red light. These include argon/dye or metal vapor lasers. More recently, diode lasers have been used (Fig. 5) (12,102). Diode lasers for other photosensitizers are available as well. The light generated and emitted by the laser is delivered to the

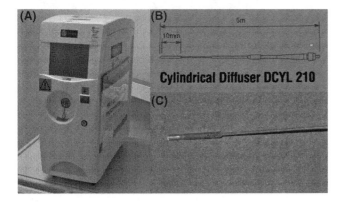

Figure 5 Laser system and cylindrical diffusing tip used for photodynamic therapy. The figure shows a Diomed 630 PDT system (DIOMED Inc., Andover, Massachusetts, U.S.), which is used in conjunction with porfimer sodium (Photofrin®) (**A**). The diode laser provides up to 2000 mW of 630-nm continuous wave laser radiation to the tip of a flexible delivery fiber optic. The optical diffuser fiber (Optiguide™ DCYL 210, DIOMED Inc.) (**B, C**) is a light delivery system consisting of a 400-μm core silica optical fiber, a proximal SMA-type connector (*), and a distal light diffusing tip (**C**). The fiber is designed to distribute light energy uniformly over the specified length of the diffuser tip.

endobronchial tumor by optical fibers with either a cylindrical diffusing tip or a microlens. The former distributes light circumferentially and can be used for interstitial treatment when the diffusing tip is placed within the tumor mass. The microlens emits forward-firing light and is used for surface application to treat superficial growth. The light dose at its point of delivery usually ranges from 200 to 400 J/cm of lesion (94). The optical fiber is introduced through the biopsy channel of the flexible bronchoscope. This can be done with or without previous insertion of a rigid bronchoscope. If a rigid bronchoscope is used, the procedure requires general anesthesia. Obviously, the technique using rigid bronchoscopy is associated with the usual general anesthesia risks. However, advantages are patient comfort, ease of operation, stability of the position of the optical fiber, better airway clearance, and improved ability to handle complications. As a consequence, most authors use the rigid technique for advanced disease or endobronchial obstruction involving the major airways, while the flexible approach is preferred for early and superficial lesions (12,91). The PDT unit and the cylindrical diffusing tip used at our institution are depicted in Figure 5.

Prior to performing PDT, it is crucial to examine the entire airway to evaluate for the presence of synchronous malignant lesions. Some authors use autofluorescence to better delineate the tumor and its extent (Fig. 2). This technique may also facilitate the detection of synchronous lesions that may otherwise be missed with white light bronchoscopy (103). After intravenous administration of the photosensitizer, several days are allowed for absorption and retention of the agent within the malignant tissue. The duration of this latent period is largely dependent on the type of photosensitizer used. For porfimer sodium, this is typically 48 to 72 hours. During this period, the photosensitizer is being washed out of normal tissue, while it is retained in the tumor. After the latent period, illumination is carried out. Exposure times range from 5 to 30 minutes. Interestingly, neither exposure time nor light dose has been exactly determined. After PDT, the airway may need to be cleared of secretions and debris. This step may have to be repeated a few days later, especially in the case of large endoluminal tumors. In case of extensive debris or secretions, rigid bronchoscopy may be most effective for airway clearance. At this point, the airway may also be reevaluated for the presence of residual tumor. If areas of residual tumor are present, re-illumination can be performed. However, this needs to be performed as long as the tissue concentration of the photosensitizer within the tumor is within the therapeutic window. For porfimer sodium, this is usually six to seven days. The total number of treatments that one can have is unknown.

D. Indications

PDT is usually performed for histologically confirmed malignant lesions. These may either be obstructive, endobronchial lesions or early, superficial lesions. In the case of obstructive lesions, the intent of PDT may be curative or palliative. PDT for cure is usually performed in patients with technically resectable malignancies, but who are poor surgical candidates. The most recent evidence comes from Moghissi et al. (104). These authors demonstrated that bronchoscopic PDT in early central lung cancer can achieve long disease-free survival and suggested that this technique be considered as a treatment option in patients ineligible for resection. In addition, the method may be used for detection and treatment of multifocal and synchronous early endobronchial cancer that is not amenable to resection (103). Endobronchial metastases—from lung cancer or other cancer types for that matter—may be amenable to PDT as well. It should be noted that the detection rate of early or synchronous endobronchial cancer can be improved by the use of autofluorescence bronchoscopy and/or endobronchial ultrasonography (99,103–108). Several authors have demonstrated that PDT can mediate long-term survival in patients with early superficial lung cancer. At Tokyo Medical University, where there is ample experience with the use of bronchoscopic PDT in early lung cancer, a 60% five-year survival rate and a more than 90% cancer-specific survival rate have been demonstrated (87,109). Similar results were reported in a literature review of a total of 650 patients undergoing PDT for early lung cancer (91). Multiple publications (90,95,101,110–115) describe the treatment of early NSCLC with PDT. Although these studies vary with regard to power, energy, and exposure times, as well as the definition of "early" lung cancer, current literature supports the role of PDT for lung cancer that is relatively noninvasive (<1 cm), limited in surface area, not bulky, and accessible by the bronchoscope. Taken together, the data to date indicate that patients with early lung cancer treated with PDT achieve a complete response in approximately 75% cases. The recurrence rate is approximately 30%. Complete response rates >90% can be achieved when lesions are <1 cm in diameter, superficial, and when all margins can be visualized. Not surprisingly, success rates decrease with an increase in lesion size, especially if it is ≥1 cm (116). Local recurrence at the same site is thought to be caused by residual tumor cells from deep layers, because of inadequate light penetration.

If PDT is performed with the goal of palliation, patients are usually symptomatic with dyspnea, cough, and/or hemoptysis. As with any other endobronchial technique, PDT should only be pursued if the symptoms are expected to improve after the intervention.

All histological types of lung cancer, including small cell lung cancer, are PDT sensitive (91,95,96). Previous surgeries, chemotherapy, or radiation therapy, as well as other previous bronchoscopic interventions, do not represent exclusion criteria. Survival after PDT is usually related to the stage of the disease. Two subsets of patients have been demonstrated to experience a survival benefit. These include patients with a good performance status as defined above and patients without extrathoracic metastases (96). Interestingly, the histology of the tumor does not seem to influence survival. PDT has also been successfully used in conjunction with other treatment modalities. The concomitant use with chemotherapy as well as the use of PDT after chemotherapy/radiotherapy has been reported (87,96,108). Furthermore, PDT is an elegant method of treating patients with advanced central NSCLC suffering from tumor recurrence after chemoradiation. It should also be noted that PDT has been successfully applied to patients with lesions that were unresponsive to chemotherapy or radiation therapy (96).

PDT for nonmalignant airway pathology is not well described.

E. Complications

Recent publications (12,91,96) have demonstrated the safety of PDT. The procedure in and of itself is not associated with any reported mortality. The 30-day mortality has been reported to be <1%. The most common adverse effects include skin burns (4–41%), hemorrhage/hemoptysis (0–2.3%), and respiratory complications (5–29%). Photosensitivity-induced skin burns are by far the most common adverse effect and can be substantial. However, with counseling and precautionary measures, skin burn rates of only 4% to 5% have been demonstrated (12). Precautionary measures should be undertaken for four to six weeks.

Table 1 Indications and Complications for Endobronchial Cryotherapy, Brachytherapy, and Photodynamic Therapy

	Cryotherapy	Brachytherapy	Photodynamic therapy
Malignancy/tumor[a]			
Urgent relief of life-threatening symptoms	−	−	−
Nonurgent relief of symptoms	+	+	+
Non–massive hemoptysis[b]	±	+	+
Curative treatment of early-stage NSCLC	±	+	++
Removal of foreign body, clot, mucous plugs	+	−	−
Granulation tissue	+	(+?)	−
Selected complications	Fever, tissue slough, hemoptysis	Hemoptysis, fistula, stenosis, bronchitis	Skin burn, hemoptysis, tissue slough

[a]Role of brachytherapy or photodynamic therapy in treating benign airway tumors is not well described.
[b]No role for these therapies in treating massive hemoptysis.
Abbreviation: NSCLC, non-small cell lung cancer.

Table 2 Effectiveness of Cryotherapy, Brachytherapy, and Photodynamic Therapy in Treating Endobronchial Lung Cancer

	Cryotherapy	Brachytherapy	Photodynamic therapy
Control of nonmassive hemoptysis	+	++	+
Symptom relief from obstruction, non–life threatening	+	+	+
PFT improvement related to obstruction	±	±	±±
Cure early-stage NSCLC	±	+	++

Source: Modified from Ref. 12.
Abbreviations: PFT, pulmonary function test; NSCLC, non-small cell lung cancer.

V. Conclusions

ECT, brachytherapy, and photodynamic therapy are fundamentally different modalities applicable to a variety of malignant or benign conditions. Each method has advantages and disadvantages. The modalities should be viewed as complementary. Ideally, the interventional pulmonologist has all modalities available - but this is unrealistic - so he or she must utilize what is both appropriate and available. Indications, complications, and effectiveness in lung cancer of the three methods are summarized in Tables 1 and 2. Additionally, these modalities can be combined with each other, as well as with other local or systemic treatments. However, their specific roles in combination regimens require further investigation in form of randomized, controlled, prospective trials.

References

1. Kennedy TC, McWilliams A, Edell E, et al. Bronchial intraepithelial neoplasia/early central airways lung cancer: ACCP evidence-based clinical practice guidelines (2nd edition). Chest 2007; 132:221S–233S.
2. Arnott J. On the Treatment of Cancer Through the Regulated Application of an Anaesthetic Temperature. London: J. Churchill, 1851.
3. Gage A. Cryotherapy for cancer. In: Rand R, Rinfret A, Von Leden H, eds. Cryotherapy. Springfield: Charles C. Thomas, 1968:376–387.
4. Sheski FD, Mathur PN. Cryotherapy, electrocautery, and brachytherapy. Clin Chest Med 1999; 20:123–138.
5. Eichler B, Savy FP, Melloni B, et al. [Tumoral tracheobronchial desobstruction by cryotherapy using a flexible catheter]. Presse Med 1988; 17:2138–2139.
6. Homasson JP, Thiery JP, Angebault M, et al. The operation and efficacy of cryosurgical, nitrous oxide-driven cryoprobe. I. Cryoprobe physical characteristics: their effects on cell cryodestruction. Cryobiology 1994; 31:290–304.
7. Maiwand MO, Homasson JP. Cryotherapy for tracheobronchial disorders. Clin Chest Med 1995; 16:427–443.
8. Walsh DA, Maiwand MO, Nath AR, et al. Bronchoscopic cryotherapy for advanced bronchial carcinoma. Thorax 1990; 45:509–513.
9. Mathur PN, Wolf KM, Busk MF, et al. Fiberoptic bronchoscopic cryotherapy in the management of tracheobronchial obstruction. Chest 1996; 110:718–723.
10. Forest V, Peoc'h M, Ardiet C, et al. In vivo cryochemotherapy of a human lung cancer model. Cryobiology 2005; 51:92–101.
11. Forest V, Peoc'h M, Campos L, et al. Effects of cryotherapy or chemotherapy on apoptosis in a non-small-cell lung cancer xenografted into SCID mice. Cryobiology 2005; 50:29–37.
12. Vergnon JM, Huber RM, Moghissi K. Place of cryotherapy, brachytherapy and photodynamic therapy in therapeutic bronchoscopy of lung cancers. Eur Respir J 2006; 28:200–218.
13. Gage AA, Caruana JA Jr., Montes M. Critical temperature for skin necrosis in experimental cryosurgery. Cryobiology 1982; 19:273–282.
14. Miller RH, Mazur P. Survival of frozen–thawed human red cells as a function of cooling and warming velocities. Cryobiology 1976; 13:404–414.
15. Gage AA, Guest K, Montes M, et al. Effect of varying freezing and thawing rates in experimental cryosurgery. Cryobiology 1985; 22:175–182.
16. Mazur P. The role of intracellular freezing in the death of cells cooled at supraoptimal rates. Cryobiology 1977; 14:251–272.
17. Martino MN, Zaritzky NE. Ice recrystallization in a model system and in frozen muscle tissue. Cryobiology 1989; 26:138–148.
18. Homasson JP, Renault P, Angebault M, et al. Bronchoscopic cryotherapy for airway strictures caused by tumors. Chest 1986; 90:159–164.
19. Sohrab S, Mathur PN. Management of central airway obstruction. Clin Lung Cancer 2007; 8:305–312.
20. Gilbert JC, Onik GM, Hoddick WK, et al. Real time ultrasonic monitoring of hepatic cryosurgery. Cryobiology 1985; 22:319–330.
21. Schumann C, Mattfeldt T, Hetzel M, et al. Improving the diagnostic yield of endobronchial biopsies by flexible cryoprobe in lung cancer—comparison of forceps and cryoprobe technique. Eur Respir J 2004; 24:S491.

22. Sutedja TG, Codrington H, Risse EK, et al. Autofluorescence bronchoscopy improves staging of radiographically occult lung cancer and has an impact on therapeutic strategy. Chest 2001; 120:1327–1332.

23. Reddy AJ, Govert JA, Sporn TA, et al. Broncholith removal using cryotherapy during flexible bronchoscopy: a case report. Chest 2007; 132:1661–1663.

24. Bertoletti L, Elleuch R, Kaczmarek D, et al. Bronchoscopic cryotherapy treatment of isolated endoluminal typical carcinoid tumor. Chest 2006; 130:1405–1411.

25. Noppen M, Meysman M, Van Herreweghe R, et al. Bronchoscopic cryotherapy: preliminary experience. Acta Clin Belg 2001; 56:73–77.

26. Deygas N, Froudarakis M, Ozenne G, et al. Cryotherapy in early superficial bronchogenic carcinoma. Chest 2001; 120:26–31.

27. Altin S, Dalar L, Karasulu L, et al. Resection of giant endobronchial hamartoma by electrocautery and cryotherapy via flexible bronchoscopy. Tuberk Toraks 2007; 55:390–394.

28. Nassiri AH, Dutau H, Breen D, et al. A multicenter retrospective study investigating the role of interventional bronchoscopic techniques in the management of endobronchial lipomas. Respiration 2008; 75:79–84.

29. Homasson JP, Pecking A, Roden S, et al. Tumor fixation of bleomycin labeled with 57 cobalt before and after cryotherapy of bronchial carcinoma. Cryobiology 1992; 29:543–548.

30. Vergnon JM, Schmitt T, Alamartine E, et al. Initial combined cryotherapy and irradiation for unresectable non-small cell lung cancer. Preliminary results. Chest 1992; 102:1436–1440.

31. Yankauer S. Two cases of lung tumor treated bronchoscopically. NY Med J 1922; 115:741.

32. Henschke UK. Interstitial implantation in the treatment of primary bronchogenic carcinoma. Am J Roentgenol Radium Ther Nucl Med 1958; 79:981–987.

33. Henschke UK, Hilaris BS, Mahan GD. Remote afterloading with intracavitary applicators. Radiology 1964; 83:344–345.

34. Mendiondo OA, Dillon M, Beach LJ. Endobronchial brachytherapy in the treatment of recurrent bronchogenic carcinoma. Int J Radiat Oncol Biol Phys 1983; 9:579–582.

35. Moylan D, Strubler K, Unal A, et al. Work in progress. Transbronchial brachytherapy of recurrent bronchogenic carcinoma: a new approach using the flexible fiberoptic bronchoscope. Radiology 1983; 147:253–254.

36. Seagren SL, Harrell JH, Horn RA. High dose rate intraluminal irradiation in recurrent endobronchial carcinoma. Chest 1985; 88:810–814.

37. Gaspar LE. Brachytherapy in lung cancer. J Surg Oncol 1998; 67:60–70.

38. Bergner A, Stief J, Holdenrieder S, et al. Effects of single-dose irradiation on bronchial epithelium: a comparison of BEAS 2B cell monolayers, human organ cultures, and Goettinger minipigs. Radiat Res 2003; 160:647–654.

39. Kotsianos D, Bach D, Gamarra F, et al. High-dose-rate brachytherapy: dose escalation in three-dimensional miniorgans of the human bronchial wall. Int J Radiat Oncol Biol Phys 2000; 46:1267–1273.

40. Miller JI Jr., Phillips TW. Neodymium: YAG laser and brachytherapy in the management of inoperable bronchogenic carcinoma. Ann Thorac Surg 1990; 50:190–195; discussion 195–196.

41. Spratling L, Speiser BL. Endoscopic brachytherapy. Chest Surg Clin North Am 1996; 6:293–304.

42. Nag S, Abitbol AA, Anderson LL, et al. Consensus guidelines for high dose rate remote brachytherapy in cervical, endometrial, and endobronchial tumors. Clinical Research Committee, American Endocurietherapy Society. Int J Radiat Oncol Biol Phys 1993; 27:1241–1244.

43. Nag S, Kuske RR, Vicini FA, et al. Brachytherapy in the treatment of breast cancer. Oncology (Williston Park) 2001; 15:195–202, 205; discussion 205–197.

44. Huber RM, Fischer R, Hautmann H, et al. Palliative endobronchial brachytherapy for central lung tumors. A prospective, randomized comparison of two fractionation schedules. Chest 1995; 107:463–470.

45. Scarda A, Confalonieri M, Baghiris C, et al. Out-patient high-dose-rate endobronchial brachytherapy for palliation of lung cancer: an observational study. Monaldi Arch Chest Dis 2007; 67:128–134.

46. Escobar-Sacristan JA, Granda-Orive JI, Gutierrez Jimenez T, et al. Endobronchial brachytherapy in the treatment of malignant lung tumours. Eur Respir J 2004; 24:348–352.

47. Speiser B, Spratling L. Intermediate dose rate remote afterloading brachytherapy for intraluminal control of bronchogenic carcinoma. Int J Radiat Oncol Biol Phys 1990; 18:1443–1448.

48. Aygun C, Weiner S, Scariato A, et al. Treatment of non-small cell lung cancer with external beam radiotherapy and high dose rate brachytherapy. Int J Radiat Oncol Biol Phys 1992; 23:127–132.

49. Hernandez P, Gursahaney A, Roman T, et al. High dose rate brachytherapy for the local control of endobronchial carcinoma following external irradiation. Thorax 1996; 51:354–358.

50. Schray MF, McDougall JC, Martinez A, et al. Management of malignant airway compromise with laser and low dose rate brachytherapy. The Mayo Clinic experience. Chest 1988; 93:264–269.

51. Taulelle M, Chauvet B, Vincent P, et al. High dose rate endobronchial brachytherapy: results and complications in 189 patients. Eur Respir J 1998; 11:162–168.

52. Mallick I, Sharma SC, Behera D. Endobronchial brachytherapy for symptom palliation in non-small cell lung cancer—analysis of symptom response, endoscopic improvement and quality of life. Lung Cancer 2007; 55:313–318.

53. Miller KL, Shafman TD, Anscher MS, et al. Bronchial stenosis: an underreported complication of high-dose external beam radiotherapy for lung cancer? Int J Radiat Oncol Biol Phys 2005; 61:64–69.

54. Huber RM, Fischer R, Hautmann H, et al. Does additional brachytherapy improve the effect of external irradiation? A prospective, randomized study in central lung tumors. Int J Radiat Oncol Biol Phys 1997; 38:533–540.

55. Saito M, Yokoyama A, Kurita Y, et al. Treatment of roentgenographically occult endobronchial carcinoma with external beam radiotherapy and intraluminal low dose rate brachytherapy. Int J Radiat Oncol Biol Phys 1996; 34:1029–1035.

56. Yokomise H, Nishimura Y, Fukuse T, et al. Long-term remission after brachytherapy with external irradiation for locally advanced lung cancer. Respiration 1998; 65:489–491.

57. Ung YC, Yu E, Falkson C, et al. The role of high-dose-rate brachytherapy in the palliation of symptoms in patients with non-small-cell lung cancer: a systematic review. Brachytherapy 2006; 5:189–202.

58. Bastin KT, Mehta MP, Kinsella TJ. Thoracic volume radiation sparing following endobronchial brachytherapy: a quantitative analysis. Int J Radiat Oncol Biol Phys 1993; 25:703–707.

59. Harms W, Krempien R, Grehn C, et al. Electromagnetically navigated brachytherapy as a new treatment option for peripheral pulmonary tumors. Strahlenther Onkol 2006; 182:108–111.

60. Lee JS, Komaki R, Morice RC, et al. A pilot clinical laboratory trial of paclitaxel and endobronchial brachytherapy in patients with non-small cell lung cancer. Semin Radiat Oncol 1999; 9:121–129.

61. Marsiglia H, Baldeyrou P, Lartigau E, et al. High-dose-rate brachytherapy as sole modality for early-stage endobronchial carcinoma. Int J Radiat Oncol Biol Phys 2000; 47:665–672.

62. Sutedja G, Baris G, van Zandwijk N, et al. High-dose rate brachytherapy has a curative potential in patients with intraluminal squamous cell lung cancer. Respiration 1994; 61:167–168.

63. Tredaniel J, Hennequin C, Zalcman G, et al. Prolonged survival after high-dose rate endobronchial radiation for malignant airway obstruction. Chest 1994; 105:767–772.

64. Perol M, Caliandro R, Pommier P, et al. Curative irradiation of limited endobronchial carcinomas with high-dose rate brachytherapy. Results of a pilot study. Chest 1997; 111:1417–1423.

65. Vonk-Noordegraaf A, Postmus PE, Sutedja TG. Bronchoscopic treatment of patients with intraluminal microinvasive radiographically occult lung cancer not eligible for surgical resection: a follow-up study. Lung Cancer 2003; 39:49–53.

66. Macha HN, Wahlers B, Reichle C, et al. Endobronchial radiation therapy for obstructing malignancies: ten years' experience with iridium-192 high-dose radiation brachytherapy afterloading technique in 365 patients. Lung 1995; 173:271–280.

67. Nori D, Allison R, Kaplan B, et al. High dose-rate intraluminal irradiation in bronchogenic carcinoma. Technique and results. Chest 1993; 104:1006–1011.

68. Sheski FD, Mathur PN. Endobronchial electrosurgery: argon plasma coagulation and electrocautery. Semin Respir Crit Care Med 2004; 25:367–374.

69. Kramer MR, Katz A, Yarmolovsky A, et al. Successful use of high dose rate brachytherapy for non-malignant bronchial obstruction. Thorax 2001; 56:415–416.

70. Kennedy AS, Sonett JR, Orens JB, et al. High dose rate brachytherapy to prevent recurrent benign hyperplasia in lung transplant bronchi: theoretical and clinical considerations. J Heart Lung Transplant 2000; 19:155–159.

71. Tendulkar RD, Fleming PA, Reddy CA, et al. High-dose-rate endobronchial brachytherapy for recurrent airway obstruction from hyperplastic granulation tissue. Int J Radiat Oncol Biol Phys 2008; 70:701–706.

72. Madu CN, Machuzak MS, Sterman DH, et al. High-dose-rate (HDR) brachytherapy for the treatment of benign obstructive endobronchial granulation tissue. Int J Radiat Oncol Biol Phys 2006; 66:1450–1456.

73. Halkos ME, Godette KD, Lawrence EC, et al. High dose rate brachytherapy in the management of lung transplant airway stenosis. Ann Thorac Surg 2003; 76:381–384.

74. Kelly JF, Delclos ME, Morice RC, et al. High-dose-rate endobronchial brachytherapy effectively palliates symptoms due to airway tumors: the 10-year M. D. Anderson cancer center experience. Int J Radiat Oncol Biol Phys 2000; 48:697–702.

75. Cox JD, Yesner R, Mietlowski W, et al. Influence of cell type on failure pattern after irradiation for locally advanced carcinoma of the lung. Cancer 1979; 44:94–98.

76. Miller RR, McGregor DH. Hemorrhage from carcinoma of the lung. Cancer 1980; 46: 200–205.

77. Hara R, Itami J, Aruga T, et al. Risk factors for massive hemoptysis after endobronchial brachytherapy in patients with tracheobronchial malignancies. Cancer 2001; 92:2623–2627.

78. Langendijk JA, Tjwa MK, de Jong JM, et al. Massive haemoptysis after radiotherapy in inoperable non-small cell lung carcinoma: is endobronchial brachytherapy really a risk factor? Radiother Oncol 1998; 49:175–183.

79. Speiser BL, Spratling L. Remote afterloading brachytherapy for the local control of endobronchial carcinoma. Int J Radiat Oncol Biol Phys 1993; 25:579–587.

80. Finsen NF. Phototherapy. London: Arnold, 1901.

81. Lipson RL, Gray MJ, Blades EJ. Haematoporphyrin derivative for detection and management of cancer. Abstr Proc 9th Int Cancer Congress Tokyo 1966; Section, II-01-a:50696.

82. Dougherty TJ, Grindey GB, Fiel R, et al. Photoradiation therapy. II. Cure of animal tumors with hematoporphyrin and light. J Natl Cancer Inst 1975; 55:115–121.

83. Kelly JF, Snell ME. Hematoporphyrin derivative: a possible aid in the diagnosis and therapy of carcinoma of the bladder. J Urol 1976; 115:150–151.

84. Dougherty TJ, Kaufman JE, Goldfarb A, et al. Photoradiation therapy for the treatment of malignant tumors. Cancer Res 1978; 38:2628–2635.

85. Dougherty TJ, Lawrence G, Kaufman JH, et al. Photoradiation in the treatment of recurrent breast carcinoma. J Natl Cancer Inst 1979; 62:231–237.

86. Hayata Y, Kato H, Konaka C, et al. Fiberoptic bronchoscopic laser photoradiation for tumor localization in lung cancer. Chest 1982; 82:10–14.

87. Kato H. Photodynamic therapy for lung cancer—a review of 19 years' experience. J Photochem Photobiol B 1998; 42:96–99.
88. Hayata Y, Kato H, Konaka C, et al. Hematoporphyrin derivative and laser photoradiation in the treatment of lung cancer. Chest 1982; 81:269–277.
89. Balchum OJ, Doiron DR, Huth GC. Photoradiation therapy of endobronchial lung cancers employing the photodynamic action of hematoporphyrin derivative. Lasers Surg Med 1984; 4:13–30.
90. Edell ES, Cortese DA. Bronchoscopic phototherapy with hematoporphyrin derivative for treatment of localized bronchogenic carcinoma: a 5-year experience. Mayo Clin Proc 1987; 62:8–14.
91. Moghissi K, Dixon K. Is bronchoscopic photodynamic therapy a therapeutic option in lung cancer? Eur Respir J 2003; 22:535–541.
92. Cecic I, Minchinton AI, Korbelik M. The impact of complement activation on tumor oxygenation during photodynamic therapy. Photochem Photobiol 2007; 83:1049–1055.
93. Dougherty TJ. Photodynamic therapy. Clin Chest Med 1985; 6:219–236.
94. Edell ES, Cortese DA. Photodynamic therapy. Its use in the management of bronchogenic carcinoma. Clin Chest Med 1995; 16:455–463.
95. McCaughan JS Jr., Williams TE. Photodynamic therapy for endobronchial malignant disease: a prospective fourteen-year study. J Thorac Cardiovasc Surg 1997; 114:940–946; discussion 946–947.
96. Moghissi K, Dixon K, Stringer M, et al. The place of bronchoscopic photodynamic therapy in advanced unresectable lung cancer: experience of 100 cases. Eur J Cardiothorac Surg 1999; 15:1–6.
97. Allison R, Downie G, Cuenca R, et al. Photosensitisers in clinical PDT. Photodiagnosis Photodyn Ther 2004; 1:27–42.
98. Kato H, Furukawa K, Sato M, et al. Phase II clinical study of photodynamic therapy using mono-L-aspartyl chlorin e6 and diode laser for early superficial squamous cell carcinoma of the lung. Lung Cancer 2003; 42:103–111.
99. Usuda J, Tsutsui H, Honda H, et al. Photodynamic therapy for lung cancers based on novel photodynamic diagnosis using talaporfin sodium (NPe6) and autofluorescence bronchoscopy. Lung Cancer 2007; 58:317–323.
100. Piotrowski WJ, Marczak J, Nawrocka A, et al. Inhalations of 5-ALA in photodynamic diagnosis of bronchial cancer. Monaldi Arch Chest Dis 2004; 61:86–93.
101. Imamura S, Kusunoki Y, Takifuji N, et al. Photodynamic therapy and/or external beam radiation therapy for roentgenologically occult lung cancer. Cancer 1994; 73:1608–1614.
102. Mang TS. Lasers and light sources for PDT: past, present and future. Photodiagnosis Photodyn Ther 2004; 1:43–48.
103. Moghissi K, Dixon K. Photodynamic therapy for synchronous occult bronchial cancer 17 years after pneumonectomy. Interact Cardiovasc Thorac Surg 2005; 4:327–328.
104. Moghissi K, Dixon K, Thorpe JA, et al. Photodynamic therapy (PDT) in early central lung cancer: a treatment option for patients ineligible for surgical resection. Thorax 2007; 62: 391–395.
105. Lam S, Kennedy T, Unger M, et al. Localization of bronchial intraepithelial neoplastic lesions by fluorescence bronchoscopy. Chest 1998; 113:696–702.
106. Herth F, Becker HD. Endobronchial ultrasound of the airways and the mediastinum. Monaldi Arch Chest Dis 2000; 55:36–44.
107. Herth F, Becker HD, LoCicero J 3rd, et al. Endobronchial ultrasound in therapeutic bronchoscopy. Eur Respir J 2002; 20:118–121.
108. Takahashi H, Sagawa M, Sato M, et al. A prospective evaluation of transbronchial ultrasonography for assessment of depth of invasion in early bronchogenic squamous cell carcinoma. Lung Cancer 2003; 42:43–49.

109. Kato H, Harada M, Ichinose S, et al. Photodynamic therapy (PDT) of lung cancer: experience of the Tokyo Medical University. Photodiagnosis Photodyn Ther 2001; 1:49–55.
110. Hayata Y, Kato H, Konaka C, et al. Photoradiation therapy with hematoporphyrin derivative in early and stage 1 lung cancer. Chest 1984; 86:169–177.
111. Kato H, Kawate N, Kinoshita K, et al. Photodynamic therapy of early-stage lung cancer. Ciba Found Symp 1989; 146:183–194; discussion 195–197.
112. Edell ES, Cortese DA. Photodynamic therapy in the management of early superficial squamous cell carcinoma as an alternative to surgical resection. Chest 1992; 102:1319–1322.
113. Balchum OJ, Doiron DR. Photoradiation therapy of endobronchial lung cancer. Large obstructing tumors, nonobstructing tumors, and early-stage bronchial cancer lesions. Clin Chest Med 1985; 6:255–275.
114. Cortese DA, Edell ES, Kinsey JH. Photodynamic therapy for early stage squamous cell carcinoma of the lung. Mayo Clin Proc 1997; 72:595–602.
115. Corti L, Toniolo L, Boso C, et al. Long-term survival of patients treated with photodynamic therapy for carcinoma in situ and early non-small-cell lung carcinoma. Lasers Surg Med 2007; 39:394–402.
116. Furukawa K, Kato H, Konaka C, et al. Locally recurrent central-type early stage lung cancer <1.0 cm in diameter after complete remission by photodynamic therapy. Chest 2005; 128:3269–3275.

4
Airway Stents

PYNG LEE
Singapore General Hospital, Singapore

ELIF KUPELI
Mesa Hospital, Ankara, Turkey

ATUL C. MEHTA
Sheikh Khalifa Medical City, managed by Cleveland Clinic, Abu Dhabi, UAE

I. Introduction

A stent is a hollow, cylindrical prosthesis that maintains luminal patency and provides support for a graft or anastomosis. It is named after Charles Stent, a British dentist who was the first to create dental splints in the nineteenth century. Airway stenting has been practiced for over a century. Indications for stent placement can be for its barrier effect by protecting the airway lumen from tumor or granulation tissue ingrowth, for splinting effect by counterbalancing the extrinsic pressure exerted on the airway, or both (1). The covering of the stent provides the barrier effect while dynamic and static properties determine the splinting effect (2).

The first stents were implanted surgically by Trendelenburg (3) and Bond (4) for the treatment of airway strictures, which quickly progressed to endoscopic application by Brunings and Albrecht in 1915 (5). In 1965, Montgomery designed a T-tube with an external side limb made of silicone and rubber for treatment of subglottic stenosis. Since then, silicone has become the most commonly used material for stents (6). However, the designs of the silicone stents at that time abolished the innate mucociliary mechanisms essential to clear the airway of secretions. Thus the real breakthrough in airway stenting was achieved when Dumon presented a dedicated tracheobronchial prosthesis that could be introduced with a rigid bronchoscope (7). These straight stents are made up of silicone with studs on the outer wall that minimize interference to the ciliary action, are relatively inexpensive, and can be easily removed and exchanged when needed. However, limitations and disadvantages of silicone stents and their counterparts should be appreciated, of which an important factor is the need for rigid bronchoscopy for placement. On the basis of a recent ACCP survey, only 5% of pulmonologists in North America are trained with the procedure of rigid bronchoscopy (8). Moreover, the silicone stent is poorly tolerated in the subglottis and tends to migrate when deployed to treat for complex tracheal strictures. These limitations have led to the modification of metal stents originally developed for the vascular system for use in the tracheobronchial tree (9,10). Although metal stents are easy to apply with the flexible bronchoscope, they are also fraught with problems such as tumor or granulation tissue ingrowth around the struts and epithelialization into the airway wall, which make removal difficult and challenging (10).

45

Table 1 Characteristics of an Ideal Stent

Is easy to insert
Is available in different sizes and lengths appropriate to relieve airway obstruction
Reestablishes the luminal patency with minimal morbidity and mortality
Has sufficient expansive strength to resistive compressive forces and elasticity to conform to
    airway contours
Maintains luminal patency without causing ischemia or erosion into adjacent structures
Has minimal migration but can be easily removed if necessary
Is made of inert material that will not promote infection or granulation tissue formation
Preserves mucociliary function of the airway for mobilization of secretions
Is affordable

Therefore, the search for an ideal stent, which has all the characteristics mentioned in Table 1, has become the holy grail for the interventional pulmonologists, radiologists, thoracic surgeons, and otolaryngologists involved in the management of patients with central airway obstruction.

II. Indications for Airway Stenting

Approximately 30% of patients with lung cancer will present with central airway obstruction, of which 35% will die as a result of asphyxia, hemoptysis, and post-obstructive pneumonia (11). Stent placement is a valuable adjunct to other therapeutic bronchoscopic techniques used to relieve central airway obstruction; the indications are primarily to reestablish patency of the compressed or stenosed airway, to support weakened cartilages in tracheobronchomalacia as well as seal tracheobronchial esophageal fistula (11,12). Although primary tumor resection and airway reconstruction provide the most reliable treatment option, most central airway obstructions because of malignancy are advanced at the time of presentation. Therapeutic bronchoscopy coupled with stent placement not only results in rapid relief of symptoms and improved quality of life, importantly it also allows time for administration of adjuvant chemoradiotherapy that might lead to prolonged survival (1,11–14). In fact Chhajed and coworkers have demonstrated no difference in survival between those with advanced malignancy receiving palliative chemotherapy but without central airway obstruction (median survival 8.4 months) compared with others who had airway obstruction treated with laser (25%), stent (25%), or both (50%) followed by chemotherapy (median survival 8.2 months, $p = 0.395$). Contrary to previous perception, airway obstruction is not a poor prognostic sign if treated appropriately (15).

Benign strictures secondary to postintubation injury, and inflammatory and infectious disease may require stent placement if the patient's underlying disease or associated comorbidity prohibits definitive surgical repair. Lung transplant recipients who develop airway dehiscence in the immediate postoperative period may benefit from placement of endobronchial stents. The Cleveland Clinic experience of using uncovered metal stent as an alternative treatment for high-grade anastomotic dehiscence after lung transplantation in seven patients deemed high risk for a second operation has demonstrated not only satisfactory airway healing, but also that stent removal is not difficult if performed within eight weeks of placement before epithelialization with the airway wall occurs (16). Table 2 details the indications for stent placement.

Table 2 Indications for Airway Stenting of Malignant and Benign Diseases

Airway obstruction from extrinsic compression or submucosal disease
Obstruction from endobronchial tumor when patency is <50% after bronchoscopic laser therapy
Aggressive endobronchial tumor growth and recurrence despite repetitive laser treatments
Loss of cartilaginous support from tumor destruction
Sequential insertion of airway and esophageal stents for tracheoesophageal fistulas

Benign airway disease	
Fibrotic scar or bottleneck stricture following:	Posttraumatic: intubation, tracheostomy, laser, balloon bronchoplasty
	Postinfectious: endobronchial tuberculosis, histoplasmosis-fibrosing mediastinitis, herpesvirus, diphtheria, *Klebsiella rhinoscleroma*
	Postinflammatory: Wegener's granulomatosis, sarcoidosis, inflammatory bowel disease, foreign body aspiration
	Post–lung transplantation: anastomotic complications
Tracheobronchomalacia	Diffuse: idiopathic, relapsing polychrondritis, tracheobronchomegaly (Mounier-Kuhn syndrome)
	Focal: tracheostomy, radiation therapy, post–lung transplantation
Benign tumors	Papillomatosis
	Amyloidosis

Table 3 Characteristics of Tube Stents

Montgomery T-tube	Designed for treatment of subglottic and mid-tracheal stenosis
	Introduced through a tracheostomy with the side tube protruding through the stoma; the proximal limb within the stenosis and the distal limb into the distal trachea
Dumon	Silicone tube with external studs to prevent migration, most widely used silicone stent. Y-shaped and right main bronchus designs are available
Hood	Smooth silicone tube with flanges to prevent migration. L- or Y-shaped designs available
Noppen	Screw-thread cylindrical silicone prosthesis, more rigid than regular silicone tubes. Needs a special introducer, and cannot be folded into an applicator for bronchoscopic insertion
Dynamic	Silicone Y-stent with the anterior and lateral wall reinforced by steel struts to simulate tracheal wall. Requires special forceps and rigid laryngoscope
Polyflex	Self-expandable stent made of polyester wire mesh with a thin layer of silicone
Alveolus	Hybrid stent that conforms to airway tortuosity without foreshortening upon deployment. It can be deployed with the rigid or flexible bronchoscope

III. Types of Stents

A myriad of stents are available for application in the tracheobronchial tree, and the biomechanical properties depend on the materials used as well as how they are constructed (Tables 3 and 4). They are divided into three groups: (*i*) made of polymer,

Table 4 Characteristics of Metallic Stents

Balloon expandable	
Strecker	Tantalum monofilament knitted into a wire –mesh; most useful in narrow stenoses
Palmaz	Stainless steel tube with rectangular slots along the long axis; may collapse with strong external pressure, e.g., vigorous cough
Self-expanding	
Wallstent	Wire mesh made of cobalt-based alloy filaments and coated with silicone; uncovered metallic ends prevent migration
Ultraflex	Cylindrical wire mesh of nitinol, available in covered and uncovered form

which include the Montgomery T-tube, Dumon, Polyflex, Noppen, and Hood stents; (*ii*) made of metal (covered or uncovered version) such as Gianturco, Palmaz, and Ultraflex stents; and (*iii*) hybrid comprising of Orlowski, Dynamic, and Alveolus stents made of silicone and reinforced by metal rings (Figs. 1 and 2).

The major advantages of tube stents are that they allow repositioning and removal without difficulty, and are relatively inexpensive. Disadvantages include stent migration, granuloma formation, mucus plugging, unfavorable wall to inner diameter thickness, insufficient flexibility to conform to irregular airways, difficult to position in distal airways, interference with mucociliary clearance, and need for rigid bronchoscopy for placement (Table 5). Rigid bronchoscopy expertise to deploy and remove tube stents poses a major obstacle, limiting their use, since pulmonologists' training in rigid bronchoscopy has dramatically declined worldwide (8).

A. Tube Stents
Montgomery T-Tube
Since 1965, the Montgomery T-tube has undergone only slight modifications and continues to be used for the treatment of subglottic and tracheal stenosis (6). Early models made of acrylic were later replaced by silicone rubber. They are available in different diameters and variable lengths for the three limbs. The prerequisite for this stent is a tracheostomy, and it can be placed during the initial operation or via rigid bronchoscopy. The limb protruding out of the tracheostoma is left open for cricoid or glottic stenosis, unplugged transiently for bronchial toilet or closed to allow speech. Migration is rarely encountered as one limb is fixed in the tracheostomy opening. High mucosal pressure is not required to hold the stent in position, and blood and lymphatic flows to the sensitive upper trachea are not compromised, thereby making the Montgomery T-tube especially safe for high tracheal stenosis.

Dumon Stent
Dumon initially described his experience with a new dedicated tracheobronchial pros-thesis made of silicone with studs (7). A multicenter trial (17) followed where 1574 stents were placed in 1058 patients, of which 698 were for malignant airway obstruction. Stent migration occurred in 9.5%, granuloma formation in 8%, and stent obstruction by mucus in 4% during mean follow-up of 4 months for malignant and 14 months for benign stenoses. In a similar study conducted by Diaz-Jimenez and colleagues, 125

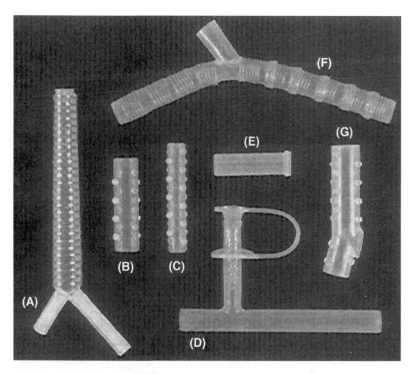

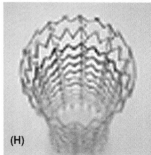

Figure 1 Types of tube and hybrid stents. (**A**) Dynamic (Rusch) stent; (**B**) Dumon tracheal stent; (**C**) Dumon bronchial stent; (**D**) Montgomery T-tube; (**E**) Hood bronchial stent; (**F**) Orlowski stent; (**G**) Hood custom tracheobronchial stent; (**H**) Hybrid stent (Alveolus) that can be deployed with flexible or rigid bronchoscope without foreshortening.

silicone stents were placed in 60 patients with malignant and 30 with benign tracheobronchial disease. Migration was observed in 13%, granuloma in 6%, and mucus plugging in 2% (18). Lower complication rates were observed by Cavaliere et al. where a series of 393 silicone stents were placed in 306 patients with malignant airway strictures. Stent migration was observed in 5% and granuloma formation in 1% (11).

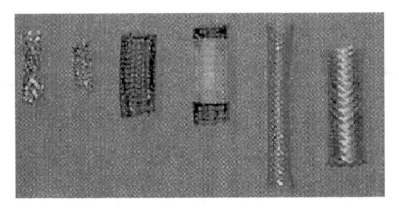

Figure 2 Types of metallic stents. From left to right: Palmaz stent, Tantalum Strecker stent, uncovered Ultraflex stent, covered Ultraflex stent, uncovered Wallstent, and covered Wallstent.

Table 5 Comparison of the Dumon Stent and the Covered Ultraflex Stent

Characteristics	Dumon stent	Covered Ultraflex stent
Mechanical considerations		
High internal to external diameter ratio	−	+++
Resistant to recompression when deployed	+	++
Radial force exerted uniformly across stent	+	++
Absence of migration	−	++
Flexible for use in tortuous airways	−	+++
Removable	+++	−
Dynamic expansion	−	++
Can be customized	+++	−
Tissue-stent interaction		
Biologically inert	++	++
Devoid of granulation tissue	+	−
Tumor ingrowth	++	+
Ease of use		
Can be deployed with FB	−	+++
Deployed under local anesthesia with conscious sedation	−	++
Radiopaque for position evaluation	−	+++
Can be easily repositioned	++	−
Cost		
Inexpensive	+	−

−, poor; +, fair; ++, good; +++, best.

After its introduction, the Dumon stent (Novatech, France) has become the most frequently used stent worldwide and is considered the "gold standard" by many experts. Different diameters and lengths are available for structural stenoses of the trachea, main stem bronchus, and bronchus intermedius of adults and children. A recent addition is a bifurcated model known as Dumon Y stent (Tracheobronxane Y, Novatech, France) which can be applied to palliate lower tracheal and/or main carinal stenoses. However, as good contact pressure between the airway wall and the studs is required to prevent stent migration, it is not ideal for tracheobronchomalacia or to bridge tracheoesophageal fistula.

Noppen Stent

The Noppen stent is made of Tygon (Reynders Medical Supplies, Belgium) and has a corkscrew-shaped outer wall that prevents migration by generating friction between the airway and stent. Results of a study that compared the use of Noppen stents with the Dumon stents demonstrated lower migration rate for benign tracheal stenoses with use of the former (19).

Polyflex Stent

The Polyflex stent (Boston Scientific, Massachusetts, U.S.) is a self-expanding stent made of cross-woven polyester threads embedded in silicone. Its walls are thinner than the Dumon or Noppen stents. This stent can be used to treat benign and malignant strictures as well as tracheobronchial fistula. Different lengths and diameters as well as tapered models for sealing stump fistula are available. Incorporation of tungsten into the stent makes it radio-opaque; however, the outer surface is smooth, which increases the risk for migration. In a small series of 12 patients where 16 Polyflex stents were used for benign airway disorders such as anastomotic stenosis following lung transplantation, tracheal stenosis, tracheobronchomalacia, tracheobronchopathia osteochondroplastica, relapsing polychondritis, and bronchopleural fistula, the reported complication rate was alarmingly high at 75%, even though immediate palliation was achieved in most cases (90%). Stent migration was the most common complication that occurred between 24 hours and 7 months after deployment. Notably, all four patients with lung transplant–related anastomotic stenoses encountered complications with the Polyflex stents; two had significant mucus plugging requiring emergent bronchoscopy while the stents migrated in the other two patients. The authors have since abandoned the use of Polyflex stent in their practice (20).

Hood Stent

The Hood stent (Hood Laboratories, Pembroke, U.S.) is made of silicone and can be dumbbell-shaped for bronchial anastomosis or tube with flanges customized to L or Y shape.

Dynamic Stent

The dynamic stent (Rüsch Y stent, Rüsch AG Duluth, GA) is a bifurcated silicone stent that is constructed to simulate the trachea. It is reinforced anteriorly by horseshoe-shaped metal rings that resemble tracheal cartilages and a soft posterior wall that behaves like the membranous trachea by allowing inward bulge during cough. Stent fracture from fatigue and retained secretions are rarely encountered, and the stent is used for strictures of the trachea, main carina and/or main bronchi; tracheobronchomalacia; tracheobronchomegaly, and esophageal fistula.

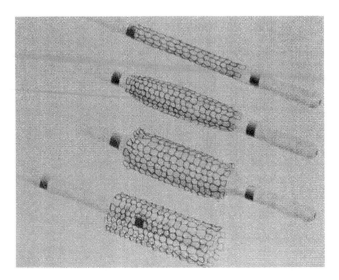

Figure 3   Balloon-expandable stents: Palmaz and Strecker. A balloon expandable stent consists of a stent balloon assembly and relies on the balloon to dilate the stent to its correct diameter.

B.   Metallic Stents

Metallic stents are gaining popularity because of their ease of insertion. They can be placed via FB in patients under local anesthesia and conscious sedation and even at an outpatient setting (21,22). They can be categorized by the method of deployment: balloon expandable and self-expanding. A balloon-expandable stent consists of a stent balloon assembly and relies on the balloon to dilate it to its correct diameter at the target site (Fig. 3). A self-expanding stent has a shape memory that enables it to assume its predetermined configuration, when released from a constraining delivery catheter (Fig. 4).

Advantages of metallic stents for the management of malignant tracheobronchial obstruction include their radio-opaque nature, greater airway cross-sectional diameters because of thinner walls, ability to conform to tortuous airways, preservation of mucociliary clearance and ventilation when placed across a lobar bronchial orifice, and their ease of insertion compared to tube stents. Major disadvantages, however, include granulation tissue formation within the stent and difficulty in removal or repositioning following stent epithelialization, which occurs in six to eight weeks (Table 5).

Palmaz and Strecker Stents

The balloon-expandable stents (Palmaz and Strecker) can be dilated to diameters 11 to 12 mm, and are primarily restricted to use in children. The Palmaz stent is not indicated for adults, as it is a device that exhibits plasticity without radial force, such that when the yield point is crossed, permanent deformity ensues. Thus, a strong external force from a vigorous cough, compression from an enlarging tumor, or adjacent vascular structure can lead to its collapse, resulting in obstruction and migration (23).

The Strecker stents are available in lengths of 20 to 40 mm and can be used in adults for precise stenting of short segment stenoses since they do not foreshorten on

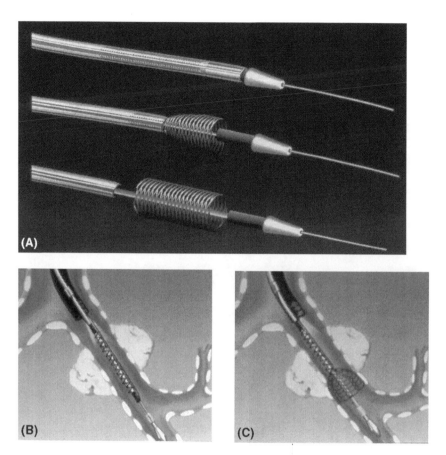

Figure 4 Self-expanding stents: (**A**) Wallstent and Ultraflex stent. (**B**) Wallstent deployment system. (**C**) Ultraflex stent deployment system. Ultraflex stent is mounted on introduction catheter with crochet knots; pulling the thread releases the stent.

deployment (24). Both Palmaz and Strecker stents are uncovered and unsuitable for malignant lesions, as they do not protect against tumor ingrowth, and may become loose when these stenoses improve following chemoradiotherapy.

The Wallstent and Ultraflex Stents (Boston Scientific) are self-expanding stents. They do not require hooks to prevent migration, as they have outward radial force that is uniformly applied over the bronchial wall, which stabilizes the stent and reduces the risk of mucosal perforation. They are easy to deploy and are available in covered forms.

The Wallstent is a self-expandable wire mesh made of cobalt-based superalloy monofilaments (Fig. 5). Dasgupta and coworkers reported their experience using 52 uncovered Wallstents in 37 patients: 20 with malignant airway obstruction and 17 with benign disease. Stent-related obstructive granuloma occurred in 11% of patients, two patients developed Staphylococcal bronchitis, which necessitated stent removal in one patient. Stent migration and mucus plugging were, however, not observed (9).

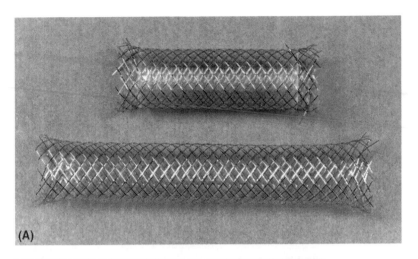

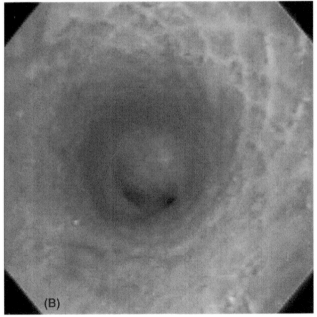

Figure 5   (**A**) Covered and uncovered Wallstents. (**B**) Wallstent in main bronchus.

The Ultraflex is a second-generation self-expanding stent made of nitinol (Fig. 6). Nitinol is an alloy with shape memory, which deforms at low temperature and regains its original shape at higher temperatures. Miyazawa and coworkers deployed 54 Ultraflex stents in 34 patients with inoperable malignant airway stenoses via flexible or rigid bronchoscopy. Immediate relief of dyspnea was achieved in 82% of the patients who

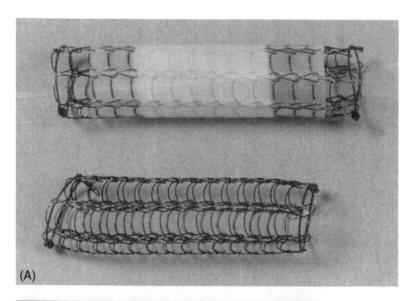

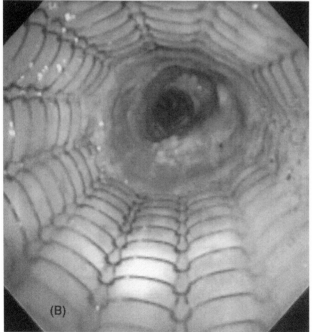

Figure 6 (**A**) Covered and uncovered Ultraflex stents. (**B**) Ultraflex stent in trachea.

demonstrated corresponding improvements in spirometry. Retained secretions and migration were not observed. Stent removal and repositioning was possible in one case of misplacement, and the Ultraflex stent was found to be safe for subglottic stenosis (25). Herth and colleagues further demonstrated that the Ultraflex stents could be placed satisfactorily without fluoroscopy, minimizing radiation exposure to patients and staff (26) (Fig. 6).

Long-term outcome of patients with malignant and benign airway strictures treated with Wallstents and Ultraflex stents was analyzed. Median follow-up for patients with lung cancer was 42 days, 329 days for lung transplant recipients, and 336 days for other benign conditions. No cases of mucus plugging, fistulous formation, or fatal hemoptysis were observed. Overall observed complication rate was 0.06 complications per patient-month. The most common complication (15.9%) was infectious tracheo-bronchitis and one patient had the stent removed because of persistent *Staphylococcus aureus* tracheobronchitis. Obstructing granuloma (14.6%) was the second most common complication necessitating multiple interventions to restore airway patency. Tumor ingrowth was seen in 6.1%, early migration in four patients treated with Wallstents, and metal mesh fatigue in one patient after two years (27). Although data on long-term complications of Ultraflex stent and its application in benign airway stenoses are limited, it proves to be a good prosthesis for complex malignant airway stricture, because of ease of placement, excellent flexibility, and biocompatibility. However, it should not be used in patients with benign airway conditions, until options of tube stent placement or surgery have been exhausted.

Alveolus Stent
Alveolus stent (Alveolus Inc., Charlotte, North Carolina, U.S.) is a new self-expanding, completely polyurethane-covered metallic stent that has been designed for use even in non-neoplastic airway strictures as it can be easily removed. Accurate sizing for the stent can be achieved with an Alveolus stent-sizing device (Alveolus Inc.), which can be introduced through the working channel of a therapeutic FB. It consists of a sliding external sheath and an inner wire. The device has a measuring tool on one end and a handle on the other. When the internal wire is retracted from the handle, the wings of the measurement device open and are capable of measuring diameters between 6 and 20 mm. Once tissue contact is made, the color bars that code for specific lumen diameters will show, which aid the bronchoscopists in the selection of appropriate stents.

Moreover, the Alveolus stent is laser constructed from a single piece of nitinol with concentric rings held in position by nitinol strands. Because of its structure, investigators have found it amenable to length modification. Since it does not fore-shorten with deployment, and is completely covered in polyurethane coating, even when customized, the stent keeps to its trimmed length and structural integrity (28). Despite its advantages, stent collapse causing hemoptysis and dyspnea in a woman who was treated for postintubation tracheal stenosis was reported (29).

IV.   Choice of a Stent
Besides the site, shape, and length of stenosis, presence or absence of malacia or fistula determine choice of a stent. The underlying cause of airway pathology is also an important consideration. Proper sizing of the stent (length and diameter) in relation to

the dimensions of the trachea or bronchus is important to avoid stent-related complications such as migration, mucus plugging, granulation, and tumor ingrowth.

Tube stent placement requires specialized equipment, training, and competency in rigid bronchoscopy, while metal stents can be inserted via an FB and in an outpatient setting. The ease of placement should not lead to the erroneous choice of the easiest stent over the best one to treat a given condition. Considering the immediate and long-term complications associated with indwelling stents, the endoscopist should run through a checklist: (*i*) Is a stent required? (*ii*) Will the patient benefit from stent placement in terms of quality of life or prognosis? (*iii*) Does the stent interfere or prohibit a curative surgical procedure later? (*iv*) Do I have the expertise, equipment, and team to place and more importantly, if required, to remove the stent? (*v*) What is the underlying airway pathology and which stent is ideal? (*vi*) Is it safe to place a stent in this anatomical site? (*vii*) What are the required stent dimensions (length and diameter)? (*viii*) Do I have the optimal stent or should I order a more appropriate one?

For benign strictures, stents that are easy to remove and replace (e.g., tube stent) are preferred to minimize mucosal damage that might otherwise preclude subsequent surgery. For malacia because of relapsing polychondritis or tracheomegaly syndrome, uncovered wire mesh stents are preferred, as they do not interfere with mucociliary clearance and have a low migration rate (30,31). In expiratory dynamic airway collapse associated with chronic obstructive pulmonary disease, a removable stent is considered only after standard therapy including noninvasive ventilation fails (32), while covered metal and tube stents are indicated in malignant stenoses (11,17,18,21,28) and tracheoesophageal fistulae (33,34).

V. Stent Insertion Techniques

Prior to stent insertion, dilatation of the stricture to its optimal diameter should be attempted using a rigid bronchoscope, bougie, or balloon. Tumor tissue should be removed either with laser or electrocautery. The largest possible prosthesis should be selected, and even if it does not completely unfold, it can be opened with a balloon or forceps.

Placement of tube stents requires rigid bronchoscopy while metal stents can be deployed using the flexible bronchoscope. Special catheters and deployment systems have been developed for metal stents. The Palmaz and Strecker stents are mounted on balloon catheters. These stents are deployed over the stenotic areas and expanded to their specified dimensions by means of balloon inflation (Fig. 3). The Ultraflex stent is a self-expanding stent that is mounted on an introduction catheter with crochet knots. Pulling on a thread unravels the knots and releases the stent. The distal release model is easier to deploy than the proximal release design (Fig. 4).

The Polyflex stent with its pusher system is deployed with the help of a rigid bronchoscope. Insertion of the Dumon stent is facilitated by the use of the dedicated Dumon-Efer rigid bronchoscope and stent applicator set (Efer, France). Placement of dynamic and other bifurcated stents is facilitated with dedicated forceps.

A stent alert card detailing the type and dimensions of the stent as well as its location in the tracheobronchial tree should be given to the patient. It should also indicate appropriate size of endotracheal tube to use if emergency intubation is required with the stent in situ.

VI. Tracheal Transplantation with Aortic Allografts

Primary tracheal tumors can arise from the respiratory epithelium, salivary glands, and mesenchymal structure of the trachea. Primary tracheal tumors account for up to 0.4% of malignant diseases, with 2.6 new cases per million people every year (35,36). In adults 90% are malignant with squamous cell carcinoma and adenoid cystic carcinoma accounting for two-thirds of these tumors (36). The adult trachea measures 12 cm in length, and is 1.5 to 2.5 cm wide. Depending on individual's anatomic and physiological factors, up to 50% of the trachea (i.e., not more than 7 cm) can be resected. Tracheal resection with end-to-end anastomosis is the treatment of choice unless the tumor involves more than 50% of trachea or invades mediastinal structures, lymph nodes, distant metastases, or the mediastinum, or the patient has received maximum radiation of more than 60 Gy (37,38). In these the circumstances, patients do not undergo surgery but receive palliation with endotracheal stents, debridement, external beam radiation, or brachytherapy (39).

Preliminary animal studies using allogenic aortic allografts to replace the trachea have demonstrated promise, as there were no occurrences of anastomotic leak, dehiscence, stenosis, or rejection over a period of 1 to 16 months (40,41). In fact recipient cells colonized the aortic graft. The tracheal epithelium that developed comprised of basal, secretory, and ciliated cells. A posterior membrane and cartilage rings could also be detected.

Recently tracheal transplantation is shown to be feasible in humans. Two patients with chemoradiotherapy-resistant mucoepidemoid and adenoid cystic carcinomas underwent tracheal resection and replacement with aortic allografts. Silicone Y-stents were left in place postoperatively to prevent collapse of the aortic grafts. Biopsy specimens of the aortic allografts in both patients at one year showed development of respiratory epithelium although it was unclear whether host mesenchymal stem cells had engrafted the aortic allograft and undergone cartilaginous differentiation. No complications of graft ischemia, suture dehiscence, infection, or graft rejection were observed despite notable omission of immunosuppressive therapy (42).

VII. Conclusion

Airway stenting is a valuable adjunct to other therapeutic bronchoscopic techniques used for relieving central airway obstruction. However, clinical studies are needed to identify patients who will derive the greatest benefit from stenting as well as in the search of the ideal stent. Tracheal replacement therapy with aortic allograft offers promise for patients with extensive tracheal tumors.

Summary

Stent placement is commonly used as a method of palliation for patients with central airway obstruction because of malignancy. Stents are used to maintain airway patency following dilatation of postinflammatory and infectious strictures, for airway dehiscence after lung transplantation as well as in the management of tracheobronchomalacia. Covered stents can be applied to seal fistulas between trachea or bronchi and the esophagus, and dehiscence of pneumonectomy stump. Careful patient selection, characteristics of the airway stenosis, physician's expertise, and availability of equipment determine the type of stent used. Placement of tube stents requires rigid bronchoscopy and is preceded by dilatation of the strictures, while metal stents can be placed using a flexible bronchoscope (FB). This chapter discusses the advantages and disadvantages of commonly used airway stents as well as future role of allogenic aortic grafting for the tracheobronchial tree.

References

1. Bolliger CT, Sutedja TG, Strausz J, et al. Therapeutic bronchoscopy with immediate effect: laser, electrocautery, argon plasma coagulation and stents. Eur Respir J 2006; 27:1258–1271.
2. Freitag L. Tracheobronchial stents. In: Bolliger CT, Mathur PN, eds. Interventional Bronchoscopy, Progress in Respiratory Research. Vol 30. Basel: Karger, 2000; 171–186.
3. Trendelenburg F. Beitrage zu den Operationen an den Luftwegen. Langenbecks Arch Chir 1872; 13:335.
4. Bond CJ. Treatment of tracheal stenosis by a new T-shaped tracheostomy tube. Lancet 1891; I:539–540.
5. Brunings W, Albrecht W. Direkte Endoskopie der Luft und Speisewege. Stuttgart: Enke 1915; 134–138.
6. Montgomery WW. T-tube tracheal stent. Arch Otolaryngol 1965; 82:320–321.
7. Dumon JF. A dedicated tracheobronchial stent. Chest 1990; 97:328–332.
8. Colt HG, Prakash UB, Offord KP. Bronchoscopy in North America: survey by the American Association for Bronchology. J Bronchology 2000; 7:8–25.
9. Dasgupta A, Dolmatch BC, Abi-Saleh WJ, et al. Self-expandable metallic airway stent insertion employing flexible bronchoscopy: preliminary results. Chest 1998; 114:106–109.
10. Lemaire A, Burfeind WR, Toloza E, et al. Outcomes of tracheobronchial stents in patients with malignant airway disease. Ann Thorac Surg 2005; 80:434–438.
11. Cavaliere S, Venuta F, Foccoli P, et al. Endoscopic treatment of malignant airway obstruction in 2008 patients. Chest 1996; 110:1536–1542.
12. Colt HG, Harrell JH. Therapeutic rigid bronchoscopy allows level of care changes in patients with acute respiratory failure from central airways obstruction. Chest 1997; 112:202–206.
13. Bolliger CT, Probst R, Tschopp K, et al. Silicone stents in the management of inoperable tracheobronchial stenoses. Indications and limitations. Chest 1993; 104:1653–1659.
14. Lee P, Kupeli E, Mehta AC. Therapeutic bronchoscopy in lung cancer. Laser therapy, electrocautery, brachytherapy, stents, and photodynamic therapy. Clin Chest Med 2002; 23:241–256.
15. Chhajed PN, Baty F, Pless M, et al. Outcome of treated advanced non-small cell lung cancer with and without airway obstruction. Chest 2006; 130:1803–1807.
16. Mughal MM, Gildea TR, Murthy S, et al. Short-term deployment of self-expanding metallic stents facilitates healing of bronchial dehiscence. Am J Respir Crit Care Med 2005; 172:768–771.
17. Dumon J, Cavaliere S, Diaz-Jimenez JP, et al. Seven experience with the Dumon prosthesis. J Bronchol 1996; 31:6–10.
18. Diaz-Jimenez JP, Farrero Munoz E, Martinez Ballarín JI, et al. Silicone stents in the management of obstructive tracheobronchial lesions: 2 year experience. J Bronchol 1994; 1:15–18.
19. Noppen M, Meysman M, Claes I, et al. Screw-thread vs Dumon endoprosthesis in the management of tracheal stenosis. Chest 1999; 115:532–535.
20. Gildea TR, Murthy SC, Sahoo D, et al. Performance of a self-expanding silicone stent in palliation of benign airway conditions. Chest 2006; 130:1419–1423.
21. Mehta AC, Dasgupta A. Airway stents. Clin Chest Med 1999; 20:139–151.
22. Rafanan AL, Mehta AC. Stenting of the tracheobronchial tree. Radiol Clin North Am 2000; 38:395–408.

23. Slonim SM, Razavi M, Kee S, et al. Transbronchial Palmaz stent placement for tracheobronchial stenosis. J Vasc Interv Radiol 1998; 9:153–160.
24. Strecker EP, Liermann D, Barth KH, et al. Expandable tubular stents for treatment of arterial occlusive diseases: experimental and clinical results. Radiology 1990; 175:87–102.
25. Miyazawa T, Yamakido M, Ikeda S, et al. Implantation of Ultraflex nitinol stents in malignant tracheobronchial stenoses. Chest 2000; 118:959–965.
26. Herth F, Becker HD, LoCicero J, et al. Successful bronchoscopic placement of tracheobronchial stents without fluoroscopy. Chest 2001; 119(6):1910–1912.
27. Saad CP, Murthy S, Krizmanich G, et al. Self-expandable metallic airway stents and flexible bronchoscopy. Chest 2003; 124:1993–1999.
28. Hoag JB, Juhas W, Morrow K, et al. Predeployment length modification of a self-expanding metallic stent. J Bronchol 2008; 15:185–190.
29. Trisolini R, Paioli D, Fornario V, et al. Collapse of a new type of self-expanding metallic tracheal stent. Monaldi Arch Chest Dis 2006; 65:56–58.
30. Dunne JA, Sabanathan S. Use of metallic stents in relapsing polychondritis. Chest 1994; 105:864–867.
31. Collard PH, Freitag L, Reynaert MS, et al. Terminal respiratory failure from tracheobronchomalacia. Thorax 1996; 51:224–226.
32. Murgu SD, Colt SD. Complications of silicone stent insertion in patients with expiratory central airway collapse. Ann Thorac Surg 2007; 84:1870–1877.
33. Colt HG, Meric B, Dumon JF. Double stents for carcinoma of the esophagus invading the tracheobronchial tree. Gastrointest Endosc 1992; 38:485–489.
34. Freitag L, Tekolf E, Steveling H, et al. Management of malignant esophago-tracheal fistulas with airway stenting and double stenting. Chest 1996; 110:1155–1160.
35. Gelder CM, Hetzel MR. Primary tracheal tumors: a national survey. Thorax 1993; 48: 688–692.
36. Bhattacharyya N. Contemporary staging and prognosis for primary tracheal malignancies: a population-based analysis. Otolaryngol Head Neck Surg 2004; 131:639–642.
37. Gaissert HA, Grillo HC, Shadmehr MB, et al. Long-term survival after resection of primary adenoid cystic and squamous cell carcinoma of the trachea and carina. Ann Thorac Surg 2004; 78:1889–1896.
38. Grillo HC. Development of tracheal surgery: a historical review. Part 2: treatment of tracheal diseases. Ann Thorac Surg 2003; 75:1039–1047.
39. Macchiarini P. Primary tracheal tumors. Lancet Oncol 2006; 7:83–91.
40. Martinod E, Seguin A, Holder-Espinasse M, et al. Tracheal regeneration following tracheal replacement with an allogenic aorta. Ann Thorac Surg 2005; 79:942–949.
41. Jaillard S, Holder-Espinasse M, Hubert T, et al. Tracheal replacement with allogenic aorta in the pig. Chest 2006; 130:1397–1404.
42. Wurtz A, Porte H, Conti M, et al. Tracheal replacement with allogenic aorta. N Engl J Med 2006; 355:1938–1940.

5

High-Resolution Bronchoscopy: Bringing These Modalities into Focus

DAVID RIKER

Department of Pulmonary and Critical Care Medicine, University of California, San Diego, San Diego, California, U.S.A.

I. Introduction

Flexible bronchoscopy was initially introduced in 1966 by Dr Shigeto Ikeda, who is regarded by many to be the "father" of fiberoptic bronchoscopy. This revolutionary pulmonary tool was established in clinical practice in 1968 and became available in the United States in 1972 (1).

Since that time, the bronchoscope has evolved into a highly technical instrument with true color video capability in a variety of scope diameters. Bronchoscopy allows direct visual access to larger airways and bronchioles and extended instrument access to the alveolar level. Along with these advancements, bronchoscope resolution has been enhanced, providing remarkable clarity of human airway, blood vessels, and mucosa. High-resolution bronchoscopy has been used to describe modalities such as auto-fluorescence (AF), narrow band imaging (NBI), fibered confocal microscopy (FCFM), and optical coherence tomography (OCT). While high-resolution techniques continue to be useful for research purposes, their application in clinical practice is innovative yet underutilized. There persists a need for optical tissue conformation through rapid diagnostic imaging. We will explore high-resolution bronchoscopy and provide a framework for current practice and future potential.

II. Autofluorescence Bronchoscopy
A. Introduction

Fluorescence is a luminescence optical phenomenon in which absorption of light energy photons triggers excitation and emission of another photon with a longer wavelength. Usually the initial photon is in the ultraviolet range with the emitted light being within the visible range. A fluorophore is a component of a molecule that causes fluorescensce (Table 1). Absorption occurs at a specific wavelength energy, and visible light energy is reemitted.

Fluorescence can be created with 380- to 490-nm light exposure, which excites the natural human airway fluorophores, collagen, and elastin (2). Exogenous compounds such as indocyanine green or fluorescein also fluoresce in the presence of light stimulation, allowing observation of airway mucosal changes. Novel research is currently ongoing to determine the use of fluorescein dye in airway cancer detection (Fig. 1).

AF, however, is the fluorescence of substances other than the fluorophore of interest (3). Of specific importance are early airway changes consistent with dysplasia,

Table 1 Common Fluorophores

Chlorophyll
Collagen
Elastin
Fibrillin
Flavin
Indolamine
Indolamine dimer
Indolamine trimer
Lipofuscin
NADH (reduced form only)
Plant polyphenols
Tryptophan

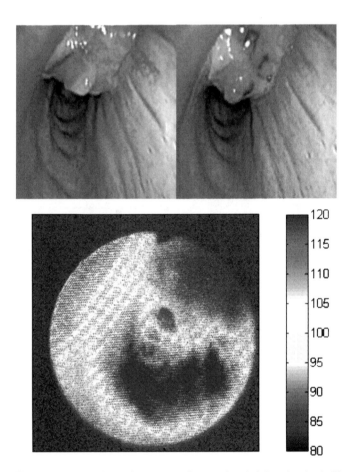

Figure 1 Pre– and post–intravenous fluorescein administration (*top*). Photo showing poor fluorescein uptake in tumor (*bottom*). *Source*: Photo courtesy of Dr David Riker and Dr Melissa Suter.

carcinoma in situ or invasive cancer. These changes occur in the cell and tissue state during a pathologic process, resulting in modifications of the amount and distribution of endogenous fluorophores and chemical-physical properties of their microenvironment. Abnormal AF signal may be useful as a diagnostic indicator in early airway cancer detection.

B. Literature

Several AF systems are available including DAFE (Richard Wolf GmbH, Knittlingen, Germany), AFI (Olympus Optical Co., Ltd, Tokyo, Japan), Storz D-Light (Storz, Tuttlingen, Germany), Novadaq Pinpoint (Novadaq Technologies Inc., Ontario, Canada), ONCOLIFE (Xillix Technologies, Vancouver, Canada), and Pentax Safe-3000 (Pentax Corp., Tokyo, Japan) (4). Each system uses a different source of light excitation energy including laser, high-arc mercury bulb, or xenon bulb. Most systems use a blue light energy wavelength between 380 and 460 nm (5). Review of the in-depth optical and operating differences between each system is beyond the scope of this chapter.

Much published trials on autofluorescence bronchoscopy (AFB) pertain to the LIFE (Xillix Technologies) device. White light bronchoscopy (WLB) is performed prior to AFB in a majority of trials, resulting in a calculated relative sensitivity between the two modalities. All abnormal regions on WLB are confirmed using AFB, while subsequent suspicious areas not identified with WLB are detected by AF. Biopsies are then required to document pathologic tissue changes consistent with invasive or preinvasive conditions. Regions felt to exhibit visible features of normal airway mucosa are used as comparison "controls."

A 1.3- to 6.3-fold increase in the detection of dysplasia and carcinoma in situ (CIS) has been reported with the LIFE device (6–11). The most recent trial by Chhajed et al. described 158 consecutive high-risk individuals undergoing mass screening for lung cancer and having abnormal sputum cytology screened by LIFE and WLB (11). All patients underwent fiberoptic bronchoscopy followed by LIFE. While LIFE improved dysplasia or malignancy detection by 1.3-fold, specificity was reduced by 2.3-fold.

Less published data exist for other systems including Karl Storz D-Light. Two Storz D-Light trials were performed in the last five years. In 2004, Beamis et al. enrolled 300 patients having known, suspected, or resected lung cancer to undergo D-Light surveillance (12). Bronchoscopic findings were stratified into four classes with biopsies only obtained in class III (abnormal/premalignant) lesions. Adding AF to WLB increased preinvasive disease detection by 5.8-fold (Fig. 2). No difference in specificity was observed between the two modalities. Häußinger et al. included 1173 smokers randomized to D-Light AFB + WLB or WLB alone (5). The combination of AFB and WLB had a 1.42-fold increased sensitivity for detecting dysplasia and CIS over WLB alone. Specificity was decreased, however, owing to higher false positive findings.

Varying prospective AFB studies have used different AF systems. Currently, few data exist in head-to-head systems comparison. Herth et al. published the largest prospective study comparing two AF systems, Storz D-Light and LIFE, in 332 patients with known or suspected non–small cell lung cancer. No clinical difference between LIFE and D-Light were observed; however, exam length was four minutes longer with LIFE (13). It is difficult to determine superiority between AF systems. The choice of AF equipment should be determined by operator preference, video optics, cost, and ease of integration into a preexisting bronchoscopy system.

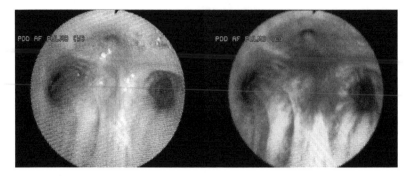

Figure 2 White light and Storz D-Light image of abnormal carinal mucosa. *Source*: Photo courtesy of Dr John Beamis.

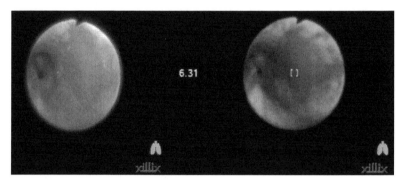

Figure 3 Elevated ONCOLIFE red/green ratio (Right side of photo, dark gray/light gray respectively) (6.31) indicating blood from acute mucosal trauma. This observation with AFB can lead to false-positive results. *Source*: Photo courtesy of Dr David Riker.

C. Limitations

Criticism of these studies includes introduced sensitivity bias resulting from initial WLB preceding AFB. AFB showed greater sensitivity for distinguishing intraepithelial neoplastic lesions compared to invasive carcinomas. Autopsy, the gold standard, does not exist in these trials for obvious reasons. Therefore, accuracy of WLB and AFB must be compared with one another. The resulting comparison measures relative sensitivity and specificity. Mucosal trauma is one example of false positive findings observed with AFB (Fig. 3).

It is difficult to completely rely on decade-old studies using older generation AF/fiberoptic bronchoscopes to extrapolate data from newer, improved resolution color videobronchoscopes. It is unclear what impact optic limited AF/fiberoptic bronchoscopes contribute to overall test sensitivity. Newer generation color videobronchoscopes have improved resolution up to 38 μm, far greater than fiberoptic bronchoscopes. On the basis of data gathered with fiberoptic AF systems, there is not a strong role for AFB + WLB when visible cancers are detected using WLB alone. This is likely true using white light color videobronchoscopy as well. Pentax Safe-3000 is the only available AF system compatible for use with color videobronchoscopy. It is approved for research in the United States, but may be purchased for clinical use in other countries. Ongoing small trials are being conducted to compare Safe-3000 with its AF/fiberoptic predecessors.

The role of AFB in generalized lung cancer screening is highly controversial. One of the central criticisms of AFB for mass screening arises from the poorly understood prevalence and natural progression of airway dysplasia and CIS. Dysplasia II-III can be found in 3.9% of the smoking population, while CIS is observed in only 1% of high-risk individuals (8). Preinvasive progression to invasive disease is rarely reported or confirmed by biopsy-proven pathology (14–17).

Sputum cytology suggests that up to 46% of severe dysplasia could progress to CIS (18). Venmans et al. discovered CIS in 9 of 144 patients undergoing AFB surveillance over three years (17). Despite local endobronchial therapy, 56% progressed to invasive carcinoma. These findings were supported by Bota et al. who found 416 lesions in 104 high-risk patients followed by AFB over two years (19). At three months 70% of dysplasia regressed and 37% stabilized or progressed at two years. Overall, 41% regressed to normal after two years and 22% regressed to a low-grade dysplasia. However, CIS persisted with 78% of the lesions remaining as severe dysplasia or CIS at three months.

It is not entirely clear that treating dysplasia is helpful, as a majority of lesions tend to regress over time. Detection of CIS by AFB raises an important question of appropriate management and future surveillance. No large long-term study has confirmed the widely held belief that CIS represents premalignancy. Consideration for AFB surveillance at three-month intervals is reasonable with endobronchial treatment performed if lesions persist for three or more months.

D. Conclusions

Fluorescence bronchoscopy shows promise, providing a valuable opportunity to understand the natural progression of bronchial dysplasia and CIS. It may be possible to combine AFB with tumor marker sputum cytology and other advanced high-resolution bronchoscopy techniques, facilitating a shift in the current paradigm of lung cancer screening. However, it will ultimately be necessary to demonstrate use of these new tools associated with a significant reduction in lung cancer mortality before integration of fluorescence bronchoscopy can be recommended for lung cancer screening.

While AFB cannot be recommended for mass screening, several defined populations may benefit from screening and surveillance. Those patients who are symptomatic smokers have a history of prior head and neck cancers; post–lung resection for lung cancer or preresection candidates should be considered for AFB. Nonsurgical candidates or patients with advanced stage IIIB/IV lung cancer have the option of endobronchial tumor resection. There exists the possibility to define endobronchial tumor margins using bronchoscopy including AFB. AFB-detected tumors without confirmed cartilage invasion are ideal for endobronchial therapy. Recommendations for the treatment and surveillance of dysplasia and CIS include AFB at three-month intervals to determine stability of either lesion. If dysplastic regions show no signs of progression, further surveillance could be performed as needed. Routine bronchoscopy and endobronchial therapy should be applied to CIS lesions proven to persist three months or greater.

Future research should concentrate on mortality end points, further defining the role of AFB in select population screening. Combining endobronchial diagnostic multimodalities, including AFB, endobronchial ultrasound, and OCT, may provide accurate depth and resection margins for submucosal disease.

III.   Narrow-Band Imaging
A.   Introduction

Narrow-band imaging (NBI) is an optical filter technology that radically improves the visibility of capillaries, veins, and other tissue structures by optimizing the absorbance and scattering characteristics of light. NBI is based on the principle that the depth of light penetration depends on its wavelength: The longer the wavelength, the deeper the penetration. A typical bronchoscope system uses white light from a Xenon lamp passing through a rotary RGB filter that separates the light into the colors red, green, and blue. Light is detected by a charged coupled device at the endoscope tip, and three images are integrated into a single color image by the video processor. When a light filter is used, the red spectrum is removed, leaving a blue and green spectrum. These two discrete bands of light, blue at 415 nm and green at 540 nm, then enhance the surrounding airway tissue. Blue light penetrates only superficially, whereas green light penetrates into deeper layers. Narrow-band blue light is absorbed by hemoglobin displaying superficial capillary networks, while green light displays subepithelial vessels (20) (Fig. 4). The end result is an extremely high contrast image of the mucosa and submucosal surfaces. Capillaries within the mucosa are visualized in brown and the submucosal veins are depicted in cyan (blue).

B.   Rationale

The continuing development of pulmonary NBI results from the current disheartening paradigm surrounding lung cancer screening and early lung cancer detection. Prior studies have confirmed the futility of lung cancer screening with chest X ray alone or in concert with sputum cytology (21,22). Despite larger lung cancer screening trials using CT scans in high-risk patients, there has been no distinct progress toward improved lung cancer screening sensitivity. ELCAP screened 1000 asymptomatic patients who had a

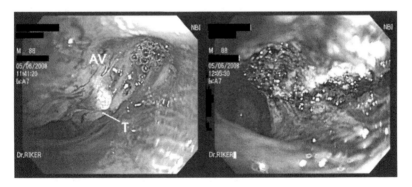

Figure 4   NBI mode showing endobronchial tumor (T) and abnormal vascularity (AV) pre- and postelectrocautery. *Source*: Photo courtesy of Dr David Riker.

$\geq$10 pack-year smoking history with low-dose spiral chest CT (23). I-ELCAP looked at 31,567 asymptomatic participants with baseline CT scans (24). Annual screening scans and follow-up were accomplished on 27,456 patients. Screening in asymptomatic smokers yielded a high prevalence of lung cancer; however, there is debate surrounding uncontrolled overdiagnosis and lead-time bias in addition to the inability to determine lung cancer–specific and overall mortality rates (25).

The question has been posed whether bronchoscopic surveillance or screening can be accomplished. Most accept the cancerization hypothesis associated with cigarette use (26). Earlier postmortem studies documented premalignant airway pathology occurring in extensive areas of bronchial tissue. These preinvasive bronchial changes were seen in heavy smokers (27,28). Since early airway cancer exists and early cancer detection may improve mortality, there is a substantial need to define a screening tool capable of identifying these lesions.

C. NBI Systems

Combination color videobronchoscopes are available with the NBI feature. The only commercially available NBI devices are the Olympus EVIS EXERA II models BF1T180, BF-Q180, and BF-P180 bronchoscopes combined with the CLV 180 light source, CV-180 video processor, and OEV-191H LCD monitor (Olympus Optical). Bronchoscope sizes for the three models are a 6.0-mm outer tube diameter design with a large 3.0-mm working channel, 5.1 mm diameter at the insertion tube and 5.5 mm and the distal end with 2.0-mm working channel, or a 4.9-mm tube size with a 2.0-mm working channel. A separate operator button allows smooth transition from white light mode to NBI mode.

D. Literature

Most studies using NBI technology are targeting upper gastrointestinal pathology including Barrett's esophagus, metaplasia, and GERD (29). However, newer studies have used NBI to detect colon adenomas along with dysplasia in patients with ulcerative colitis (30,31). Unfortunately, these studies have relatively small patient numbers and have been performed in highly specialized centers.

Classification systems have been proposed describing various mucosal patterns. Systematic image and biopsies were performed in nearly 200 selected areas of 63 Barrett's esophagus cases (32). Metaplasia was associated with normal vascular and mucosal patterns combined with flat mucosa devoid of pits or villi. Those regions exhibiting irregular vascular or mucosal patterns and abnormal blood vessels were associated with high-grade intestinal neoplasia.

Other authors described three categories for mucosal patterns (ridged/villous, circular, and irregular/distorted) and two categories for vascular patterns (normal and abnormal) (33,34). Prospective evaluation of 51 patients was completed. Sensitivity is 94% for detecting intestinal metaplasia while the irregular/distorted pattern had a sensitivity of 100% for high-grade intestinal neoplasia.

Additional classification systems are based on regular, irregular, and absent microstructural patterns, and regular and irregular microvascular patterns (35).

NBI may provide the observation of early tumor neovascularization through abnormal mucosal vessel patterns. Increased vessel density in the submucosa can be observed in bronchial dysplasia, indicating that angiogenesis occurs early on during lung cancer proliferation (36–38). Shibuya et al. studied patients undergoing AFB with normal and abnormal epithelium using high-magnification bronchovideoscopy (HMB) (39). Sixteen specimens with normal AFB and bronchial epithelium, 22 with bronchitis, and 21 dysplasia specimens with abnormal fluorescence were observed. Bronchitis specimens had a twofold increase in mean vascular ratios compared with normal epithelium, and a threefold increase in mean vascular ratios was observed with dysplastic specimens compared with normal epithelium. Those with dysplasia had mucosal vascular patterns described as "complex networks of tortuous vessels."

While this chapter previously discussed AFB, there are a paucity of studies confirming the utility of combining NBI and AFB in detecting preinvasive bronchial changes and invasive lung carcinoma. The additional role of NBI added to AFB was observed in a small 48-patient study by Shibuya et al (40). All patients with sputum cytology specimens suspicious or positive for malignancy were entered into the study. Angiogenic squamous dysplasia (ASD) was imaged by combined HMB and NBI. ASD is thought to be a premalignant condition in lung cancer pathogenesis. HMB can enlarge an image up to 100 times. Mass screening of sputum cytologic examinations identified high-risk lung cancer cases. 48 patients were included in the high-risk group comprising 46 males and 2 females. Majority of patients were current smokers. WLB was performed followed by AFB using the LIFE lung system (Xillix Technologies). HMB was directed toward regions with abnormal fluorescence and examination repeated by NBI. Bronchial biopsy specimens were sampled from all abnormal areas. Abnormal dotted vessels, in addition to increased vessel growth and complex networks of tortuous vessels, were associated with dysplasia. Among the vascular networks with abnormal fluorescence without dotted vessels, 98% did not show dysplasia. The dotted vessels were observed in 18 abnormal fluorescence sites, in which 14 (78%) exhibited dysplasia. There was a significant association between NBI-observed dotted vessel frequency and ASD pathology ($p = 0.002$). Dotted vessel diameter observed by NBI was similar to capillary blood vessel size on pathology. Further studies are needed to confirm the clinical role for NBI in preneoplastic or invasive cancer screening.

Few studies have concentration on NBI compared to WLB alone. Silvestri et al. studied 22 patients in a prospective partially blinded trial using WLB and NBI. WLB was performed first, followed by NBI. There was no significant improvement in diagnostic yield with NBI; however, a significant greater detection in dysplasia was observed ($p = 0.005$) (41).

E. Limitations

NBI may be complimentary to AFB, but advantages are less clear combined with WLB. Tumor angiogenesis can be observed in endobronchial disease, but not all tumors are vascular, adding to potential false-negative NBI findings. In NBI mode, acute bleeding appears very dark in color and obscures vascular tissue findings. Minimal airway blood and mucous is essential for optimal NBI surveillance. It is common to observe increased submucosal vascularity in emphysema patients and former and active smokers. Unfortunately, there is no accepted or well-defined clinical description and classification of abnormal airway vascularity. If NBI is performed and vascularity is observed, distinct pathologic vessel alterations may be missed without high-magnification bronchoscopy.

F. Conclusions

NBI seems to have a superior role combined with AFB and WLB, compared to WLB alone. This is not surprising as AFB has improved sensitivity in detecting early dysplasia compared with WLB. Future studies will need to focus on a multimodal bronchoscopic approach to lung cancer screening and surveillance. Perhaps NBI combined with AFB and WLB could reduce the false positives associated with AFB and WLB alone. NBI and AFB may improve localization of tumor and tumor margins post–endobronchial resection. Both AFB and NBI improve dysplasia detection; however, there is no data suggesting an acceptable reduction in false negatives and positives needed to support lung cancer screening with NBI, even in surgical cure patients.

IV. Raman Spectroscopy
A. Introduction

Raman spectroscopy (RS) is a vibrational spectroscopic technique that can be used to optically probe molecular changes associated with diseased tissues. The technique relies on the scattering of monochromatic light, usually delivered by a near-infrared (NIR) laser having a wavelength of 750 to 1400 nm (42).

Laser light interacts with phonons that are responsible for physical properties of solids such as thermal or electrical conductivity. Energy is then "shifted" and detected as a Raman signal. Depth of penetration can vary between 0.5 and 1 mm depending on the system used (43).

B. History

Inelastic scattering of light was first theorized by Smekal in 1923, but was not observed in experiments until 1928. While several individuals discovered the Raman effect, an Indian scientist, Sir C. V. Raman, was credited as the major founder. In 1928 Raman, Landsberg, and Maldelstam observed this effect by means of sunlight (44). For this discovery, Raman was awarded the Nobel Prize in physics in 1930. Using sunlight and a photographic filter, monochromatic light was created. Monochromatic light passing through a second blocking filter underwent frequency alterations, but "blocked" light frequency was unchanged.

C. Rationale

The Raman effect exploits differences between the incident and scattered frequencies that correspond to the vibrational modes of molecules participating in the interaction. Scattered photon intensity plotted as a function of frequency shift is depicted as Raman spectra. The spectra results in a "light-induced" fingerprint of specific molecular species, with the potential to be used for biomedical applications. Raman-active scattering can be observed in many biologic molecules, each exhibiting a unique spectral fingerprint. Raman spectra usually exhibit sharp spectral features that are characteristic for specific molecular structures and conformations of tissue, thus providing more specific molecular information about a given tissue or disease state (45,46). NIR-RS has certain advantages, such as relative insensitivity to tissue water contents and deeper penetration depth into the tissue, that justify its increasing popularity for biomedical applications (47,48). A laser beam is used to irradiate a spot on the sample under investigation (Fig. 5). The resulting Raman effect is analogous to an optical tissue biopsy, identifying particular atoms or ions that comprise the tissue molecules (49).

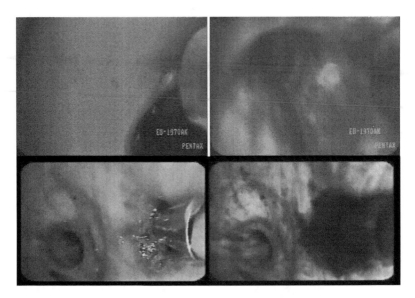

Figure 5 White light and autofluorescence images of the tissue contact sensor laser beam indicating the aiming point of the Raman probe (*upper row*). White light and autofluorescence mode with suspected malignant endobronchial disease analyzed by Raman probe (*lower row*). *Source*: Photo courtesy of Dr John Beamis.

D. Literature

A paucity of Raman data exists for lung cancer detection, which is discussed below. However, RS has been used to identify numerous nonpulmonary tumors such as stomach, colon, laryngeal, cervical, ovarian, and skin cancers (50–52). In 2000, Ling et al. investigated a combined total of 40 normal and malignant gastric samples (53). Malignant molecular bonds differed compared with normal mucosa. Water and protein variation within malignant tissue may allow RS to detect these differences. Mizuno et al. performed an ex vivo study with 251 biopsy specimens of gastric carcinoma and normal mucosa obtained from 49 gastric cancer patients undergoing endoscopy (54). Immediate Raman measurements were taken and principal component analysis of gastric cancer and normal tissue completed. Sensitivity, specificity, and accuracy of Raman spectra for gastric cancer were 66%, 73%, and 70% respectively. Gastric dysplasia has also been analyzed using RS. In a study conducted by Teh et al., a total of 76 gastric samples in 44 patients undergoing endoscopy or gastric resection were included (55). All specimens underwent histopathologic examination yielding 55 normal and 21 dysplastic samples. Diagnostic sensitivity was 85.7% and specificity 80.0%.

RS in colon cancer has been explored. Molckovsky et al. used 54 ex vivo and 10 in vivo colon polyp samples, without normal controls (56). Ex vivo samples included 34 adenomatous and 20 hyperplastic polyps. Spectral algorithms yielded 91% sensitivity and 95% specificity with 93% accuracy for ex vivo adenomatous polyps. In vivo adenomas were diagnosed with 100% sensitivity, 89% specificity, and 95% accuracy. There appeared to be a clear distinction between normal and malignant gastric tissue.

Stone et al. biopsied suspected laryngeal cancer and observed Raman spectral changes in seven normal, four dysplastic, and four cancer samples (57). Sensitivity and specificity were 92% and 90% for carcinoma, 76% and 91% for dysplasia, and 83% and 94% for identifying normal tissue.

The largest study involving Raman and lung cancer was described by Yamakazi et al., in which 35 ex vivo lungs with 210 spectral measurements of normal and cancerous tissue were performed (58). The majority of cancer types were adenocarcinoma, followed by squamous cell, large cell, and adenosquamous carcinomas. All specimens were naïve to cancer treatment. Specimens of 5 mm diameter were excised from native lungs and Raman measurements obtained from three separate positions in each sample. The identical procedure was carried out for the noncancerous analysis. Overall sensitivity of cancer detection was 91%, with 97% specificity. Two unique spectral peaks were observed at 1448/cm and 1662/cm, signifying the presence of malignant tissue compared to nonmalignant controls.

These results were further supported by Huang et al. in an ex vivo study comprising 28 total bronchial tissue samples from 10 patients with suspected lung cancer (59). AFB was performed using the LIFE system (Xillix Technologies) and biopsies obtained from areas displaying abnormal fluorescence signal. Surgical specimens were also included. Histopathology showed 10 squamous cell carcinoma, 6 adenocarcinoma, and 12 normal samples. All samples were free from observed necrosis. Although malignant tissue had several bands discovered by Raman spectra, two peaks were consistently appreciated. Using a ratio of the two bands, 1445/cm and 1655/cm, tumor tissue was separated from normal tissue with a sensitivity and specificity of 94% and 92%. Observed Raman signal was stronger with larger tissue samples.

E. Limitations

Raman spectra can provide immediate confirmation of abnormal tissue changes. However, a large drawback surrounds the small sampling area of the probe and penetration depth. Most newer generation probes are 2.0 mm or less and can investigate tissue, resulting in rapid spectral analysis. Depth of tumor invasion may not be accurately measured; however, conformation of malignancy, CIS, or dysplasia is feasible. The optimal number of sample sites that maximize spectral sensitivity is unclear. Probe size is not an issue with ex vivo studies; however, future in vivo analysis will be more challenging. It is impossible to scan large areas of bronchial tissue using a miniprobe. Therefore, Raman cannot provide tumor confirmation without the aid of high-resolution bronchoscopy tools such as AFB or NBI. Current in vivo studies investigating Raman combined with AFB may yield promising results.

Accurate sampling requires direct tissue contact without interference from surrounding light. The patient must experience excellent anesthesia to accomplish adequate sampling in the central airways. Blood, mucous, tissue AF, and mucosal irregularities can disrupt successful Raman spectral analysis (58).

Human airway tissue AF results from laser light exposure. Most Raman cancer studies used laser wavelengths of 700 to 800 nm or YAG wavelength of 1064 nm to cause tissue excitation. Increasing laser wavelength to NIR may improve tissue penetration depth; however, documented changes in AF occur. Kaminaka et al. reported a reduction in background AF as wavelength approaches the NIR region (60).

Tumors may exhibit profound necrosis with tissue debris or surface epithelialization, which sequesters the advancing neoplasm. The ability of RS to distinguish necrosis or epithelial changes from normal tissue or tumor has not been determined (59).

Initial spectral lung cancer studies described a weak Raman scattering signal and a need for improved sensitivity of photon counting equipment. As technology of the Raman technique progresses, catheter and detector advancements may allow routine use in cancer screening bronchoscopy (58).

F. Conclusions

RS is a tool confined to ongoing research protocols with current in vivo studies under investigation. The rationale for spectral analysis combined with bronchoscopy has the potential to add optical biopsy confirmation of malignant or premalignant tissue. The probe can be integrated into a current endoscopic system and has applications in gastrointestinal, dermatologic, and gynecologic subspecialities. Raman is not suited for independent lung cancer applications but should be considered an option for histopathologic tissue verification once a region of interest is identified. AFB integrated with RS could improve the specificity and perhaps sensitivity compared with AFB alone. Spectroscopy will continue to develop into a clinical tool for rapid and noninvasive diagnosis of lung cancers. Presently the technique could provide an adjunct to AFB + WLB, directing biopsies for histopathologic investigation of recurrent and primary preinvasive or invasive bronchial disease.

V. Optical Coherence Tomography
A. Introduction

OCT is a technique for obtaining mucosal and submucosal images at a resolution similar to low power microscopy (61). OCT uses a laser light source, usually in the NIR range, capturing reflected images. These images are created by "optical ultrasound" using light instead of ultrasound waves. This technology has the capability of providing tissue images with superior resolution to ultrasound or magnetic resonance imaging. Given the dramatic resolution of OCT images, this technology has a strong potential as a clinical tool for preinvasive or invasive lung cancer.

B. Background

Initial OCT evolved from white light inferometry used for ocular measurements (62). Professor Naohiro Tanno developed OCT in 1990 along with Huang in 1991, providing substantial gains in tissue image resolution and cross-sectional abilities (63–65). Well suited for ophthalmic applications, this modality has spread to GI, cardiac, vascular, and pulmonary fields. OCT imaging does not require direct tissue contact unlike other competing technologies such as ultrasound, FCFM, and RS. Morphologic tissue imaging is superior to ultrasound, magnetic resonance imaging, spectroscopy, and FCFM as OCT has 1- to 3-mm penetration depth and advanced resolution of 4 to 15 μm (66–68). Up to 20-fold increase in resolution is observed with OCT imaging compared with medical ultrasound (66). Contrasted with conventional interferometry where interference of laser light occurs over several meters, OCT interference is reduced to micrometers. Broad bandwidth light is created using short pulse lasers, usually in the NIR 1000 to 1310 nm range, since longer wavelength light affords deeper tissue penetration (62,69).

OCT image construction is based on principles of reflected scattered and coherent light (70). Scattered light has gone awry and cannot be utilized for imaging. However, the small amount of reflected coherent light is captured by the OCT optical interferometer. The interferometer separates incoherent, unusable light and the desired coherent light, resulting in image generation. It also provides depth and intensity specifics from the light reflected within cartilage, mucosal, and submucosal layers. Images are stacked, or built on one another, similar to medical ultrasound. Additionally, images are captured in real time with speeds up to 10 frames per second.

Imaging depth is 1 to 3 mm, as reflected light traveling greater than 3 mm is largely incoherent, resulting in image deterioration. Noncontact images are easily acquired with low laser output without subsequent tissue damage.

C. Literature

Medical OCT applications, first introduced in ophthalmology, included retinal mapping, retinal artery flow measurements, and a diagnostic tool for diabetic retinopathy (71,72).

OCT has been used in coronary imaging and in support of GI malignancy detection (73,74). Newer advances in OCT technology have been directed toward laryngeal disease. In 2005, Wong et al. described a prospective observational study with 115 patients undergoing laryngeal, esophageal, or tracheobronchial endoscopy and OCT (75). Patients had at least one laryngeal subsite evaluated by OCT, with 60 and 23 patients having laryngeal and vocal chord biopsies, respectively. Malignancy was confirmed by histopathology in 16 patients. Consistent identification of laryngeal epithelium and lamina propria was observed in normal patients. Exceptional tissue layer demarcation may further distinguish tumor invasion of the basement membrane in laryngeal cancer patients. Armstrong et al. studied OCT in 133 patients, 22 of who had a diagnosis or history of laryngeal cancer (76). All patients underwent endoscopy and 21 patients had tissue biopsies. OCT successfully identified the basement membrane in those with invasive disease; however, OCT penetration was limited in several cases, resulting in an incomplete investigation of basement membrane integrity.

More recently, there has been a resurgence of interest in pulmonary OCT applications. Feasibility studies were initially done on cadaver specimens to provide OCT airway proof of concept. Costas et al. described an early observational study using OCT in cadaver epiglottis, vocal chord, trachea, bronchus, and secondary bronchus specimens (77).

Well-delineated epithelium and submucosal structures were identified including glands, cartilage, and supporting tissue. Except for recent trachea trauma from intubation, all specimens were considered "normal" tissue without specific pathology. OCT scanning depth was 2 to 3 mm and resolution 10 to 20 μm. As a result, further in vivo studies of airway pathology would be needed to determine the role of OCT in central airway disease imaging. Jung et al. performed an animal observational study using OCT in a septic rabbit model (78). Several rabbits with normal tracheas and those with sepsis-induced tracheal injury were examined by gross and pathologic specimen collection. Tissue was imaged by two systems: a moving stage and fiberoptic OCT catheter. OCT images of normal and septic tracheas exhibited excellent correlation with histopathology. Both OCT systems demonstrated equivalent image findings.

Further studies support OCT imaging in pleural and tracheobronchial disease. In a combined in vivo and ex vivo study, Hanna et al. used a septic rabbit model with induced pleural and parenchymal tumor implantation and observed OCT findings (79).

Airway injury was clearly demonstrated by OCT, resulting in observed mucosal thickening, airway edema, and hyperemia. Pleural tumors were well demarcated by OCT along with visualized subpleural tumor invasion. Human patients with known or suspected airway disease had in vivo OCT imaging at 1 to 2 mm penetration depth and 20 to 30 μm resolution. Thickened mucosa and disorganized tissue layers identified areas of suspected tumor.

Similar finding were observed by Whiteman et al. in an ex vivo 15-patient study (80). All patients underwent lung resection for lung cancer. OCT images were obtained from gross specimens followed by histopathologic analysis. Across all sections, OCT imaging penetrated 2 to 3 mm within the tissue with a resolution of 10 μm. OCT clearly demonstrated discernable tissue layers including epithelium, lamina propria, smooth muscle, perichondrium, and cartilage. Inflamed tissue was recognized by intact epithelium and lamina propria with difficulty distinguishing deep lamina propria from cartilage. Absorption of laser light, because of increased vascularity, also reduced image quality leading to backscatter. Tumor clearly effaced normal tissue boundaries, creating a disordered multilayer appearance.

Tsuboi et al. (81) described a preliminary study with seven ex vivo human lung specimens and five in vivo airway cancers imaged by OCT. Ex vivo pathology included two central squamous cancers and five peripheral adenocarcinomas. In vivo cases comprised four squamous cancers and one small-cell cancer. Several regions of normal bronchial mucosa also underwent OCT interrogation. Normal bronchial mucosa and submucosa appeared homogeneous with increased submucosal reflection largely resulting from extracellular matrix. Increased scatter occurred in cartilageous areas. Bronchial walls contained epithelial layers and membranes. In contrast, tumor displayed uneven backscatter, submucosal thickening, and loss of structure layering. The results suggest a role for real-time OCT in the clinical evaluation of preinvasive and invasive central airway cancers.

The largest in vivo study performed by Lam et al. included 138 volunteer heavy smokers participating in a chemoprevention trial along with 10 known lung cancer patients (66). All underwent surveillance WLB and AFB using the ONCOLIFE system (Xillix Technologies). Endobronchial regions with abnormal AF signal had further real-time imaging by a 1.5-mm OCT probe with 3 mm depth of penetration (Fig. 6). Biopsies were performed from normal and abnormal sites, allowing for pathologic correlation; 281 OCT images were obtained, including 145 normal/hyperplasia, 61 metaplasia, 39 mild dysplasia, 10 moderated dysplasia, 6 severe dysplasia, 7 CIS, and 13 invasive malignancies. Quantitative epithelial thickness measurements obtained by OCT were compared. Invasive cancer significantly differed from CIS and dysplasia differed from metaplasia and hyperplasia. Darker cellular nuclei were seen in pathology specimens with moderate dysplasia up to invasive cancer. OCT was unable to determine grades of dysplasia on the basis of epithelial thickness alone.

D. Conclusion

OCT is a diagnostic tool with the potential to identify preinvasive or invasive lung cancer. The technique is limited to imaging 1 to 3 mm below the tissue surface; however, penetration depth is sufficient to detect invasive cancer. OCT image generation does not require the probe to directly contact tissue, reducing operator error and

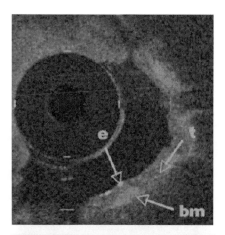

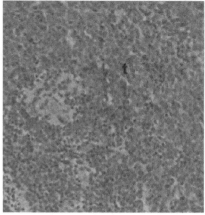

Figure 6 OCT image showing carcinoma (t) with invasion through the epithelium (e) and basement membrane (bm), resulting in loss of layered structure. *Source*: Photo courtesy of Dr Stephen Lam.

improving image quality. Current resolution is remarkable at 10 to 20 μm with future generation systems predicted to improve resolution to 5 μm. The low-output laser light source is not sufficient to cause tissue damage, making OCT a safe adjunct to standard bronchoscopy. Real-time images are acquired, providing the clinician with rapid tissue interrogation without significantly extending procedure time. Large airway scanning is not yet feasible given the 1.5 to 2 mm probes; nevertheless, OCT can be successfully combined with AFB and WLB. Blood and dense mucous result in image distortion and poor light penetration into airway tissues. Frequency domain OCT is being developed that enables faster imaging speeds, while the reduced losses during a single scan improve the signal-to-noise ratio (82).

VI. Fibered Confocal Microscopy

A. Introduction

Confocal imaging is partially based on the principles of conventional fluorescence microscopy. Usually, a light source illuminates the entire specimen. All regions of the specimen are excited by a light source and a photodetector captures the image. In contrast, confocal imaging uses pinpoint illumination, eliminating out-of-focus images (83). Confocal refers to the condition where two lenses are arranged to focus on the same point. Only focal plane light can be captured, enhancing image quality compared to conventional microscopy (84). Tissue scanning is required to create a three-dimensional image, using parallel scanning lines.

B. Background

Initially pioneered by Marvin Minsky in 1955, the confocal technique was later patented in 1959 (85). Newer FCFM systems can acquire bronchial mucosa tissue images with a 600 × 500–µm field of view, providing visualization of intracellular structures. This technique is currently employed by cell biologists, gastroenterologists, and dermatologists, providing vivid images and cellular characteristics of abnormal tissue. Medical confocal systems use laser scanning microscopes that yield improved image quality and provide near real-time frame rate speeds of 10 to 15 frames per second. Confocal microscopy utilizes the natural AF of airway elastin and collagen to obtain exceptional images of human tracheobronchial and alveolar tissue. Endoscopic FCFM represents a minimally invasive method to study specific in vivo airway basement membrane alterations associated with premalignant bronchial lesions. The technique may also be useful to investigate bronchial wall remodeling in nonmalignant chronic bronchial diseases and alveolar septal changes in interstitial lung diseases.

C. FCFM Systems

The only FDA-approved medical FCFM system is Cellvizio® made by Mauna Kea Technologies (Cambridge, Massachusetts, U.S.). This system adapts to GI or pulmonary applications, capturing confocal images using a 1.4-mm-diameter pulmonary probe. Field of view is 600 × 500 µm, with lateral resolution of 10 µm and scanning depth up to 50 µm. Tissue AF is created using a 488-nm laser and images are visualized at 12 frames per second. For GI applications laser wavelength is 488 or 660 nm and three separate probes can be chosen with different resolution, size, and tissue penetration depth.

D. Literature

Studies using applied confocal microscopy for medical imaging appeared in the early 1990s. Initially, Koester et al. demonstrated confocal microscopy in optical sectioning by the use of confocal slits (86). Sectioning allowed the observation of weakly scattered structures within the cornea. Structures described included epithelial cells, keratocytes, endothelial cells, nerve fiber bundles, and inflammatory cells. Dermal confocal applications were described by Rajadhyaksha et al. during an in vivo study involving human skin (87). Prior to biopsy, normal skin, nevi, and vitiliginous skin were imaged using 400 to 700 nm and 800 to 900 nm light sources. Imaging depth was confined to the superficial papillary dermis and deep capillaries, respectively. There was good correlation between histology and confocal cellular and morphologic features. Confocal microscopy may provide noninvasive optical biopsy information that is rapid and compares favorably to histopathology.

Cervical tissue has also been interrogated by confocal microscopy. Drezek et al. used confocal imaging on cervical cells and colposcopically normal and abnormal cervical biopsy specimens (88). Images were obtained before and after the application of 6% acetic acid. Observed specimen subcellular image quality was present throughout the epithelial thickness. Two years later Sung et al. successfully applied an in vivo confocal catheter to image lip tissue (89). Real-time imaging was possible obtaining data at 15 frames per second. Cell morphology and tissue architecture were observed at superior resolution.

Microcatheter confocal devices were improved, extending the ability of endoscopic applications. In 2004 Rouse reduced the size of an FCFM catheter from 7 mm to 3 mm (90). Tissue image depth was approximated at 25 μm. The catheter was successfully tested in an Olympus CF-100L colonoscope (Olympus Optical) with a 3.2-mm-diameter instrument channel. While confocal microscopy of the GI tract was now feasible, the size of this catheter did not permit its use in standard bronchoscopes with 2.0- to 2.8-mm working channels.

Confocal exploration in tracheobronchial imaging has recently evolved. In 2004, Wang et al. used FCFM to image rabbit airway receptors (91). Ten rabbits were sacrificed with soft tissues harvested from the trachea and large airways. Confocal imaging of various receptor types was observed. Imaged tissue layers were identified including smooth muscle, lamina propria, and epithelium. Airway receptors showed distinct structural differences determined by tissue layer location. Ex vivo confocal airway imaging provided detailed morphology of airway tissues and structures.

Bronchoscopy using FCFM has only recently been publicized. In 2006, Thiberville illustrated successful in vivo endoscopic analysis of the bronchial structure using FCFM (92). He later described the first in vivo study usually a commercially available FCFM system in 29 high-risk individuals scheduled for bronchoscopy to detect preinvasive lesions (93). White light and AFB were performed using the ONCOLIFE system (Xillix Technologies). AFB was first conducted with subsequent FCFM performed with a 1.4-mm direct contact probe. Five different trachea and bronchial areas were imaged per patient. A total of 71 and 32 FCFM samples were collected from biopsy of naive and previous biopsy sites. Five distinct microscopic patterns were described in the normal areas from the trachea to respiratory bronchi. AF microstructure alterations were observed in 19 of 22 metaplastic and dysplastic samples and all CIS and invasive cancers. Disorganization of the fibered network was observed in 1/3 of preinvasive pathology indicating basement membrane disruption (Fig. 7).

E. Limitations

Image resolution for FCFM is excellent; however, several issues limit routine application in pulmonary diseases. As with newly applied technology, FCFM-observed tissue needs to be accurately described to discern normal and abnormal features. This has been initiated along with describing images collected from pathologic conditions. Once a library of image data can be compiled, improvements in FCFM applications can be constructed. Laser light is of low power and poses no significant injury risk to tissue. Current pulmonary probes are compatible with bronchoscopes having at least 2.0-mm working channels. Tissue penetration is superficial and does not allow scanning to the cartilage which may not be appropriate to investigate and diagnose depth of cancer

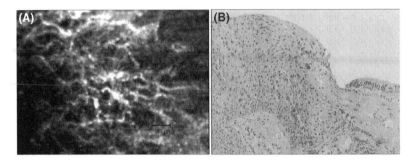

Figure 7 FCFM-observed CIS (*left*) identified by disorganized pattern with defects in micro-autofluorescence compared with histopathology (*right*). *Source*: Photo courtesy of Dr Luc Thiberville and Mauna Kea Technologies Inc.

invasion. Since cellular changes in CIS and dysplasia occur less than 1 mm in depth, FCFM may provide sufficient optical conformation for preinvasive disease. Similar to OCT and RS, FCFM must be coupled with inspection bronchoscopy, either white light or a combination of WLB and AFB.

F. Conclusion
The role of FCFM in the diagnosis and posttreatment surveillance for interstitial lung disease, lung cancer, and alveolar disease remains unclear. Superficial tissue imaging may be well suited toward identifying premalignant lung disease versus determining depth of tumor invasion. Pulmonary FCFM applications show promise, but are in the initial stages of clinical research. This technology must be adapted and synchronized with AFB surveillance to enhance rapid optical assessment of endobronchial disease. Current FCFM images are being collected and a library constructed of normal confocal airway anatomy. The largest publication to date is an observational study with known pathology and the inability to clearly define specific image criteria, distinguishing different pathologic conditions. In addition, the true extent of confocal image differences observed in natural airway structure and tissue variations is unknown. Future studies on high-risk cancer patients may be feasible once applied image criteria are validated in a large population and compared with biopsy-proven histopathology. FCFM strengths include excellent resolution, and the potential for real-time optical imaging without additional patient risk.

VII. Chapter Conclusion
Current lung cancer screening guidelines strongly discourage sputum cytology, routine chest X rays and CT scans in high-risk patients who are asymptomatic unless in the context of a clinical trial (94,95). Bronchoscopy has a well-defined position as a diagnostic and therapeutic clinical tool. This instrument allows the pulmonary clinician the opportunity to navigate and detect pathology. The marriage of technology and medicine continues to stimulate growth of ideas, striving to improve the current lung cancer paradigm. Clinical research is gaining momentum, but continued support from device company–sponsored and investigator-initiated trials is required. This chapter has focused

on advanced high-resolution imaging modalities that can be delivered by bronchoscopy. It is unlikely for one modality to establish sole precedence in lung cancer screening. However, combination high-resolution bronchoscopy has great potential to provide superior optical tissue images, revealing a window into early cancer pathogenesis.

Success can start by developing a model for cancer detection in high-risk patients having a history of lung cancer. This model could be applied to surgical cure patients with early stage lung disease. Postresection radiographic surveillance guidelines are neither evidence based nor uniform (96,97). Bronchoscopy is not advocated for cancer surveillance in this population. Indeed, future clinical research with high-resolution bronchoscopy may provide the optimism needed to detect preinvasive malignancy in a patient population facing a 1% to 4% yearly risk of recurrent cancer (98). To focus on the future role of high-resolution bronchoscopy, we must reflect on the past. Dr Shigeto Ikeda's ideals remain true today. "We will never give up" because, after all, "there is more hope with the bronchoscope" (99).

References

1. Ikeda S, Tsuboi E, Ono R, et al. Flexible bronchofiberscope. Jpn J Clin Oncol 1971; 1:55–65.
2. Battaglia M. Fluorescein angiography and indocyanine green videoangiography in the iris of pseudoexfoliation syndrome. Metab Pediatr Syst Ophthalmol 1998; 21(1–4):7–13.
3. Monici M. Cell and tissue autofluorescence research and diagnostic applications. Biotechnol Annu Rev 2005; 11:227–256.
4. Kennedy T, McWilliams A, Edell E, et al. Bronchial intraepithelial neoplasia/early central airways lung cancer. Chest 2007; 132:221S–233S.
5. Häußinger K, Becker H, Stanzel F, et al. Autofluorescence bronchoscopy with white light bronchoscopy compared with white light bronchoscopy alone for the detection of precancerous lesions: a European randomised controlled multicentre trial. Thorax 2005; 60:496–503.
6. Lam S, MacAulay C, Le Riche J. Early localisation of bronchogenic carcinoma. Diagnost Therapeut Endoscopy 1994; 1:75.
7. Lam S, MacAulay C, Hung J, et al. Detection of dysplasia and carcinoma in situ with a lung imaging fluorescence endoscope device. J Thorac Cardiovasc Surg 1993; 105(6):1035–1040.
8. Lam S, Kennedy T, Unger M, et al. Localization of bronchial intraepithelial neoplastic lesions by fluorescence bronchoscopy. Chest 1998; 113(3):696–702.
9. Weigel TL, Kosco PJ, Dacic S, et al. Postoperative fluorescence bronchoscopic surveillance in non-small cell lung cancer patients. Ann Thorac Surg 2001; 71(3):967–970.
10. Chhajed PN, Shibuya K, Hoshino H, et al. A comparison of video and autofluorescence bronchoscopy in patients at high risk of lung cancer. Eur Respir J 2005; 25:951–955.
11. Khanavkar B, Gnudi F, Muti A, et al. Basic principles of LIFE—autofluorescence bronchoscopy. Results of 194 examinations in comparison with standard procedures for early detection of bronchial carcinoma—overview. Pneumologie 1998; 52(2):71–76.
12. Beamis JF Jr., Ernst A, Simoff M, et al. A multicenter study comparing autofluorescence bronchoscopy to white light bronchoscopy using a non-laser light stimulation system. Chest 2004; 125:148S–149S.
13. Herth F, Ernst A, Becker H. Autofluorescence bronchoscopy—a comparison of two systems (LIFE and D-Light). Respiration 2003; 70:395–398.
14. Thiberville L, Payne P, Vielkinds J. Evidence of cumulative gene losses with progression of premalignant epithelial lesions to carcinoma of the bronchus. Cancer Res 1995; 55:5133.
15. Satoh Y, Ishikawa Y, Nakagawa K. A follow-up study of progression from dysplasia to squamous cell carcinoma with immunohistochemical examination of p53 protein overexpression in the bronchi of ex-chromate workers. Br J Cancer 1997; 75:678.

16. Breuer RH, Pasic A, Smit EF. The natural course of preneoplastic lesions in bronchial epithelium. Clin Cancer Res 2005; 11:537.

17. Venmans BJ, van Boxem TJ, Smit EF, et al. Outcome of bronchial carcinoma in situ. Chest 2000; 117(6):1572–1576.

18. Risse EK, Vooijs GP, van't Hof MA. Diagnostic significance of "severe dysplasia" in sputum cytology. Acta Cytol 1988; 32:629–634.

19. Bota S, Auliac JB, Paris C, et al. Follow-up of bronchial precancerous lesions and carcinoma in situ using fluorescence endoscopy. Am J Respir Crit Care Med 2001; 164(9):1688–1693.

20. Gono K, Obi T, Yamaguchi M, et al. Appearance of enhanced tissue features in narrow-band endoscopic imaging. Biomed Opt 2004; 9(3):568–577.

21. Brett GZ. The value of lung cancer detection by six-monthly chest radiographs. Thorax 1968; 23:414.

22. Brett GZ. Earlier diagnosis and survival in lung cancer. Br Med J 1969; 4:260.

23. Henschke CI, McCauley DI, Yankelevitz DF, et al. Early lung cancer action project: overall design and findings from baseline screening. Lancet 1999; 354(9173):99–105.

24. Henschke CI, Yankelevitz D, Libby DM, et al. Early lung cancer action project: annual screening using single-slice helical CT. Ann NY Acad Sci 2001; 952:124–134.

25. Welch HG, Woloshin S, Schwartz LM, et al. Overstating the evidence for lung cancer screening: the international early lung cancer action program (I-ELCAP) study. Arch Intern Med 2007; 167(21):2289–2295.

26. Johnson B. Second lung cancers in patients after treatment for an initial lung cancer. J Natl Cancer Inst 1998; 90(18):1335–1345.

27. Sharma P, Bansal A, Mathur S, et al. The utility of a novel narrow band imaging endoscopy system in patients with Barrett's esophagus. Gastrointest Endosc 2006; 64(2):167–175.

28. Sharma P, Weston AP, Topalovski M, et al. Magnification chromoendoscopy for the detection of intestinal metaplasia and dysplasia in Barrett's oesophagus. Gut 2003; 52(1): 24–27.

29. Prateek S, Sachin W, Ajay B, et al. A feasibility trial of narrow band imaging endoscopy in patients with gastroesophageal reflux disease. Gastroenterology 2007; 133:454–464.

30. Matsumoto T, Kudo T, Jo Y, et al. Magnifying colonoscopy with narrow band imaging system for the diagnosis of dysplasia in ulcerative colitis: a pilot study. Gastrointest Endosc 2007; 66(5):957–965.

31. Adler A, Pohl H, Papanikolaou IS, et al. A prospective randomised study on narrow-band imaging versus conventional colonoscopy for adenoma detection: does narrow-band imaging induce a learning effect? Gut 2008; 57(1):59–64.

32. Kara MA, Ennahachi M, Fockens P, et al. Detection and classification of the mucosal and vascular patterns (mucosal morphology) in Barrett's esophagus by using narrow band imaging. Gastrointest Endosc 2006; 64(2):155–166.

33. Auerbach O, Forman JB, Gere JB. Changes in the bronchial epithelium in relation to smoking and cancer of the lung: a report of progress. N Engl J Med 1957; 256:97.

34. Auerbach O, Stout AP, Hammond EC, et al. Changes in bronchial epithelium in relation to cigarette smoking and in relation to lung cancer. N Engl J Med 1961; 265:253.

35. Anagnostopoulos GK, Yao K, Kaye P, et al. Novel endoscopic observation in Barrett's oesophagus using high resolution magnification endoscopy and narrow band imaging. Aliment Pharmacol Ther 2007; 26(3):501–507.

36. Fontanini G, Calcinai A, Boldrini L. Modulation of neoangiogenesis in bronchial preneoplastic lesions. Oncol Rep 1999; 6:813–817.

37. Fisseler-Eckhoff A, Rothstein D, Muller KM. Neovascularization in hyperplastic, metaplastic and potentially preneoplastic lesions of the bronchial mucosa. Virchows Arch 1996; 429:95–100.

38. Gazdar AF, Minna JD. Angiogenesis and the multistage development of lung cancers. Clin Cancer Res 2000; 6:1611–1612.

39. Shibuya K, Hoshino H, Chiyo M, et al. Subepithelial vascular patterns in bronchial dysplasias using a high magnification bronchovideoscope. Thorax 2002; 57(10):902–907.
40. Shibuya K, Hoshino H, Chiyo M, et al. High magnification bronchovideoscopy combined with narrow band imaging could detect capillary loops of angiogenic squamous dysplasia in heavy smokers at high risk for lung cancer. Thorax 2003; 58(11):989–995.
41. Vincent BD, Fraig M, Silvestri GA. A pilot study of narrow-band imaging compared to white light bronchoscopy for evaluation of normal airways and premalignant and malignant airways disease. Chest 2007; 131(6):1794–1799.
42. International Union of Pure and Applied Chemistry. "Phonon" Compendium of Chemical Terminology Internet edition. Available at: http://www.iupac.org/goldbook/T065299.pdf
43. Matousek P, Draper ERC, Goodship AE, et al. Non-invasive Raman spectroscopy of human tissue in vivo. Central Laser Facility Annual Report 2005/2006:133–135.
44. Gardiner DJ. Practical Raman Spectroscopy. Springer-Verlag Publishing, 1989.
45. Jeanmaire D, van Duyne R. Surface Raman electrochemistry. Part I. Heterocyclic, aromatic and aliphatic amines adsorbed on the anodized silver electrode. J Electroanal Chem 1977; 84:1–20.
46. Matousek P, Clark IP, Draper ERC, et al. Subsurface probing in diffusely scattering media using spatially offset Raman spectroscopy. Appl Spectrosc 2005; 59:393.
47. Choo-Smith LP, Edwards HG, Endtz HP, et al. Medical applications of Raman spectroscopy: from proof of principle to clinical implementation. Biopolymers 2002; 67(1):1–9.
48. Eikje NS, Ozaki Y, Aizawa K, et al. Fiber optic near-infrared Raman spectroscopy for clinical noninvasive determination of water content in diseased skin and assessment of cutaneous edema. J Biomed Opt 2005; 10(1):14013.
49. Ellis DI, Goodacre R. Metabolic fingerprinting in disease diagnosis: biomedical applications of infrared and Raman spectroscopy. Analyst 2006; 131:875–885.
50. Maheedhar K, Bhat R, Malini R, et al. Diagnosis of ovarian cancer by Raman spectroscopy: a pilot study. Photomed Laser Surg 2008; 26(2):83–90.
51. Jess P, Smith D, Mazilu M, et al. Early detection and diagnosis early detection of cervical neoplasia by Raman spectroscopy. Int J Cancer 2007; 121(12):2723–2728.
52. Nijssen A, Maquelin K, Santos LF, et al. Discriminating basal cell carcinoma from perilesional skin using high wave-number Raman spectroscopy. J Biomed Opt 2007; 12(3):034004.
53. Ling X, Li W, Song Y, et al. FT-Raman spectroscopic investigation on stomach cancer. Guang Pu Xue Yu Guang Pu Fen Xi 2000; 20(5):692–693.
54. Kawabata T, Mizuno T, Okazaki S, et al. Optical diagnosis of gastric cancer using near-infrared multichannel Raman spectroscopy with a 1064-nm excitation wavelength. J Gastroenterol 2008; 43(4):283–290.
55. Teh SK, Zheng W, Ho KY, et al. Diagnostic potential of near-infrared Raman spectroscopy in the stomach: differentiating dysplasia from normal tissue. Br J Cancer 2008; 98(2):457–465.
56. Molckovsky A, Song LM, Shim MG, et al. Diagnostic potential of near-infrared Raman spectroscopy in the colon: differentiating adenomatous from hyperplastic polyps. Gastrointest Endosc 2003; 57(3):396–402.
57. Stone N, Stavroulaki P, Kendall C, et al. Raman spectroscopy for early detection of laryngeal malignancy: preliminary results. Laryngoscope 2000; 110(10 pt 1):1756–1763.
58. Yamazaki H, Kaminaka S, Kohda E, et al. The diagnosis of lung cancer using 1064-nm excited near-infrared multichannel Raman spectroscopy. Radiat Med 2003; 21(1):1–6.
59. Huang Z, McWilliams A, Lui H, et al. Near infrared Raman spectroscopy for optical diagnosis of lung cancer. Int J Cancer 2003; 107:1047–1052.
60. Kaminaka S, Yamazaki H, Ito T, et al. Near-infrared Raman spectroscopy of human lung tissues: possibility of molecular level cancer diagnosis. J Raman Spectrosc 2001; 32:139–141.
61. Zysk AM, Nguyen FT, Oldenburg AL, et al. Optical coherence tomography: a review of clinical development from bench to bedside. J Biomedical Optics 2007; 12(5):051403.

62. Fercher AF, Mengedoht K, Werner W. Eye-length measurement by interferometry with partially coherent light. Opt Lett 1988; 13:186–188.

63. Naohiro T, Tsutomu I, Akio S. Lightwave reflection measurement. Japanese Patent # 2010042, 1990.

64. Shinji C, Naohiro T. Backscattering optical heterodyne tomography. Prepared for the 14th Laser Sensing Symposium, 1991.

65. Huang D, Swanson EA, Lin CP, et al. Optical coherence tomography. Science 1991; 254 (5035):1178–1181.

66. Lam S, Standish B, Baldwin C, et al. In vivo optical coherence tomography imaging of preinvasive bronchial lesions. Clin Cancer Res 2008; 14(7):2006–2011.

67. Fujimoto JG, Brezinski ME, Tearney GJ, et al. Biomedical imaging and optical biopsy using optical coherence tomography. Nat Med 1995; 1:970–972.

68. Tearney GJ, Brezinski ME, Bouma BE, et al. In vivo endoscopic optical biopsy with optical coherence tomography. Science 1997; 276:2037–2039.

69. Riederer SJ. Current technical development of magnetic resonance imaging. IEEE Eng Med Biol Mag 2000; 19(5):34–41.

70. Bourquin S, Seitz P, Salathé RP. Optical coherence topography based on a two-dimensional smart detector array. Opt Lett 2001; 26(8):512–514.

71. Massin P, Vicaut E, Haouchine B, et al. Reproducibility of retinal mapping using optical coherence tomography. Arch Ophthalmol 2001; 119:1135–1142.

72. Yazdanfar S, Rollins A, Izatt J. In vivo imaging of human retinal flow dynamics by color doppler optical coherence tomography. Arch Ophthalmol 2003; 121:235–239.

73. Fujimoto JG, Boppart SA, Tearney GJ, et al. High resolution in vivo intra-arterial imaging with optical coherence tomography. Heart 1999; 82:128–133.

74. Costas P, Jesser C, Boppart S, et al. Feasibility of optical coherence tomography for high-resolution imaging of human gastrointestinal tract malignancies. J Gastroenterol 2000; 35:87–92.

75. Wong B, Jackson R, Guo S, et al. In vivo optical coherence tomography of the human larynx: normative and benign pathology in 82 patients. Laryngoscope 2005; 115:1904–1911.

76. Armstrong W, Ridgway J, Vokes D, et al. Optical coherence tomography of laryngeal cancer. Laryngoscope 2006; 116:1107–1113.

77. Costas P, Brezinski M, Bouma B, et al. High resolution imaging of the upper respiratory tract with optical coherence tomography: a feasibility study. Am J Respir Crit Care Med 1998; 157:1640–1644.

78. Jung W, Jun Zhang J, Mina-Araghi R, et al. Feasibility study of normal and septic tracheal imaging using optical coherence tomography. Lasers Surg Med 2004; 35:121–127.

79. Hanna N, Saltzman D, Mukai D, et al. Two-dimensional and 3-dimensional optical coherence tomographic imaging of the airway, lung, and pleura. J Thorac Cardiovasc Surg 2005; 129:615–622.

80. Whiteman S, Yang Y, van Pittius D, et al. Optical coherence tomography: real-time imaging of bronchial airways microstructure and detection of inflammatory/neoplastic morphologic changes. Clin Cancer Res 2006; 12(3):813–818.

81. Tsuboi M, Hayashi A, Ikeda N, et al. Optical coherence tomography in the diagnosis of bronchial lesions. Lung Cancer 2005; 49:387–394.

82. Fercher AF, Hitzenberger CK, Kamp CK, et al. Measurement of intraocular distances by backscattering spectral interferometry. Opt Commun 1995; 117(1–2):43–48.

83. Goldie RG, Rigby PJ, Pudney CJ, et al. Confocal microscopy and the respiratory tract. Pulm Pharmacol Ther 1997; 10:175–188.

84. Rigby PJ, Goldie RG. Confocal microscopy in biomedical research. Croat Med J 1999; 40:346–352.

85. Minsky M. Memoir on inventing the confocal scanning microscope. Scanning 1988; 10:128–138.

86. Koester CJ, Auran JD, Rosskothen HD, et al. Clinical microscopy of the cornea utilizing optical sectioning and a high-numerical-aperture objective. J Opt Soc Am 1993; 10(7): 1670–1679.

87. Rajadhyaksha M, Grossman M, Esterowitz D, et al. In vivo confocal scanning laser microscopy of human skin: melanin provides strong contrast. J Invest Dermatol 1995; 104(6):946–952.

88. Drezek RA, Collier T, Brookner CK, et al. Laser scanning confocal microscopy of cervical tissue before and after application of acetic acid. Am J Obstet Gynecol 2000; 182(5):1135–1139.

89. Sung KB, Liang C, Descour M, et al. Fiber-optic confocal reflectance microscope with miniature objective for in-vivo imaging of human tissues. IEEE Trans Biomed Eng 2002; 49(10):1168–1172.

90. Rouse A, Kano A, Udovich J, et al. Design and demonstration of a miniature catheter for a confocal microendoscope. Appl Opt 2004; 43(31):5763–5771.

91. Wang YF, Yu J. Structural survey of airway sensory receptors in the rabbit using confocal microscopy. Acta Physiol Sin 2004; 56(2):119–129.

92. Thiberville L, Bourg-Heckly G, Peltier E, et al. In vivo endoscopic analysis of the bronchial structure using fluorescence fibered confocal microscopy [abstract]. Eur Respir J 2006; 28(suppl 50):155S.

93. Thiberville L, Moreno-Swirc S, Vercauteren T, et al. In vivo imaging of the bronchial wall microstructure using fibered confocal fluorescence microscopy. Am J Respir Crit Care Med 2007; 175(1):22–31.

94. Humphrey LL, Teutsch S, Johnson M. Lung cancer screening with sputum cytologic examination, chest radiography, and computed tomography: an update for the U.S. Preventive Services Task Force. Ann Intern Med 2004; 140(9):740–753.

95. U.S. Preventive Services task Force. Lung cancer screening: recommendation statement. Ann Intern Med 2004; 140(9):738–739.

96. Pfister DG, Johnson DH, Azzoli CG, et al. American society of clinical oncology treatment of unresectable non-small-cell lung cancer guideline: update 2003. J Clin Oncol 2004; 22(2): 330–353.

97. National Comprehensive Cancer Network (NCCN) guidelines. Available at: www.nccn.org/ physician_gls/index.htm. Accessed May 13, 2008.

98. Naama R, Bogot N, Quint L. Imaging of recurrent lung cancer. Cancer Imaging 2004; 4:61–67.

99. Udaya P. "Never give up": professor Shigeto Ikeda, 1925–2001. J Bronchol 2002; 9(2): 83–84.

6

Endoscopic Staging of Lung Cancer

KAZUHIRO YASUFUKU

Toronto General Hospital, University Health Network, Toronto, Ontario, Canada

I. Introduction

Lung cancer is the leading cause of cancer-related death in the Western world (1). Accurate staging is important to not only determine the prognosis but also decide the most suitable treatment plan for both operable and inoperable patients with non–small cell lung cancer (NSCLC) (1). Noninvasive imaging techniques such as computed tomography (CT) and positron emission tomography (PET) are inaccurate in the diagnosis of mediastinal lymph node metastasis (2). The sensitivity and specificity of CT for identifying mediastinal lymph node metastasis are 51% (range: 47–54%) and 85% (range: 84–88%), respectively; thus, CT has limited ability to either rule in or exclude mediastinal metastasis (2). PET scanning is more accurate than CT scanning, with a pooled sensitivity and specificity of 74% (range: 69–79%) and 85% (range: 82–88%), respectively (2). Furthermore, distant metastasis can be detected by PET scanning. With either CT or PET, abnormal findings must be confirmed by tissue biopsy. Surgical staging by mediastinoscopy, the gold standard for mediastinal staging, has a high sensitivity (80%) and specificity (100%) (3). The false-negative rate of mediastinoscopy is approximately 10% (3) with even lower rates with video-mediastinoscopy (7%). However, it is an invasive procedure that requires general anesthesia. Complications cannot be ignored.

Recent advances in technology have enabled real-time guidance for needle aspirations of mediastinal lymph nodes during bronchoscopy and esophagoscopy (4). Endoscopic techniques for mediastinal staging provide a minimally invasive alternative for surgical staging. In this chapter, the different endoscopic techniques for mediastinal staging in lung cancer will be discussed in details.

II. Transbronchial Needle Aspiration

Transbronchial needle aspiration (TBNA is performed through the flexible bronchoscope under local anesthesia. However, the first report of TBNA was described through the rigid bronchoscope (5). After the introduction of the flexible needle that could be used through the flexible bronchoscope (6), the use of TBNA for mediastinal lymph node sampling using the flexible bronchoscope was first described in 1983 (7–9). The utility of TBNA for the diagnosis of endobronchial and peripheral lesions has been confirmed by subsequent publications and now has spread as a useful procedure that can be performed as an outpatient procedure with no significant morbidity (7–12).

A. Equipment

The needle systems available for TBNA come in different sizes. For cytological specimens, 20- to 22-gauge needles are usually used. 19-gauge needles are used to obtain core biopsy for histological examination (13). Flexibility of the bronchoscopes necessary for TBNA depends on the outer diameter of the TBNA needle and the diameter of the channel of the bronchoscope.

B. Procedure

Before the procedure, a thorough review of the CT scan is mandatory for the selection of proper site for needle insertion (14). After localization of landmarks for needle insertion, the needle catheter is passed through the working channel of the bronchoscope and guided to the area of interest. The bronchoscope should be kept at a straight position, with its distal tip in the neutral position to prevent damage to the working channel of the bronchoscope. The tip of the needle must be secured within the metal hub before passing it through the channel. The needle is advanced and locked in place after the metal hub is visible beyond the tip of the bronchoscope. The scope is then advanced to the target area and the needle is anchored in the tracheobronchial wall into the lymph node. The needle should be kept as perpendicularly as possible. TBNA can be performed from the hilar and mediastinal lymph nodes adjacent to the airway (Fig. 1) (15,16).

While the needle is inserted in the lesion, suction is applied and the catheter is moved up and down. The needle is withdrawn from the lymph node after the suction is released. The bronchoscope is then straightened and the needle is pulled out of the channel (16). The aspirated specimen is blown out to the slide using a 50-mL syringe before smearing it with two slides. Rapid onsite cytologic evaluation of the aspirates improves

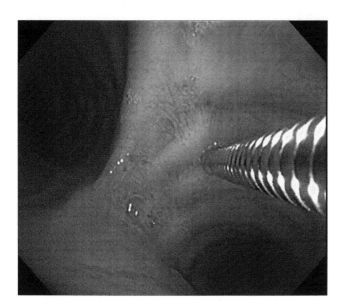

Figure 1 Bronchoscopic view of a transbronchial needle aspiration of a subcarinal lymph node.

the yield, is cost-effective, and eliminates unnecessary passes during the procedure (17). For obtaining histology specimen, the 19-gauge needle is oftentimes used.

Penetrating Techniques

Different techniques can be used alone or in combination to penetrate the needle through the tracheobronchial wall: (*i*) the "jabbing method," whereby the bronchoscope is held stationary while the needle is jabbed forward through the intercartilaginous space; (*ii*) the "piggyback method," whereby the bronchoscope and the needle are moved forward as a unit; (*iii*) the "hub against the wall method," whereby the distal end of the catheter is placed directly in contact with the airway wall with the needle in the retracted position, while the needle is pushed out of the catheter for penetration; and (*iv*) the "cough method," whereby the patient is asked to cough while the bronchoscope and needle are held stationary, which forces the tracheobronchial wall over the needle (16).

C. Results

The diagnostic yield of TBNA for lymph node staging in lung cancer varies greatly in the published literature with the overall sensitivity of 78%, with values ranging from 14% to 100% (3). The false-negative rate ranges from 0% to 66% with an average of 28%. The specificity and false-positive rate reported are 100% and 0%, respectively. One of the factors that may explain the wide variety of yield of TBNA may be the blindness of the procedure preventing target visualization of lymph nodes. The studies of TBNA in lung cancer staging have generally had a high prevalence of mediastinal lymph node involvement. The high false-negative rate makes TBNA less useful for staging of the mediastinum especially in patients without extensive mediastinal involvement. Therefore, TBNA would probably be the preferred minimal invasive method for patients with radiographic evidence of enlarged mediastinal lymph nodes adjacent to the airways, since bronchoscopy is usually performed in lung cancer patients and assessment for endobronchial lesions can be performed during the same procedure. Positive results are reliable, but negative TBNA results cannot exclude mediastinal nodal involvement.

D. Complications

Complications following TBNA are uncommon if appropriate precautions are taken. The literature to date supports the safety of TBNA in lung cancer staging. Furthermore, mortality related to the procedure has not been described yet. Complications that have been reported include pneumothorax, pneumomediastinum, hemomediastinum, bacteremia, and pericarditis, but these are rare (9,18–20). Although various complications have been reported, damage to the working channel of the bronchoscope is by far the most important and major complication.

III. Endobronchial Ultrasound

Two types of EBUS are available for clinical use during flexible bronchoscopy. The radial probe EBUS (RP-EBUS) was first introduced in 1992. The miniaturized 20-MHz radial probe fitted with a catheter that carries a water-inflatable balloon at the tip allows visualization of detailed images of the surrounding structures as well as the bronchial wall structure (21,22). By visualization of mediastinal and hilar lymph nodes, EBUS guidance has increased the yield of TBNA for lymph node staging of lung cancer (23,24). However because of the nature of the probe, it is not a real-time procedure with

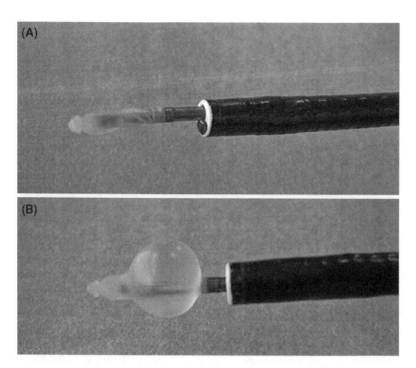

Figure 2 The radial probe EBUS. (**A**) 20-MHz miniaturized radial probe (UM-BS20-26R) inserted through a 2.8-mm working channel of a flexible bronchoscope. (**B**) The balloon sheath (MAJ-643R) on the tip inflated with water.

target visualization. The convex probe EBUS (CP-EBUS) was first described in 2004 (25). The bronchoscope integrated with a linear scanning ultrasound transducer allows real-time EBUS-guided TBNA (EBUS-TBNA) under direct ultrasound guidance. Multiple studies have shown the usefulness of EBUS-TBNA in the assessment of mediastinal and/or hilar lymph nodes, especially for staging of lung cancer (25–33). The results of the use of the two types of EBUS in mediastinal lymph node staging will be discussed in this section.

A. Radial Probe EBUS–Guided TBNA
Equipment
The miniaturized 20-MHz radial probe EBUS (UM-BS20-26R, Olympus Medical Systems Corporation, Tokyo, Japan) fitted with a catheter that carries a water-inflatable balloon at the tip (Fig. 2) is used for the assessment of central airways. The probe rotates 360° to obtain detailed images of the surrounding structures as well as the bronchial wall structure. The 20-MHz EBUS has a resolution of less than 1 mm and a penetration of 5 cm. The probe can be used from the trachea to the subsegmental bronchus. A bronchoscope with a working channel of 2.8 mm is necessary for using this probe.

Smaller ultraminiature radial probes are also available for detection of peripheral lung nodules (UM-S20-17S, Olympus Medical Systems). It is also a 20-MHz radial probe that has an external diameter of 1.4 mm. The probe is placed into a guide sheath (GS) and the GS-covered probe can be inserted into a 2.0-mm working channel of a regular flexible bronchoscope.

Procedure
Prior to the procedure, the radial probe is fitted with the balloon catheter and primed with a 20-mL syringe filled with normal saline. Air bubbles must be discarded from the balloon to assure clear ultrasound imaging. After observation of the airway with the bronchoscope with a 2.8-mm working channel, the lesion of interest is located. The radial probe EBUS fitted with the balloon catheter is inserted through the working channel. The probe is positioned near the target area and the balloon is filled with saline in order to obtain full contact with the airway. It is important for the bronchoscopist to understand the anatomy of the mediastinum in order to understand the EBUS image and also to identify the lymph node station they are looking at. A 360° EBUS image is obtained with the anechoic space of the saline-filled balloon in the center. Detailed images of the parabronchial structures such as lymph nodes and vessels as well as the airway structure are obtained. Once the lymph node of interest is identified, the probe is removed and a needle is inserted through the working channel to perform TBNA. The radial EBUS assists the bronchoscopist for visualization of lymph nodes prior to TBNA, but the actual TBNA is a blind procedure (23,24).

Results
The indications for the radial probe EBUS-guided TBNA is similar to the conventional TBNA. Two important studies have been reported on the use of the radial probe EBUS for lymph node assessment. The first report enrolled 242 patients for the diagnosis of enlarged lymph nodes and cancer staging (23). Lymph nodes were successfully sampled in 86% of the cases that were independent of lymph node size and location. Diagnosis was obtained in 72% without complications (23). A randomized study comparing the yield of TBNA under EBUS guidance to conventional TBNA showed that the overall yield of EBUS-guided TBNA was higher compared to conventional TBNA (85% vs. 66%) (24). Patients with subcarinal lymph nodes (group A) were additionally randomized and analyzed separately from all other lymph node stations (group B). In group A, the yield of conventional TBNA was 74% compared to 86% in the EBUS-guided group, and there were no significant difference between the two procedures. However in group B, the yield of conventional TBNA (58%) was significantly improved to 84% by using EBUS guidance.

Although the yield of TBNA can be improved by the use of the radial probe EBUS, patients included in the studies generally had enlarged mediastinal lymph nodes. As so with conventional TBNA, negative results should still be confirmed by other staging procedures. The experience with this technique is limited to only a few centers, and whether it can be applied to normal-sized nodes is not known.

B. Convex Probe EBUS–Guided TBNA (Real-Time EBUS-TBNA)
Equipment
The convex probe endobronchial ultrasound (CP-EBUS), an ultrasound puncture bronchoscope with a 7.5-MHz convex transducer placed at the tip of a flexible bron-choscope (BF-UC160F-OL8, Olympus Medical Systems), is used to perform real-time

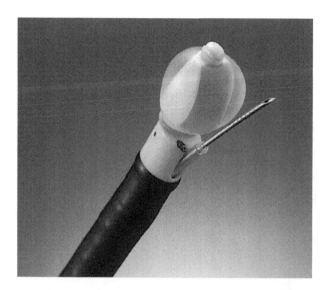

Figure 3 Tip of the convex probe endobronchial ultrasound (CP-EBUS, BF-UC160F-OL8, Olympus Medical Systems). The outer diameter of the insertion tube of the flexible bronchoscope is 6.2 mm. CP-EBUS has a linear curved array ultrasonic transducer of 7.5 MHz. The balloon attached to the tip of the bronchoscope is inflated with normal saline. The dedicated 22-gauge TBNA needle is inserted through the working channel.

EBUS-TBNA (Fig. 3). The CP-EBUS is a linear curved array transducer that scans parallel to the insertion direction of the bronchoscope. Images can be obtained by directly contacting the probe or attaching a balloon on the tip and inflating with saline. The outer diameter of the insertion tube of the CP-EBUS is 6.2 mm and that of the tip is 6.9 mm. The angle of view is 80° and the direction of view is 35° forward oblique. With the built-in CCD in the control section, it allows sharp images similar to those of regular video bronchoscopes. The inner diameter of the instrument channel is 2.0 mm.

The ultrasound image is processed in a dedicated ultrasound processor (EU-C60/EUC2000, Olympus Medical Systems). The display mode includes the B-mode as well as the Color Power Doppler mode. The display range covers 2 to 24 cm. The ultrasound images can be frozen and the size of lesions can be measured in two dimensions by the placement of cursors. The area and the circumference enclosed by calliper tracking can be measured as well.

The dedicated 22-gauge needle is used to perform EBUS-TBNA (Fig. 4). This needle has various adjuster knobs that work as a safety device to prevent damage of the channel. The maximum extruding stroke is 40 mm, and to prevent excessive protrusion, a safety mechanism stops the needle at the stroke of 20 mm. The needle is also equipped with an internal sheath that is withdrawn after passing the bronchial wall, avoiding contamination during EBUS-TBNA. This internal sheath is also used to clear out the tip of the needle after passing the bronchial wall.

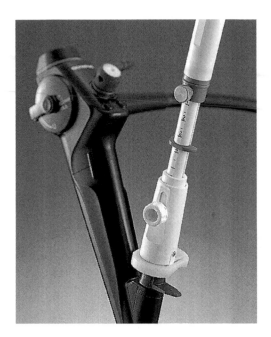

Figure 4 The dedicated 22-gauge TBNA needle attached onto the convex probe endobronchial ultrasound.

Procedure

EBUS-TBNA can be performed on an outpatient basis under conscious sedation. The bronchoscope is usually inserted orally, since the ultrasound probe on the tip will limit nasal insertion. Some investigators prefer the use of the endotracheal tube or rigid bronchoscopy under general anesthesia. An endotracheal tube larger or equal to size 8 is required because of the size of the EBUS-TBNA scope. The disadvantage of the endotracheal tube is that it causes the bronchoscope to lie in the central position within the airway that creates difficulty to bring its tip in proximity to the trachea or bronchus.

After achieving local anesthesia and conscious sedation, the CP-EBUS is inserted orally into the trachea. Once the bronchoscope is introduced into the airway until the desired position is reached for EBUS imaging, the balloon is inflated with normal saline to achieve a maximum contact with the tissue of interest. The tip of the CP-EBUS is flexed and gently pressed onto the airway. Ultrasonically visible vascular landmarks are used to identify the specific lymph node stations according to the Mountain classification system (12). The Doppler mode is used to confirm and identify surrounding vessels as well as the blood flow within lymph nodes (Fig. 5).

Once the lymph node of interest is identified, the dedicated 22-gauge TBNA needle is fastened onto the working channel of the bronchoscope. The sheath adjuster knob is loosened and the length of the sheath is adjusted so that the sheath can be visualized on endoscopic image. The tip of the bronchoscope is flexed up for contact and the lymph node is visualized again on ultrasound image. After the needle adjuster knob is loosened,

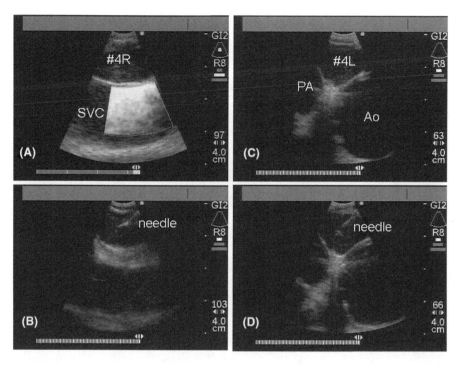

Figure 5 Representative cases of EBUS-TBNA. (**A**) EBUS image of enlarged right lower paratracheal lymph node (#4R) and SVC. (**B**) EBUS-TBNA of lymph node station #4R. The needle can be seen within the lymph node. (**C**) EBUS image of enlarged left lower paratracheal lymph node (#4L) between the aorta and pulmonary artery (PA). (**D**) EBUS-TBNA of lymph node station #4L.

EBUS-TBNA can be performed. In case a cartilage ring is encountered during TBNA, the bronchoscope is moved a little bit up or down so that the needle will go through the intercartilage space. After the initial puncture, the internal stylet is used to clear out the internal lumen, which may become clogged with bronchial membrane. The internal stylet is then removed and negative pressure is applied with the VacLok™ syringe. After the needle is moved back and forth inside the lymph node, the needle is retrieved and the internal stylet is used once again to push out the histological core. With this method, histological cores as well as cytological specimens can be obtained. The aspirated material is smeared onto glass slides, and smears are air-dried and immediately stained using Diff-Quik for immediate interpretation by an onsite cytopathologist to confirm adequate cell material. Furthermore, Papanicolaou staining and light microscopy is performed. Histological cores are fixed with formalin and stained with hematoxylin and eosin. Immunohistochemistry can also be performed if needed (26). All of the mediastinal lymph nodes except for the subaortic and paraesophageal lymph nodes (stations 5, 6, 8, and 9) are assessable by EBUS-TBNA (12). To avoid contamination and upstaging, EBUS-TBNA should be performed from the N3 nodes, followed by N2 nodes and N1 nodes.

Results

Ever since the first report of EBUS-TBNA in 2004 (25), this minimally invasive approach for the sampling of the mediastinum has gradually spread into the clinical practice of pulmonologists as well as thoracic surgeons. Case series of EBUS-TBNA for lymph node staging in lung cancer have reported a high yield ranging from 89% to 98% (25–32). The first article to report the diagnostic yield of EBUS-TBNA in a prospective study for mediastinal staging of lung cancer showed not only the high yield and safety of the procedure, but also the impact of this procedure in patient management (28). In 105 patients, EBUS-TBNA was successfully performed to obtain samples from 163 lymph nodes. With respect to the correct prediction of lymph node stage, EBUS-TBNA had a diagnostic accuracy rate of 96.3%. In the 20 suspected lung cancer cases, mediastinal lymph node was used for tissue diagnosis of malignancy as well as staging. In addition, as a result of EBUS-TBNA, 29 mediastinoscopies, 8 thoracotomies, 4 VATS, and 9 CT-guided PCNB were avoided. EBUS-TBNA spared invasive staging procedures that had a major impact on patient management in lung cancer.

A study comparing EBUS-TBNA to conventional imaging for lymph node staging of lung cancer showed a high yield by the use of the CP-EBUS (29). One hundred and two potentially operable patients with proven ($n = 96$) or radiologically suspected ($n = 6$) lung cancer were included in the study. CT, PET, and EBUS-TBNA were performed prior to surgery for the evaluation of mediastinal and hilar lymph node metastasis. EBUS-TBNA was successfully performed in all 102 patients from 147 mediastinal and 53 hilar lymph nodes. The sensitivities of CT, PET, and EBUS-TBNA for the correct diagnosis of mediastinal and hilar lymph node staging were 76.9%, 80.0%, and 92.3%, respectively. Specificities were 55.3%, 70.1%, and 100%. The diagnostic accuracies were 60.8%, 72.5%, and 98.0%. EBUS-TBNA was proven to have a high sensitivity as well as specificity compared to CT or PET, for mediastinal staging in patients with potentially resectable lung cancer.

The largest study to date looked at the yield of EBUS-TBNA in 502 patients with lung cancer and enlarged mediastinal nodes on CT (30). A total of 572 lymph nodes were punctured and 535 (94%) resulted in a diagnosis. In this series, a sensitivity of 94% and specificity of 100% for mediastinal staging was reported. From the evidence, EBUS-TBNA has been newly introduced in the *ACCP Evidence-Based Practice Guideline* (second edition) for invasive staging of lung cancer (3).

Although the reported yield of EBUS-TBNA is high and similar to the "gold standard" mediastinoscopy, there have been no studies directly comparing the mediastinoscopy and EBUS-TBNA for lymph node staging. There is an ongoing prospective trial comparing the yield of mediastinoscopy and EBUS-TBNA for mediastinal lymph node staging in patients with confirmed or suspected lung cancer (33). Patients with resectable lung cancer who require a mediastinoscopy for mediastinal staging underwent EBUS-TBNA followed by mediastinoscopy under general anesthesia in the same setting. The diagnostic yield was compared between the two procedures. Out of 45 patients enrolled in the study, the diagnostic accuracy of EBUS-TBNA and mediastinoscopy for analysis of each lymph node stations were 95.6% and 96.6%. The sensitivity, specificity, and diagnostic accuracy for the correct mediastinal lymph node staging for EBUS-TBNA and mediastinoscopy were 76.9%, 100%, and 90.9%, and 84.6%, 100%, and 93.9% respectively. These preliminary results show that EBUS-TBNA may reduce the number of mediastinoscopy needed for the staging of the mediastinum in NSCLC.

However, because of the possibility of false-negative EBUS-TBNA results, it is not clear that EBUS-TBNA will completely replace mediastinoscopy for mediastinal staging.

Complications related to EBUS-TBNA are similar to those of conventional TBNA including pneumothorax, pneumomediastinum, hemomediastinum, mediastinitis, bacteremia, and pericarditis. We have not encountered complications related to EBUS-TBNA, and to date there are no major complications reported in the literature. Although EBUS has enabled the bronchoscopist to see beyond the airway, one must be aware of the possible complications related to the procedure.

IV. Endoscopic Ultrasound–Guided Fine-Needle Aspiration

Endoscopic ultrasound-guided fine-needle aspiration (EUS-FNA) offers a minimally invasive method of examining the posterior and inferior mediastinum in patients with lung cancer. Established as a modality to evaluate the mediastinum in the early 1990s, the role of EUS-FNA in NSCLC staging continues to evolve (34–39). The EUS scope has an ultrasound transducer on the tip that allows ultrasound imaging of structures adjacent to the gastrointestinal tract. The mediastinal levels that are accessible include the lower paratracheal to the left (station 4L), subcarinal (station 7), paraesophageal (station 8), and inferior pulmonary ligament (station 9). Upper paratracheal (station 2) and lower paratracheal to the right (station 4R) oftentimes cannot be assessed by EUS because of the anatomy.

A. Procedure and Results

The curved linear array transducers from various companies are available for performing EUS-FNA (Fig. 6). Dedicated 22-gauge needles are usually used, but smaller (25-gauge) and larger (19-gauge) needles are available. EUS-FNA is an outpatient procedure that is performed under conscious sedation. The dedicated fine aspiration needle is passed

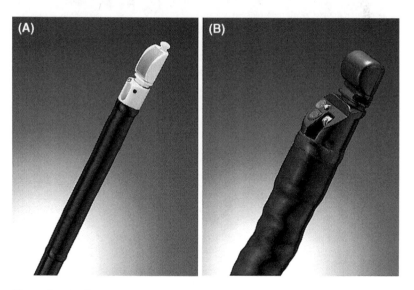

Figure 6 (**A**) The convex probe endobronchial ultrasound and (**B**) the linear transoesophageal ultrasound-guided fine-needle aspiration scope.

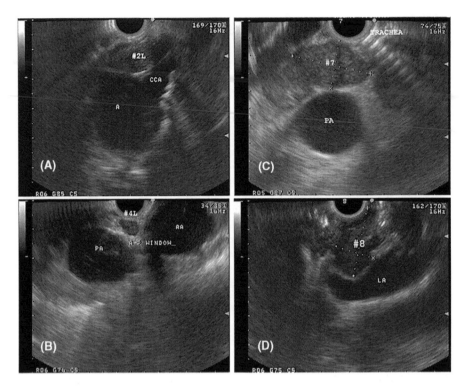

Figure 7 Representative cases of EUS-FNA. (A) EUS image of the left upper paratracheal lymph node (#2L). (B) EUS image of the left lower paratracheal lymph node (#4L) between the ascending aorta (AA) and the pulmonary artery (PA). (C) EUS image of the subcarinal lymph node (#7) along the pulmonary artery (PA). (D) EUS image of the paraesophageal lymph node (#8) along the left atrium (LA).

through a working channel and directed into the target under real-time ultrasonography (Fig. 7). There is direct visualization of the needle during the aspiration. The overall risk of EUS-FNA is approximately 0.5% and may include perforation of the bowel wall or posterior pharynx, infection, hemorrhage, and cardiac or respiratory complications related to the sedation medications (40).

The role of EUS-FNA in the lymph node staging and diagnosis of NSCLC has been well documented by multiple authors. In a meta-analysis of 14 studies, the sensitivity and specificity of EUS-FNA for the diagnosis of posterior mediastinal lymphadenopathy in NSCLC were 81% to 97% and 83% to 100%, respectively (41). As a result of EUS-FNA, surgical staging procedures such as mediastinoscopies and thoracotomies can be avoided (38). However the major drawback of EUS-FNA is the high false-negative rate. This is probably due to sampling errors or technical difficulties of small-sized lymph nodes. Therefore, EUS-FNA should be performed primarily on patients with radiologic evidence of mediastinal lymphadenopathy.

V. Conclusion

Accurate lymph node staging remains essential for management of patients with NSCLC. The recent developments in endoscopy have changed the accuracy and safety of mediastinal staging. Conventional TBNA should be performed during routine bronchoscopy for the diagnosis of enlarged lymph nodes. For tissue sampling of mediastinal and hilar nodes after a negative TBNA, EBUS-TBNA or EUS-FNA should be performed depending on the target lymph node stations. For sampling of the highest mediastinal, paratracheal, subcarinal, or hilar lymph nodes, EBUS-TBNA is ideal. For lower mediastinal lymph nodes (stations 8 or 9), EUS-FNA should be performed. Either EBUS-TBNA or EUS-FNA is capable of sampling the aortic nodes (stations 5 and 6). Therefore, other invasive procedures such as VATS, extended mediastinoscopy, or thoracoctomy should be performed for the assessment of lymph nodes outside the reach of EBUS-TBNA or EUS-FNA. If a result from cytology is negative for malignancy from either EBUS-TBNA or EUS-FNA, other staging modalities should be considered for confirmation of the absence of mediastinal involvement, since there is yet no direct comparison of endoscopic staging with the "gold standard" mediastinoscopy. However, without any doubt, the minimally invasive endoscopic methods of EBUS-TBNA and EUS-FNA will significantly reduce the need for surgical staging of lung cancer.

Summary

Tissue diagnosis of mediastinal lymph nodes is oftentimes needed for accurate lymph node staging in lung cancer. Endoscopic staging is a minimally invasive procedure that utilizes fine-needle aspiration for sampling of mediastinal and hilar lymph nodes. Transbronchial needle aspiration (TBNA) is a well-known procedure performed through the working channel of a flexible bronchoscope. It is a safe procedure that has a high impact on patient management. Despite its proven usefulness, TBNA remains to be underused among pulmonologists for various reasons. Lack of real-time needle visualization is one of the important factors that affect the yield of TBNA. The introduction of new technology, especially endoscopes with built-in ultrasound on the tip, has overcome these problems. Endobronchial ultrasound–guided TBNA (EBUS-TBNA) using the convex probe EBUS allows direct real-time TBNA under ultrasound guidance. The reach of EBUS-TBNA is similar to mediastinoscopy, the gold standard of surgical staging, but extends to the hilar lymph nodes. Paraesophageal and pulmonary ligament lymph nodes can be assessed by transesophageal ultrasound–guided fine-needle aspiration (EUS-FNA). The reach of EBUS-TBNA and EUS-FNA is complementary for assessing the different parts of the mediastinum, and recent studies suggest that the majority of the mediastinum can be staged by the combination of both procedures. Anatomically, the aortopulmonary and para-aortic lymph nodes cannot be assessed endoscopically, but need to be approached by other methods such as video-assisted thoracoscopic surgery (VATS). Nevertheless, the minimally invasive endoscopic methods of EBUS-TBNA and EUS-FNA will significantly reduce the need for surgical staging of lung cancer.

References

1. American College of Chest Physicians; Health and Science Policy Committee. Diagnosis and management of lung cancer: ACCP evidence-based guidelines. Chest 2003; 123: D-G, 1S-337S.

2. Silvestri GA, Gould MK, Margolis ML, et al. Non-invasive staging of non-small cell lung cancer: ACCP evidence-based clinical practice guidelines (2nd ed.). Chest 2007; 132: 178S–201S.
3. Detterbeck FC, Jantz MA, Wallace M, et al. Invasive mediastinal staging of lung cancer: ACCP evidence-based clinical practice guidelines (2nd ed.). Chest 2007; 132:202S–220S.
4. Yasufuku K, Fujisawa T. Staging and diagnosis of non-small cell lung cancer: invasive modalities. Respirology 2007; 12:308–310.
5. Schieppati E. Mediastinal lymph node puncture through the tracheal carina. Surg Gynecol Obstet 1958; 107:243–246.
6. Oho K, Kato H, Ogawa I, et al. A new needle for transfiberoptic bronchoscope use. Chest 1979; 76:492.
7. Wang KP, Marsh BR, Summer WR, et al. Transbronchial needle aspiration for diagnosis of lung cancer. Chest 1981; 80:48–50.
8. Wang KP, Terry PB. Transbronchial needle aspiration in the diagnosis and staging of bronchogenic carcinoma. Am Rev Respir Dis 1983; 127:344–347.
9. Wang KP, Brower R, Haponik EF, et al. Flexible transbronchial needle aspiration for staging of bronchogenic carcinoma. Chest 1983; 84:571–576.
10. Mehta AC, Kavuru MS, Meeker DP, et al. Transbronchial needle aspiration for histology specimens. Chest 1989; 96:1228–1232.
11. Schenk DA, Bower JH, Bryan CL, et al. Transbronchial needle aspiration staging of bronchogenic carcinoma. Am Rev Respir Dis 1986; 134:146–148.
12. Haponik EF, Sture D. Underutilization of transbronchial needle aspiration: experience of current pulmonary fellows. Chest 1997; 112:251–253.
13. Schenk DA, Chambers SL, Derdak S, et al. Comparison of the Wang 19 gauge and 22 gauge needles in the mediastinal staging of lung cancer. Am Rev Respir Dis 1993; 147:1251–1258.
14. Mountain CF, Dresler CM. Regional lymph node classification for lung cancer staging. Chest 1997; 111:1718–1723.
15. Mehta AC, Meeker DP. Transbronchial needle aspiration for histology specimens. In: Wang KP, Mehta AC, eds. Flexible Bronchoscopy. Cambridge: Blackwell Science, 1995:199–205.
16. Wang KP, Haponik EF, Gupta PK, et al. Flexible transbronchial needle aspiration: technical considerations. Ann Otol Rhinol Laryngol 1984; 93:233–236.
17. Baram D, Garcia RB, Richman PS. Impact of rapid on-site cytologic evaluation during transbronchial needle aspiration. Chest 2005; 128:869–875.
18. Talebian M, Recanatini A, Zuccatosta L, et al. Hemomediastinum as a consequence of transbronchial needle aspiration. J Bronchol 2004; 11:178–180.
19. White MC, Opal SM, Gilbert JG, et al. Incidence of fever and bacteremia following transbronchial needle aspiration. Chest 1986; 89:85–87.
20. Epstein SK, Winslow CJ, Brecher SM, et al. Polymicrobacterial pericarditis after transbronchial needle aspiration. Case report with an investigation on the risk of bacterial contamination during fiberoptic bronchoscopy. Am Rev Respir Dis 1992; 146:523–525.
21. Hurter T, Hanrath P. Endobronchial sonography: feasibility and preliminary results. Thorax 1992; 47:565–567.
22. Baba M, Sekine Y, Suzuki M, et al. Correlation between endobronchial ultrasonography (EBUS) images and histologic findings in normal and tumor-invaded bronchial wall. Lung Cancer 2002; 35:65–71.
23. Herth FJ, Becker HD, Ernst A. Ultrasound-guided transbronchial needle aspiration: an experience in 242 patients. Chest 2003; 123:604–607.
24. Herth F, Becker HD, Ernst A. Conventional vs endobronchial ultrasound-guided transbronchial needle aspiration: a randomized trial. Chest 2004; 125:322–325.
25. Yasufuku K, Chhajed PN, Sekine Y, et al. Endobronchial ultrasound using a new convex probe: a preliminary study on surgically resected specimens. Oncol Rep 2004; 11(2):293–296.

26. Yasufuku K, Chiyo M, Sekine Y, et al. Real-time endobronchial ultrasound guided transbronchial needle aspiration of mediastinal and hilar lymph nodes. Chest 2004; 126:122–128.

27. Krasnik M, Vilman P, Larsen SS, et al. Preliminary experience with a new method of endoscopic transbronchial real time ultrasound guided biopsy for diagnosis of mediastinal and hilar lesions. Thorax 2003; 58:1083–1086.

28. Yasufuku K, Chiyo M, Koh E, et al. Endobronchial ultrasound guided transbronchial needle aspiration for staging of lung cancer. Lung Cancer 2005; 50:347–354.

29. Yasufuku K, Nakajima T, Motoori K, et al. Comparison of endobronchial ultrasound, positron emission tomography, and computed tomography for lymph node staging of lung cancer. Chest 2006; 130:710–718.

30. Herth FJ, Eberhardt R, Vilmann P, et al. Real-time endobronchial ultrasound guided transbronchial needle aspiration for sampling mediastinal lymph nodes. Thorax 2006; 61:795–798.

31. Vincent BD, El-Bayoumi E, Hoffman B, et al. Real-time endobronchial ultrasound-guided transbronchial lymph node aspiration. Ann Thorac Surg 2008; 85:224–230.

32. Herth FJ, Ernst A, Eberhardt R, et al. Endobronchial ultrasound-guided transbronchial needle aspiration of lymph nodes in the radiologically normal mediastinum. Eur Respir J 2006; 28:910–914.

33. Yasufuku K, Quadri M, dePerrot M, et al. A prospective controlled trial of endobronchial ultrasound guided transbronchial needle aspiration compared to mediastinoscopy for mediastinal lymph node staging of lung cancer. Western Thoracic Surgical Association, 33rd Annual Meeting, 2007: abstract.

34. Kondo D, Imaizumi M, Abe T, et al. Endoscopic ultrasound examination for mediastinal lymph node metastases of lung cancer. Chest 1990; 98:586–593.

35. Hawes RH, Gress F, Kesler KA, et al. Endoscopic ultrasound versus computed tomography in the evaluation of the mediastinum in patients with non-small-cell lung cancer. Endoscopy 1994; 26:784–787.

36. Silvestri GA, Hoffman BJ, Bhutani MS, et al. Endoscopic ultrasound with fine-needle aspiration in the diagnosis and staging of lung cancer. Ann Thorac Surg 1996; 61:1441–1445.

37. Wallace MB, Silvestri GA, Sahai AV, et al. Endoscopic ultrasound-guided fine needle aspiration for staging patients with carcinoma of lung cancer. Chest 2000; 117:339–345.

38. Larsen SS, Krasnik M, Vilmann P, et al. Endoscopic ultrasound guided biopsy of mediastinal lesions has a major impact on patient management. Thorax 2002; 57:98–1034.

39. Fritscher-Ravens A. Endoscopic ultrasound evaluation in the diagnosis and staging of lung cancer. Lung Cancer 2003; 41:259–267.

40. Herth FJF, Rabe KF, Gasparini S, et al. Transbronchial and transoesophageal (ultrasound-guided) needle aspirations for the analysis of mediastinal lesions. Eur Respir J 2006; 28: 1264–1275.

41. Kramer H, Groen HJM. Current concepts in the mediastinal lymph node staging of nonsmall cell lung cancer. Ann Surg 2003; 238:180188.

7
Medical Thoracoscopy

ANDREW G. VILLANUEVA
Lahey Clinic Medical Center, Burlington, Massachusetts, U.S.A.

ANNE GONZALEZ
McGill University Health Centre, Montreal, Quebec, Canada

I. Introduction

Diseases of the pleura and the pleural space constitute a common problem in the field of chest medicine. The cause of pleural pathology—whether pleural thickening, pleural effusion, or pneumothorax—can generally be determined after obtaining a detailed history, radiographic imaging, and laboratory testing of aspirated pleural fluid. However, after initial evaluation, including thoracentesis and closed pleural biopsy, up to 25% of pleural diseases remains undiagnosed (1–5). Medical thoracoscopy is a useful diagnostic tool for these cases. In this chapter we will review the role of medical thoracoscopy, also called "pleuroscopy," in the diagnosis of pleural disorders of unclear etiology; we will discuss indications, diagnostic yield, limitations, and biopsy techniques. Medical thoracoscopy is also a useful therapeutic tool to achieve pleurodesis in conditions such as malignant pleural effusion (MPE) and spontaneous pneumothorax; we will discuss thoracoscopic talc poudrage, which is the most commonly used method for pleurodesis.

II. Diagnostic Uses of Medical Thoracoscopy
A. Indications for Diagnostic Medical Thoracoscopy

Common indications for diagnostic medical thoracoscopy are listed in Table 1 and are discussed in detail in subsequent sections of this chapter. The most frequent diagnostic indication for thoracoscopy is an unexplained recurrent or persistent pleural effusion, usually an exudative effusion, for which thoracentesis and (if used) closed pleural biopsy have been nondiagnostic (6–15). Pleuroscopy is particularly helpful in diagnosing MPEs. In cases of suspected mesothelioma, for example, the diagnosis can be difficult by cytological examination of pleural fluid and histological examination of the small samples obtained by closed-needle pleural biopsy. Medical thoracoscopy improves the diagnostic yield for mesothelioma to above 90% (6,16–19). Pleuroscopy can be used in patients with known bronchogenic carcinoma who have cytologically negative pleural effusions. Since only 6% of such patients will have completely resectable tumors (20), medical thoracoscopy can be used to identify the small group who could potentially benefit from surgical resection while preventing surgery for the majority with unresectable disease. Since the diagnostic yield of a closed-needle biopsy is 70% to 90% for tuberculous effusions (21–24), medical thoracoscopy is usually unnecessary to establish the diagnosis. Thoracoscopy may be useful, however, in difficult diagnostic situations,

Table 1 Indications for Diagnostic Medical Thoracoscopy

Recurrent or persistent exudative pleural effusions that have eluded diagnosis by other means
Suspected mesothelioma
Cytologically negative pleural effusion in a patient with known bronchogenic carcinoma
Suspected tuberculous pleural effusion not diagnosed after thoracentesis and closed pleural biopsy
Chest wall or pleural-based mass
Pleural thickening
Recurrent spontaneous pneumothorax
Interstitial lung disease

when lysis of adhesions is necessary or when larger amounts of tissue are necessary for determining drug resistance (25). Less common indications for medical thoracoscopy include the presence of a chest wall or pleural-based mass and pleural thickening without associated pleural effusions. In cases of recurrent spontaneous pneumothorax, thoracoscopy can be done to help determine the cause of the pneumothorax, to assess for the presence of blebs or bullae in the affected lung, and to plan treatment (26–28). Finally, while lung tissue is generally obtained by transbronchial biopsy or by the thoracic surgeons using video-assisted thoracic surgery (VATS), authors have reported the use of medical thoracoscopy to obtain lung tissue in patients with interstitial lung diseases (3,29–31).

B. Medical Thoracoscopy in the Diagnosis of Pleural Effusions of Unknown Etiology

Pleural effusions are a common problem worldwide with an annual incidence in the United States alone of approximately one million patients per year (2). The possible causes of pleural effusions are numerous (1,2,32), but the etiology in a particular patient can be determined without the need for medical thoracoscopy in most cases. Indeed, thoracentesis, a minimally invasive procedure, remains the most useful procedure for defining the cause of a pleural effusion. Pleural fluid cellularity, appearance, and chemistry, along with the clinical presentation, can be used to establish a presumptive or definitive diagnosis in about 75% of patients (33). When no diagnosis has been obtained after an initial thoracentesis that includes a pleural fluid marker for tuberculosis and cytology, the next steps may include observation, bronchoscopy, closed-needle biopsy of the parietal pleura, and medical thoracoscopy (34). Bronchoscopy is useful in revealing the cause of a pleural effusion only if there is a concomitant parenchymal infiltrate, hemoptysis, massive effusion, or mediastinal shift toward the side of the effusion (35,36). While closed-needle biopsy of the pleura has been considered an important diagnostic tool since its first description in 1955, its role in today's practice is diminishing because of the availability of medical thoracoscopy (21,22,37). In fact, it is no longer required for pulmonary medicine training programs in the United States to teach the technique of closed-needle pleural biopsy to trainees (38,39). Despite its waning popularity, it is still a useful technique to diagnose pleural tuberculosis since the diagnostic yield is over 75% (39).

Studies describing the diagnostic yield of medical thoracoscopy consistently show an improvement in the yield, compared with thoracentesis and closed pleural biopsy (Table 2). Loddenkemper et al. (25) prospectively compared the yield of pleural fluid

Table 2 Studies Reporting the Diagnostic Yield of Medical Thoracoscopy for Pleural Effusions of Unknown Etiology

Authors (ref)	Year	Number of cases	Diagnostic yield	Yield of thoracentesis (T) and/or CPB
Canto et al. (7)	1977	172	94% for MPE	All cases previously undiagnosed after T CPB not mentioned
Loddenkemper et al. (25)	1978	100	96% for TB or MPE	T and CPB: 73% for TB or MPE
Oldenburg and Newhouse (51)	1979	38	88%	T: All 38 nondiagnostic CPB: 16%
Boutin et al. (6)	1981	215	87.3% for MPE	T: 23% for MPE CPB: 40% for MPE
Enk and Viskum (40)	1981	387	80.1% for MPE	T: 62% for MPE CPB not mentioned
Martensson et al. (41)	1985	334	80% for MPE	T: 43% for MPE [thoracoscopy revealed tumor in 37 of 47 (79%) with MPE and negative cytology]
Menzies and Charbonneau (11)	1991	86	96% (44% MPE and 52% benign disease)	All had been undiagnosed after T and CPB
Hansen et al. (52)	1998	136	90.4%	All had been undiagnosed after three thoracenteses
Wilsher and Veale (15)	1998	58	80% overall 90% if only those in whom full pleural access was achieved (51 patients)	All patients had been undiagnosed after T and CPB
Blanc et al. (42)	2002	149	93.3%	CPB: 25%
Munavvar et al. (43)	2007	54	90.7%	T: All 54 nondiagnostic
Lee et al. (44)	2007	51	96%	T: All 51 nondiagnostic

Studies in which thoracoscopy was performed using general anesthesia were excluded.
Abbreviations: CPB, closed-needle pleural biopsy; MPE, malignant pleural effusions; TB, tuberculous effusions.

analysis and closed pleural biopsy with that of thoracoscopy in 100 patients. Of the 67 patients with either tuberculous effusions or MPEs, the yield for pleuroscopy was 96% versus 73% for pleural fluid analysis and closed pleural biopsy. Boutin et al. (6) found a sensitivity of 87% in the diagnosis of 150 MPEs compared to 23% for pleural fluid cytology and 40% for closed-needle biopsy. In a large retrospective study, Enk and Viskum (40) found that of the 387 patients undergoing medical thoracoscopy for pleural effusions, 171 had MPEs. In these patients the yield by pleuroscopy was 80%, compared to 62% by pleural fluid cytology examination. Martensson et al. (41) reported a sensitivity of 80% for MPE and noted that thoracoscopy revealed tumor in 37 of 47 patients

(79%) with MPE and negative cytology. Menzies and Charbonneau (11) performed pleuroscopy on 86 patients with pleural effusions undiagnosed after thoracentesis and pleural biopsy. Thirty-eight patients (44%) were diagnosed with cancer and 45 patients (52%) were diagnosed with benign diseases after medical thoracoscopy. The authors reported a sensitivity of 91% and a specificity of 100%. Blanc et al. (42) retrospectively compared the yield of closed-needle pleural biopsy with medical thoracoscopy and found that thoracoscopy yielded a precise diagnosis in 43 of 90 cases (48%) in which prior closed pleural biopsy was nondiagnostic and corrected the diagnosis given by needle biopsy in 11 of 30 patients (37%) thought to have pleural malignancy. Diagnostic yields of 91% and 96% were recently reported using a semirigid thoracoscope by Munavvar (43) and Lee (44), respectively. The data in these studies (Table 2) revealed diagnostic yields of 80% to 96% for exudative pleural effusions of unknown etiology and therefore support the use of medical thoracoscopy in evaluating pleural effusions that remain undiagnosed after the performance of thoracentesis and closed-needle pleural biopsy.

The increased diagnostic yield of medical thoracoscopy compared with pleural fluid cytology and closed-needle pleural biopsy is explainable by the improved visualization (Fig. 1) and larger biopsy sample size attained during pleuroscopy (3,34). Cytological examination of the pleural fluid may fail to diagnose a MPE either because there is insufficient exfoliation of cells from the pleural surfaces into the pleural effusion or because there is a lack of cytological characteristics in the collected fluid to make an accurate diagnosis. The closed-needle pleural biopsy technique is limited by restricted access and lack of direct visualization of the target lesions. In patients with metastatic pleural disease, 32% to 47% have disease inaccessible to closed-needle biopsy (3). Canto et al. (45) reported that of 78 patients with proven metastatic disease to the pleura,

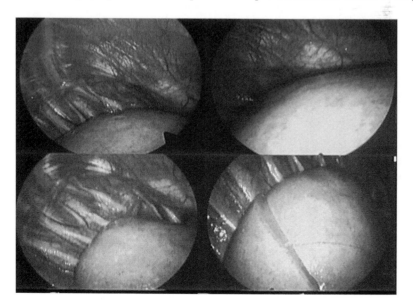

Figure 1 Normal pleura in a patient with a primary spontaneous pneumothorax.

only 53% had involvement of costoparietal pleural areas accessible to closed-needle pleural biopsy. These investigators also reported that in 84% of patients studied, the metastases were in the lower hemithorax, on the lung surface, or the diaphragm, and were poorly accessible or totally inaccessible to closed-needle biopsy (45–47). In autopsy studies, investigators have reported that the parietal pleura is less frequently involved with metastatic pleural disease than the visceral pleura (48,49). Medical thoracoscopy can overcome these limitations because of the direct access to the pleural cavity, visualization of both the parietal and visceral pleura, and larger sizes of the biopsy samples. If full visualization of the pleural space is not achieved during thoracoscopy, the diagnostic accuracy of the procedure greatly diminishes (15,42).

C. Medical Thoracoscopy in the Diagnosis of Malignant Pleural Effusions

Malignant Pleural Effusions: Carcinoma Metastatic to the Pleura

Malignant disease involving the pleura is the second leading cause of exudative pleural effusions after parapneumonic effusions and has an incidence in the United States of more than 150,000 cases annually (2). Lung cancer, breast cancer, lymphoma, and ovarian cancer account for approximately 80% of tumors metastatic to the pleura (50). Other types of neoplasms that can metastasize to the visceral or parietal pleura include sarcoma, melanoma, and carcinomas of the uterus, cervix, stomach, colon, pancreas and bladder; the primary site of malignancy is unknown in about 6% of cases (50) (Figs. 2–5). The suspicion for MPE represents the leading diagnostic indication for medical thoracoscopy (9). The yield for diagnosing MPE by medical thoracoscopy ranged from 80% to 96% in reported series (6,7,11,15,25,40,41,51,52). Loddenkemper reported that the combined yield for pleural fluid cytology, closed-needle pleural biopsy, and medical thoracoscopy was 97% (9).

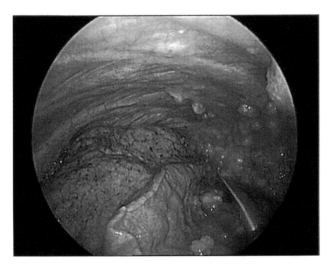

Figure 2 Parietal pleura studded with metastatic lung cancer. Anthracotic pigment can be seen on the lung surface. A chest tube is visible in the lower right of the figure.

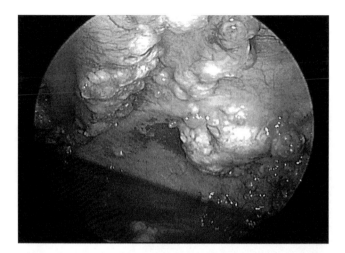

Figure 3 Metastatic adenocarcinoma of breast origin involving the parietal pleura. Pleural fluid is present.

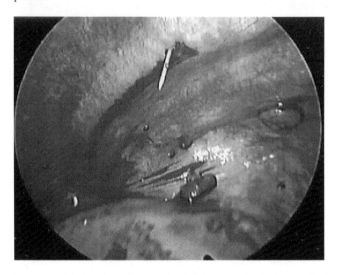

Figure 4 Metastatic melanoma involving the parietal pleura with hyperpigmented lesions. A needle used for instilling lidocaine prior to chest tube insertion is visible.

The main advantage of pleuroscopy is its ability to achieve early diagnosis of MPE when pleural fluid cytology and CPB have failed. It allows inspection of approximately 75% of the visceral pleural surface as well as of the parietal pleural surface. Boutin reported that in 85% of patients with MPE, thoracoscopy revealed visual features suggestive of malignancy, including nodules, polypoid lesions, localized masses, thickened pleural surface, and poorly vascularized pachypleuritis (53). Since appearances can be misleading—some malignancies may appear inflammatory while

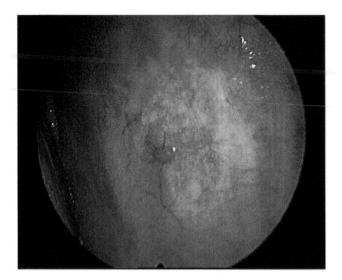

Figure 5 Single metastatic deposit on the pleural surface of a patient with a malignant pleural effusion from breast cancer.

some inflammatory lesions can look like tumors—macroscopic diagnoses must always be confirmed by histology. Biopsies can be visually directed in instances where tumor deposits appear to be localized. In addition, biopsy specimens can be obtained from multiple sites and are of greater size and depth, factors that improve the diagnostic yield (11). The larger sample sizes increases the ability of the pathologist to make an accurate diagnosis; the pathologist, for example, can better differentiate malignant mesothelioma from adenocarcinoma and can perform special studies such as hormone receptor assays or genetic marker studies on the tissue.

Malignant Pleural Effusions: Mesothelioma
In the past, pathologists found it difficult to make a definitive diagnosis of malignant mesothelioma without large samples obtained during open thoracotomy or autopsy. As the incidence of the disease has increased and with the availability of immunohistochemistry techniques, pathologists are better able to make the diagnosis. By permitting direct visualization of lesions, pleuroscopy facilitates the choice of biopsy sites and allows accurate assessment of the degree of involvement of the diaphragmatic, parietal, visceral, and mediastinal pleura (54) (Fig. 6). Boutin reported a sensitivity of thoracoscopy biopsy of 98% (185 of 188 patients) for the diagnosis of malignant mesothelioma, compared with 28% (49 of 175 patients) for pleural fluid cytology, 24% (33 of 135 patients) for closed-needle pleural biopsy, and 100% (9 of 9 patients) for surgical biopsy (17,18).

D. Medical Thoracoscopy in the Diagnosis of Tuberculous Pleural Effusions
Since tuberculous pleural effusions can be diagnosed in 70% to 90% of cases with pleural fluid analysis and closed-needle pleural biopsy (25), including culture for

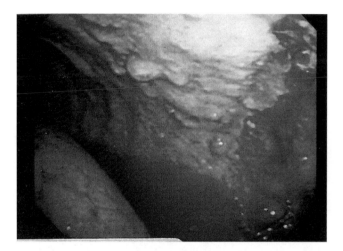

Figure 6 Diffuse involvement of the parietal pleura with malignant mesothelioma.

Mycobacterium tuberculosis, medical thoracoscopy is usually unnecessary to establish the diagnosis. Indeed, Boutin et al. reported that in their experience thoracoscopy played no significant role in the diagnosis of this disease and that the discovery of tuberculous granulomata on thoracoscopy biopsy was usually fortuitous (53). They nonetheless described the endoscopic appearance as a grayish white thickening of the whole parietal and diaphragmatic pleura, particularly along the costovertebral gutter (Fig. 7). Loddenkemper reported a diagnostic yield of 93% (30 of 32 patients) based on histology and/or culture with pleuroscopy alone and 97% (31 of 32 patients) with pleural fluid analysis plus pleuroscopy, compared with 84% (27 of 32 patients) with pleural fluid analysis plus closed-needle pleural biopsy (25).

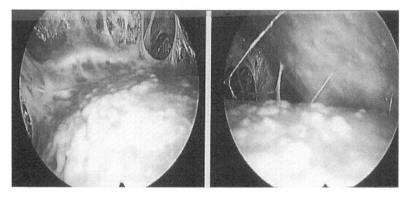

Figure 7 Characteristic grayish white thickening of the parietal pleura and diaphragmatic pleura seen in tuberculous pleurisy. Note the presence of adhesions.

E. Medical Thoracoscopy in Differentiating Benign from Malignant Causes of Pleural Effusions

In cases of pleural effusions that are neither malignant nor tuberculous, thoracoscopy may provide clues to the etiology. For example, hyaline and calcified asbestos pleural plaques have distinctive endoscopic characteristics, appearing smooth and white, and being difficult to biopsy because of their hard consistency (53). In rheumatoid effusions the visceral surface shows a nonspecific inflammation and the parietal surface has a gritty appearance (55).

The main reported value of thoracoscopy, however, is not to make a specific benign diagnosis (other than tuberculosis) but, rather, to exclude malignancy as the cause. Several authors have reviewed the benign diagnoses made during thoracoscopy and while most of them focused primarily on the short-term outcome of these patients, some reported follow-up data. Canto et al. (7) described 51 of 208 thoracoscopic biopsies showing normal pleura, acute pleurisy, or subacute chronic pleurisy; they noted eight patients in whom tumor was not found but later died of generalized carcinomatosis (a false-negative rate of 6% for MPEs). Boutin (6) reported that 65 of 215 patients undergoing thoracoscopy had benign causes such as congestive heart failure, benign asbestos effusions, infectious pleuritis, cirrhosis, and "idiopathic chronic pleural effusions" (40 patients). These patients were followed for a least one year by mail and telephone inquiry; no specific mention was made of their outcome. Enk and Viskum (40) reported 186 patients diagnosed with non-MPEs from pleurisy of unknown origin, congestive heart failure, pneumonia, rheumatic pleurisy, pulmonary infarction, uremia, and cirrhosis. Nonspecific inflammation was found on histology in 129 biopsies; no follow-up information on these patients was provided although the authors did cite a 90% sensitivity in detecting MPEs. In the series reported by Menzies and Charbonneau (11), 53 of 95 patients were diagnosed with benign disease, including asbestos-related effusion, chylothorax, Dressler's syndrome, rheumatoid effusion, lupus pleuritis, pulmonary embolism, congestive heart failure, and pneumonia; the largest cause of benign effusions was "idiopathic" (22 of 53 patients). The authors reported that 94% of these patients were alive after follow-up of at least one year. They calculated a negative predictive value of 93% for diagnosing MPE. Hansen et al. (52) found 56 of 147 patients diagnosed with benign disease after medical thoracoscopy, 45 of who had "unspecific inflammation." No follow-up data were provided. The authors reported a sensitivity of 88% and negative predictive value of 78% for malignancy. In a small series, Wilsher and Veale (15) reported that 5 of 51 patients (10%) had false-negative results for malignancy. Blanc et al. (42) retrospectively reported that 57 of 149 thoracoscopies revealed "nonspecific inflammation" and that no diagnosis other than benign pleural effusion was made during follow-up of 12 to 70 months. Ferrer et al. (56) conducted a 10-year study of 40 patients with exudative pleural effusions undiagnosed after "exhaustive evaluation" (although only 37% of these patients underwent pleuroscopy). They found that 80% of the pleural effusions remained idiopathic but that most patients had a benign course; it should, however, be noted that 2 of the 40 patients were eventually diagnosed with a MPE. Mouchantaf and Villanueva (57) retrospectively reported 25 patients who were diagnosed with non-MPEs after pleuroscopy and were followed for at least three years. The long-term survival was favorable (median five-year survival of 75%) and none of the 25 patients were subsequently diagnosed with a MPE.

Despite imperfect data, the information reported in series of patients undergoing diagnostic medical thoracoscopy suggests that while pleuroscopy often cannot give a specific histological diagnosis for nonmalignant, nontuberculous effusions, it is an effective and reliable tool in differentiating benign from malignant causes of pleural effusions. There is general agreement, however, that pleuroscopy should not replace pleural fluid chemistry, microbiology, cytology and, in appropriate cases, closed-needle pleural biopsy as initial diagnostic tests.

F. Medical Thoracoscopy in the Diagnosis of Pleural Thickening

The vast majority of patients undergoing medical thoracoscopy have pleural effusions, with or without pleural thickening. Since pleuroscopy requires the induction of a pneumothorax, the presence of pleural fluid allows this to be done safely without great risk of injuring the lung. Few series include patients undergoing thoracoscopy solely for the diagnosis of pleural thickening in the absence of a pleural effusion. Investigators reporting such patients (58,59) performed thoracoscopy under general anesthesia utilizing double-lumen intubation. Colt (58) noted that 2 of 52 patients undergoing thoracoscopy had pleural thickening but did not specify the final diagnoses in these patients. Harris et al. (59) reported that 9% of their 182 patients had a pleural mass as the indication for thoracoscopy; no specific diagnoses were noted.

G. Medical Thoracoscopy in the Diagnosis of Recurrent Pneumothorax

While the main purpose of medical thoracoscopy for spontaneous pneumothorax is therapeutic—chest tube drainage, pleurodesis, and coagulation of blebs and bullae—the technique can also be considered diagnostic since it allows inspection of the lung and pleural cavity (9,26). A complete inspection may detect a lung parenchymal laceration, a malpositioned chest tube within lung parenchyma responsible for a continued air leak, or visceral and parietal pleural abnormalities such as endometriosis, congenital cysts, and cavitating or nodular lesions in patients with granulomatous disorders (26). The most likely abnormalities are blebs and bullae, although up to 30% of patients may have normal findings (28). Using fluorescein-enhanced autofluorescence thoracoscopy (FEAT), a technique in which patients inhaled fluorescein prior to medical thoracoscopy, Noppen et al. (60) reported finding parenchymal abnormalities, which they described as "pleural porosity," more commonly in patients with primary spontaneous pneumothoraces (PSP) compared with patients without PSP; these abnormalities were evident using FEAT but not using standard white light thoracoscopy.

H. Medical Thoracoscopy in the Diagnosis of Parenchymal Lung Disease

Medical thoracoscopy has become synonymous with the term pleuroscopy because the most common indication for the procedure involves pleural diseases. Biopsy of the lung is commonly done by thoracic surgeons performing VATS, but it has also been described using cup biopsy forceps during medical thoracoscopy. Boutin et al. reported their experience with 75 patients with diffuse or localized parenchymal disease in whom thoracoscopy was used to obtain pulmonary parenchymal specimens (29). A biopsy forceps was employed and effective hemostasis was achieved by electrocautery. This thoracoscopic technique preserved the histological structure of tissues and provided biopsy specimens larger than those obtained by bronchoscopy. The overall sensitivity was 92%, ranging from 70% for peripheral lesions to 100% for diffuse diseases. Complications included pneumothorax in 8 patients and low-grade fever in 11. Another study reported successful lung biopsies with excellent hemostasis and no air leakage in 18 patients using a cryoprobe to seal the forceps biopsy site (61). Despite these reports, we cannot recommend the routine use of medical thoracoscopy for parenchymal lung biopsy until there is a larger reported experience about the yield and safety of the procedure. Patients requiring thoracoscopic lung biopsies should still be referred to the thoracic surgeons or medical thoracoscopists with extensive experience.

I. Diagnostic Limitations of Medical Thoracoscopy

Medical thoracoscopy is a safe technique in the appropriate patient. The mortality risk is 0.09% (34) and the complication rate is low; Menzies and Charbonneau reported a major complication rate of 1.9% and a minor complication rate of 5.6% (11). The major anatomic contraindication is a lack of a pleural space because of dense pleural adhesions. Medical contraindications include poor performance status, hypoxemia not due to a pleural effusion, severe pulmonary fibrosis, uncorrectable coagulation disorder, severe cardiac disease, and mechanical ventilation (34).

If the parietal and visceral pleura are well visualized during thoracoscopy, the diagnostic yield is excellent, especially for diagnosing MPEs. False-negative results are generally because of poor visualization of the pleural space because of pleural adhesions. Wilsher and Veale (15) reported a sensitivity of 80% in the diagnosis of pleural malignancy, which increased to 90% if only those cases in which full pleural access was achieved were considered. Blanc et al. (42) reported that they were unable to visualize the pleura in 6 of 149 cases; 4 were (43) later diagnosed with malignancy and 2 with tuberculous effusions. Munavvar and Lee (44) reported excellent visualization of the pleural space using a semirigid thoracoscope.

J. Techniques: Biopsy of the Parietal Pleura

Our recommended pleural biopsy technique is a standard technique that has been described in detail in previous reports (34,54,62,63). To briefly summarize, the patient is placed in a comfortable lateral decubitus position (with the affected side up) and is prepared and draped using strict aseptic technique. Moderate sedation is used for the procedure and the patient remains spontaneously breathing, with supplemental oxygen. Lidocaine is used for local anesthesia and is instilled at the chosen point of entry (usually the fourth to sixth intercostal space, mid-axillary line). After blunt dissection, a trocar is inserted and pleural fluid is evacuated using a blunt tip suction catheter. Air is allowed to enter the pleural space freely via the trocar, thus equilibrating intrapleural and atmospheric pressures. The thoracoscope is then inserted through the trocar. Once the pleural cavity is entered, almost complete visualization of the parietal and visceral pleura is possible if there are no pleural adhesions; only the posterior and the mediastinal side of the lung cannot be seen. Inspecting the pleural and performing biopsies are the two essential steps of the examination. The thoracoscopist must know about the anatomy of the thoracic cavity. In the right chest orientation can be achieved by locating the point where the three lobes meet, the junction of the oblique fissure and horizontal fissure. On the left, the oblique fissure can be used for orientation. The diaphragm can be recognized by the respiration-related movement. Rib, intercostal muscles, fat, blood vessels, and nerves are usually well distinguished. The heart and the great vessels are identified by pulsations that are occasionally transmitted to adjacent parts of the lung. In its normal state the pleura is transparent, allowing visualization of many structures through it. Variable amounts of anthracotic pigment can be seen within the visceral pleura and the surface of the lung. Fatty collections are often abundant in the pleura. These are long, yellowish plaques located along the ribs and around the pericardium and diaphragm. Malignancies often have a characteristic appearance, but it may be impossible to differentiate inflammation from malignancy on visual inspection. Multiple biopsies should therefore be taken from suspicious areas.

Parietal pleural biopsies can be performed using illuminated forceps through a single point of entry (Fig. 8). Before pleural biopsy, the rib and intercostal space should be identified with a blunt probe, such as the closed forceps; the rib will feel hard compared with the spongy intercostal space. When the pleura is thick, the biopsy is straightforward, with minimal risk of injuring the intercostal arteries. In contrast, when the pleura is thin, the biopsy should be performed against one of the ribs. Typically four to six biopsies of a suspicious pleural lesion will establish a diagnosis. When malignancy is suspected but the endoscopic findings are nonspecific, the number of biopsies should be increased to between 10 and 12, if possible, from a variety of areas on the pleural surface.

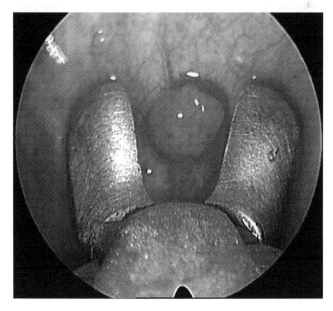

Figure 8 Optical biopsy forceps used through a single point of entry to obtain tissue samples of the parietal pleura.

K. Techniques: Biopsy of the Visceral Pleura and Lung Parenchyma

To biopsy the visceral pleura or obtain a lung biopsy using forceps, a second entry point is required so that an insulated forcep connected to electrocautery can be used. Whereas the initial trocar used to enter the pleural space is usually 7 mm in diameter and 100 mm in length, the second trocar is insulated and is 5 mm in diameter and 100 mm in length. The 5-mm double spoon–insulated coagulating forceps is used through this second trocar for visceral pleura or lung biopsies. Power should be sufficient to coagulate the cut surface of the lung without destroying the histological features of the specimen. A setting of approximately 100 W is appropriate. The forceps is used to grasp the selected site along the surface of the lung, avoiding the edges of lobes or fissures to minimize iatrogenic air leaks, and to pull the specimen through the trocar as electrocautery is applied.

L. Thoracoscopes

Medical thoracoscopy is performed using a rigid or semirigid endoscope. The use of fiberoptic bronchoscopes in the pleural space has been reported previously (64), and while it was reportedly feasible, the flexibility of the instrument made maneuvering and steering within the pleural cavity difficult. Oldenburg and Newhouse (51) compared the use of thoracoscopic examination with a flexible versus a rigid endoscope and found that the rigid instrument was superior because of the greater diagnostic accuracy. They reported that biopsy samples were significantly larger and easier to obtain using the rigid thoracoscope. Since Ernst originally reported the use of a semirigid pleuroscope (65), its utility has been verified and reported by other operators (43,44,66) and is now commercially available (Fig. 9). The advantage of the semirigid thoracoscope for pulmonologist is its similarity (handle, suction port and biopsy port) to a standard flexible bronchoscope; the proximal portion of the pleuroscope is rigid while the tip is flexible, combining the maneuverability of the rigid thoracoscope and the familiarity of a flexible bronchoscope (67).

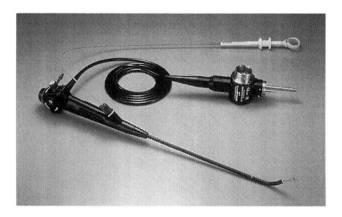

Figure 9 Semirigid thoracoscope.

III. Medical Thoracoscopy: Complications and Contraindications

In several large series, medical thoracoscopy was described as having few significant complications. Viskum and Enk (68) reported only one death in 8000 cases reviewed and Boutin et al. (6) had a mortality rate of 0.09% of 4300 cases. Major bleeding, requiring transfusion or surgical intervention, was exceedingly rare. Minor complications include a persistent air leak (approximately 2%), subcutaneous emphysema (a common result of the procedure, but not a significant complication), and postoperative fever.

Relative contraindications to pleuroscopy include poor general health of the patient, fever, unstable cardiovascular status, and hypoxemia not related to the pleural disease. Absolute contraindications include lack of pleural space, end-stage pulmonary fibrosis, mechanical ventilation, significant pulmonary hypertension, and uncontrolled coagulopathy (63).

IV. Therapeutic Uses of Medical Thoracoscopy

The major therapeutic role for pleuroscopy is to induce pleurodesis in patients with recurrent symptomatic pleural effusions, most commonly because of MPEs. Pleuroscopy can also be used to induce pleurodesis in patients with recurrent primary and secondary spontaneous pneumothoraces (Table 3).

A. Pleurodesis

Pleurodesis is the obliteration of the pleural space by the iatrogenic induction of symphysis between the parietal and visceral pleural layers, to prevent the accumulation of fluid or air within the pleural space (69). The most common indications for pleurodesis are MPEs or pneumothorax; the procedure may also be performed for recurrent non-MPEs.

Pleurodesis is accomplished by mechanical or chemical means. Mechanical pleurodesis is achieved using pleural abrasion or parietal pleurectomy, usually performed by thoracic surgeons during VATS (70). Chemical pleurodesis may be performed by the bedside instillation of a sclerosing agent via a chest tube, following drainage of the pleural cavity, or by the thoracoscopic insufflation of talc (71). Thoracoscopic talc pleurodesis (TTP) is the focus of this chapter section. Indications for TTP will first be reviewed, followed by a description of the technique of TTP and an evidence-based comparison of TTP with bedside pleurodesis via a chest tube. The side effects and complications of TTP are discussed, with attention to reports of respiratory failure and acute respiratory distress syndrome (ARDS) following talc pleurodesis, and the importance of adequate patient selection for TTP is emphasized.

Table 3 Indications for Therapeutic Thoracoscopy (Thoracoscopic Talc Poudrage) in Patients with Good Performance Status

Malignant pleural effusions causing dyspnea
Recurrence prevention for spontaneous pneumothorax
Recurrent, refractory nonmalignant pleural effusions causing dyspnea

Thoracoscopic Talc Pleurodesis: Indications

The most common indication for TTP is MPE (6,72–75). MPE is a significant source of morbidity for affected patients, with over half of them reporting dyspnea. TTP is also performed to prevent spontaneous pneumothorax recurrence (27,76,77). This is usually done in the context of a recurrent primary spontaneous pneumothorax, whether it is a second ipsilateral pneumothorax or first contralateral pneumothorax. Other indications include bilateral spontaneous pneumothorax, persistent air leak after five to seven days of tube drainage or failure to reexpand, spontaneous hemothorax, and professions at risk (e.g., divers and airline staff). Early pleurodesis is advocated for secondary spontaneous pneumothorax because of the increased risk of a recurrence, which may be life-threatening in patients with underlying lung disease (77,78). Finally, selected patients with recurrent, symptomatic non-MPE may also be treated with pleurodesis (79). The recommended selection criteria for such patients and reported success rates will be discussed.

Thoracoscopic Talc Pleurodesis: Technique

Talc is a natural, sheet-like, hydrated magnesium silicate with the chemical formula $Mg_3Si_4O_{10}(OH)_2$. There are many talc deposits worldwide and composition varies because of substitutions of magnesium with other cations and impurities. Sterilized, asbestos-free talc is used for pleurodesis (80,81). Talc insufflation (poudrage) may be performed during medical thoracoscopy.

The technique of medical thoracoscopy was reviewed earlier in this chapter. Once the thoracoscope is inserted through the trocar, the pleural space is thoroughly inspected and parietal pleural biopsies are taken when indicated. If TTP is to be done, sterile talc powder can then be insufflated using an atomizer or bulb syringe. In the United States, however, the only FDA-approved talc is supplied as an aerosol that uses dichloro-fluoromethane (CFC-12) as a propellant (Sclerosol®, Bryan Corporation). The thoracic cavity is inspected to confirm even talc distribution, and the "snowstorm" effect is observed. A chest tube is inserted and connected to suction, in order to evacuate all air and fluid, thus maintaining close apposition of pleural surfaces in order to achieve pleurodesis. Full lung reexpansion and chest tube position are verified by chest X ray, and the chest tube is removed once pleural fluid drainage decreases to less than 100 to 150 mL/day (62,63). If pleurodesis is being performed for spontaneous pneumothorax, the chest tube is removed when there is no evidence of an intrapleural air leak on bedside examination and no pneumothorax evident on chest radiograph when chest tube suction has been discontinued.

The mechanism by which talc leads to pleural fibrosis and obliteration of the pleural space is not completely understood, although a central role of the mesothelium in the cascade leading to pleurodesis is increasingly recognized (82,83). Talc rapidly induces an inflammatory response in the pleural cavity, characterized by the influx of polymorphonuclear neutrophils followed by macrophages and increased production of interleukin-8 and monocyte chemotactic protein-1 (84). In vitro, talc induces the expression of interleukin-8, monocyte chemotactic protein-1, and intercellular adhesion molecule-1 by mesothelial cells (85). Activation of the coagulation cascade and decreased fibrinolytic activity lead to the formation of a fibrin mesh that is the basis for subsequent fibrosis. There has been interest in identifying mediators of pleural fibrosis, downstream of the inflammatory process. Talc stimulates mesothelial cells to release basic fibroblast growth factor, leading to recruitment and proliferation of fibroblasts in the pleural space. In animal models, intrapleural administration of transforming growth factor-β induces pleurodesis without pleural inflammation (86,87). In the future, pleurodesis may be achieved using profibrotic cytokines, without the pain and fever associated with inflammation.

Thoracoscopic Talc Pleurodesis Vs. Bedside Pleurodesis

Chemical pleurodesis has been attempted with multiple agents other than talc including tetracycline and doxycycline, bleomycin, *Corynebacterium parvum*, quinacrine, cisplatin, and fluorouracil (71). Comparison between different sclerosing agents is rendered difficult by the lack of a standardized definition of successful pleurodesis across the various studies. Although there is no ideal pleurodesis agent, talc is widely considered to be the most effective and least expensive agent (74,88). The success rate of talc pleurodesis has been reported to be approximately 90%, although others have reported rates closer to 70% (71,80,89–97). Talc may be insufflated during medical thoracoscopy, or mixed with sterile normal saline into a slurry that is instilled via a chest tube (91).

There are several theoretical advantages to thoracoscopic talc insufflation compared with talc slurry sclerosis. Medical thoracoscopy allows complete effusion drainage under direct visualization and optimal chest tube positioning. Talc is insufflated in a manner that allows even distribution over the entire visceral and parietal pleural surfaces. In contrast, the slurry of water-insoluble talc may gravitate to the dependent part of the pleural space shortly after instillation, and rotation has not been shown to improve talc slurry distribution and pleurodesis (98). Finally, in patients with an underlying malignancy but negative fluid cytology, parietal pleural biopsies of suspicious areas can be taken at the time of medical thoracoscopy, before proceeding with pleurodesis. A systematic review comparing the various treatment options to achieve pleurodesis in patients with MPE was published in the *Cochrane Database* in 2004 (74). The comparison of TTP and talc slurry pleurodesis favored thoracoscopic pleurodesis, with a relative risk for nonrecurrence of the effusion of 1.19 (95% CI, 1.04–1.36).

A large, multicenter randomized trial comparing talc poudrage with talc slurry was conducted by the North American Cooperative Oncology Groups (91) in which a total of 482 patients were randomized to thoracoscopy with talc insufflation ($n = 242$) or tube thoracostomy with talc slurry ($n = 240$). Overall, no difference was detected in the percentage of patients with successful pleurodesis at 30 days (78% for TTP and 71% for talc slurry). However, in the subgroup of patients with primary lung or breast cancer, the success rate of TTP was found to be significantly higher than with talc slurry (82% vs. 67%, $p = 0.022$). Lung cancer and breast cancer are the first and second most common neoplasms causing malignant effusions, and these findings suggest that TTP may be a better option for a large proportion of patients with MPE.

There are little data on the role of TTP versus talc slurry in patients with primary or secondary spontaneous pneumothorax (76). For the prevention of pneumothorax recurrence, surgical referral for VATS is generally recommended (77,78). Use of medical thoracoscopy for inspection, coagulation of small blebs or bullae and talc poudrage has been advocated by some authors (9,10,27), with referral for VATS in patients with numerous large bullae. Talcage by medical thoracoscopy for primary spontaneous pneumothorax was shown to be more cost-effective than chest tube drainage in a prospective randomized study; the long-term recurrence rate of pneumothorax with thoracoscopic talc insufflation was comparable to VATS (about 5%) (99). Chest tube instillation of a sclerosing agent should be reserved for patients who are unwilling to undergo medical or surgical thoracoscopy, and have contraindications to the procedures or a poor prognosis from severe underlying disease (77,78). In a review of pleurodesis for non-MPE, Sudduth and Sahn reported an 80% success rate for chemical pleurodesis using various agents and techniques (100). Gyorik et al. (101) reported a 95% success rate of TTP for primary spontaneous pneumothorax. No formal comparison of talc slurry and TTP for the treatment of pneumothorax has been conducted.

Side Effects and Complications of Thoracoscopic Talc Pleurodesis

The most common side effects reported with TTP are pain and fever. In their detailed review of pleurodesis agents, Walker-Renard and colleagues (71) reported pain following talc insufflation in 9 of 131 patients (7%), and fever in 21 of 131 patients (16%). Fever has been described in 16% to 69% of patients undergoing talc poudrage or talc slurry pleurodesis. Froudarakis and colleagues (102) questioned whether the systemic inflammatory response associated with TTP was because of talc poudrage or thoracoscopy. The authors prospectively compared postprocedure temperature, WBC count, and C-reactive protein levels in patients undergoing TTP versus diagnostic thoracoscopy alone, and concluded that fever and systemic inflammatory reaction was because of talc and not thoracoscopy. Empyema following TTP has been reported in 0% to 3% of patients and local site infection is uncommon (80,97,103). Cardiovascular complications reported with TTP include arrhythmias, cardiac arrest, chest pain, myocardial infarction, and hypotension; these may be attributable to the procedure and not talc per se (75). Most concerning have been reports of respiratory failure following both thoracoscopic talc poudrage and talc slurry pleurodesis.

Rinaldo et al. reported (104) three patients who developed ARDS following the instillation of 10 g of talc slurry. A case of acute pneumonitis with bilateral pleural effusions after instillation of only 2 g of talc was reported by Bouchama and colleagues (105). Nandi (106) reported one death from respiratory failure, three days after talc poudrage (and another six weeks postprocedure); Todd et al. had seven cases of respiratory failure and/or pneumonia in 178 patients who underwent 197 intrapleural talc insufflations for MPE (107). In a review of 56 patients who underwent 73 talc slurry pleurodesis procedures at a single center, 3 cases of respiratory failure occurred following the procedures, with one being directly attributed to talc (108). Campos (109) reported four cases of respiratory failure 24 to 48 hours following the thoracoscopic insufflation of 2 g of talc. The same authors reviewed their 15-year experience with TTP and reported respiratory failure in 1.3% of cases (110). Rehse and colleagues (111) reported the highest rate of respiratory complications (33%) following talc pleurodesis, with 9% of patients developing ARDS. More recently, in the randomized trial of TTP versus talc slurry for MPE conducted by the Cooperative Oncology Groups, respiratory failure was observed in 4% of patients treated with talc slurry and 8% of patients randomized to TTP (91).

Interestingly, other large series of patients undergoing TTP have reported no cases of respiratory failure. Weissberg and Ben-Zeev (112) reported no procedure-related deaths in their experience of 360 patients treated with TTP. In a French series of 360 patients who underwent TTP using Luzenac talc, no cases of talc-induced acute respiratory failure were reported (97). More recently, a German group reported a consecutive series of 102 patients who underwent medical thoracoscopy and TTP for recurrent MPE; no episode of talc-induced ARDS was observed (73).

The pathogenesis of acute pneumonitis and talc-induced ARDS remains incompletely understood. The influence of talc dose on extrapleural talc dissemination following pleurodesis was examined in a rabbit model by Mones and colleagues; they found that a higher talc dose was associated with an increased risk of extrapleural talc deposition based on histopathological evaluations (113). Although the use of a maximal dose of 4 to 5 g of talc has been advocated (75), ARDS has occurred following both large and small doses of talc, and with either thoracoscopic insufflation or instillation of talc slurry. Some hypothesize that the apparent geographic variability in the occurrence of talc-induced ARDS (many of the reports of talc-induced ARDS have come from the United States) may reflect differences in the talc preparations used.

Differences in the particle size distribution and presence of contaminants were examined in eight different talc preparations used for pleurodesis, and marked variations were noted (81). The mean particle size of U.S. talc ranged from 10 to 20 μm, versus 33 μm for French talc, with a larger proportion of small particles (<10 μm) in U.S. talc preparations. Ferrer et al. also investigated the influence of talc particle size on extrapleural talc dissemination after talc slurry pleurodesis in rabbits (114). The intrapleural injection of normal talc resulted in greater pulmonary and systemic talc particle deposition than large talc. In a small randomized of mixed talc (mean particle size <15 μm) versus graded talc (most particles <10 μm removed), mixed talc was found to worsen gas exchange and induce more systemic inflammation (115). The systemic distribution of small talc particles with subsequent inflammation has been suggested as a possible mechanism for acute pneumonitis and ARDS. This hypothesis is corroborated by the autopsy finding of disseminated talc crystals in the lung, liver, kidney, heart, and skeletal muscle in a patient who died of respiratory failure after TTP (109).

The diameter of pleural stomata is reported to be approximately 6 to 7 μm (116), thus allowing the passage of talc particles of small size. Large-particle talc, also referred to as "graded" or "calibrated" talc, is talc from which the small particles (<10 μm) have been mostly removed. Two large prospective studies from Europe were recently published that attest to the safety of large-particle talc. In a multicenter, prospective cohort study (103), 558 patients with MPE underwent TTP with 4 g of calibrated French large-particle talc. There were no cases of ARDS reported. In another series of 112 patients who underwent TTP for primary spontaneous pneumothorax using French graded talc, no episodes of acute respiratory failure following pleurodesis were observed (101).

Concerns about the long-term safety of talc pleurodesis have arisen because of reports of malignancy in talc miners and millers. The possible development of restrictive lung disease as a result of diffuse pleural fibrosis was an additional consideration. The link between talc and cancer has been attributed to asbestos fibers within the talc. Lange et al. (117) reported no cases of mesothelioma after 22 to 35 years of follow-up of patients treated with talc poudrage for idiopathic spontaneous pneumothorax. In the same series, patients who received talc had a slightly lower total lung capacity than patients treated with tube thoracostomy alone (89% vs. 97%), which is unlikely to be clinically significant. In the series of patients undergoing TTP for primary spontaneous pneumothorax from Gyorik and colleagues, after a shorter median follow-up of 118 months, patients with successful pleurodesis had a median forced vital capacity of 102% and median total lung capacity of 99% of predicted (101).

Patient Selection for Thoracoscopic Talc Pleurodesis

The reported success rate of TTP varies according to the indications for the procedure, and ranges from 70% to 90% for MPE, as discussed above. For non-MPE, a success rate of 80% to 90% has been reported in small series (79,100), although the success rate may vary according to the underlying condition, with higher recurrence rates for hepatic hydrothorax (118). Kennedy and Sahn reported an overall success rate of 91% for talc pleurodesis in pneumothorax (80).

Successful pleurodesis requires contact of the visceral and parietal pleura. In patients with a symptomatic pleural effusion, the initial thoracentesis plays a key role in patient selection. The degree to which symptoms are alleviated by the pleural fluid drainage should be assessed, and lung reexpansion posttap should be demonstrated. Failure of dyspnea to improve, particularly in patients with MPE, suggests an alternate diagnosis such as pulmonary embolism, atelectasis, or lymphangitic carcinomatosis. Incomplete lung reexpansion may result from mainstem bronchus occlusion by tumor, or trapped lung because of extensive pleural infiltration.

Safe and successful medical thoracoscopy and pleurodesis, in large part, depends on judicious patient selection. Burrows et al. (119) examined predictors of survival in patients with recurrent symptomatic MPE referred for thoracoscopic pleurodesis, and found that only the Karnofsky performance status score was predictive of survival. The authors proposed that a Karnofsky score ≥ 70, which was associated with a median survival of 395 days, may be a reasonable marker for deciding which patients with MPE should undergo TTP. In patients with MPE, overall prognosis should thus be considered in the selection of patients for TTP. The median survival of patients with MPE varies from 6 to 18 months. The various management options for recurrent MPE include repeated therapeutic thoracentesis, bedside chest tube pleurodesis, TTP, placement of an indwelling pleural catheter (PleurX®), and surgical procedures such as pleurectomy or pleuroperitoneal shunting. In patients with a low performance status and limited life expectancy, placement of an indwelling pleural catheter may be the most appropriate therapeutic option; with repeated drainage, up to half of these patients may develop spontaneous pleurodesis.

V. Summary

Medical thoracoscopy has emerged as a valuable tool for the chest physician to evaluate pleural diseases. Also known as pleuroscopy, medical thoracoscopy allows thorough inspection of the pleural space and visually directed biopsies of the pleura. The main diagnostic indication for pleuroscopy is for the investigation of pleural effusions for which no cause has been found despite initial testing, including pleural fluid analysis and closed-needle pleural biopsy. Several studies have shown the increased yield that thoracoscopy provides, especially if the underlying cause is pleural malignancy; the sensitivity and specificity of pleuroscopy for the diagnosis of MPEs is high according to several studies cited in this chapter. It is also useful in differentiating benign effusions from malignant effusions with a high degree of certainty, provided that inspection of the pleural space and biopsy of the pleura were adequate. Diagnostic medical thoracoscopy should therefore be considered in those 25% of cases of pleural effusions in which the etiology is unknown.

Thoracoscopic talc poudrage is a simple and effective method of pleurodesis. On the basis of currently available data, this method should be considered the preferred technique for many patients with MPE, in particular those with underlying lung or breast cancer. It also has selected indications for the prevention of spontaneous pneumothorax recurrence and the management of refractory benign effusions. Talc insufflation is performed during medical thoracoscopy, using local anesthesia and conscious sedation, without the need for an OR (operating room). Several reports of ARDS following talc pleurodesis have emanated from the United States, and this appears related to the use of smaller size talc particles, which can be systemically absorbed. The safety of large-particle talc pleurodesis was recently confirmed in two large European studies. Future studies of the various pleurodesis agents and techniques need to use standardized definitions of pleurodesis success and failure, as recommended in the most recent ATS guidelines on the management of MPE (75).

References

1. Gunnels JJ. Perplexing pleural effusion. Chest 1978; 74:390–393.
2. Light RW. Pleural Diseases. 5th ed. Philadelphia: Lippincott Williams & Wilkins, 2007.
3. Mathur PN, Loddenkemper R. Medical thoracoscopy. Role in pleural and lung diseases. Clin Chest Med 1995; 16:487–496.
4. Poe RH, Israel RH, Utell MJ, et al. Sensitivity, specificity, and predictive values of closed pleural biopsy. Arch Intern Med 1984; 144:325–328.
5. Ryan CJ, Rodgers RF, Unni KK, et al. The outcome of patients with pleural effusion of indeterminate cause at thoracotomy. Mayo Clin Proc 1981; 56:145–149.
6. Boutin C, Viallat JR, Cargnino P, et al. Thoracoscopy in malignant pleural effusions. Am Rev Respir Dis 1981; 124:588–592.
7. Canto A, Blasco E, Casillas M, et al. Thoracoscopy in the diagnosis of pleural effusion. Thorax 1977; 32:550–554.
8. Harris RJ, Kavuru MS, Rice TW, et al. The diagnostic and therapeutic utility of thoracoscopy. A review. Chest 1995; 108:828–841.
9. Loddenkemper R. Thoracoscopy—state of the art. Eur Respir J 1998; 11:213–221.
10. Loddenkemper R, Schonfeld N. Medical thoracoscopy. Curr Opin Pulm Med 1998; 4:235–238.
11. Menzies R, Charbonneau M. Thoracoscopy for the diagnosis of pleural disease. Ann Intern Med 1991; 114:271–276.
12. Weissberg D, Kaufmann M. Diagnostic and therapeutic pleuroscopy. Experience with 127 patients. Chest 1980; 78:732–735.
13. Wang Z, Tong ZH, Li HJ, et al. Semi-rigid thoracoscopy for undiagnosed exudative pleural effusions: a comparative study. Chin Med J (Engl) 2008; 121:1384–1389.
14. Tscheikuna J. Medical thoracoscopy: experiences in Siriraj Hospital. J Med Assoc Thai 2006; 89(suppl 5):S62–S66.
15. Wilsher ML, Veale AG. Medical thoracoscopy in the diagnosis of unexplained pleural effusion. Respirology 1998; 3:77–80.
16. Martensson G, Hagmar B, Zettergren L. Diagnosis and prognosis in malignant pleural mesothelioma: a prospective study. Eur J Respir Dis 1984; 65:169–178.
17. Boutin C, Rey F. Thoracoscopy in pleural malignant mesothelioma: a prospective study of 188 consecutive patients. Part 1: Diagnosis. Cancer 1993; 72:389–393.
18. Boutin C, Rey F, Gouvernet J, et al. Thoracoscopy in pleural malignant mesothelioma: a prospective study of 188 consecutive patients. Part 2: Prognosis and staging. Cancer 1993; 72:394–404.
19. Sakuraba M, Masuda K, Hebisawa A, et al. Diagnostic value of thoracoscopic pleural biopsy for pleurisy under local anaesthesia. ANZ J Surg 2006; 76:722–724.
20. Decker DA, Dines DE, Payne WS, et al. The significance of a cytologically negative pleural effusion in bronchogenic carcinoma. Chest 1978; 74:640–642.

21. Abrams LD. A pleural-biopsy punch. Lancet 1958; 1:30–31.
22. Cope C. New pleural biopsy needle: preliminary study. J Am Med Assoc 1958; 167.
23. Defrancis N, Klosk E, Albano E. Needle biopsy of the parietal pleura: a preliminary report. N Engl J Med 1955; 252:948–951.
24. Scerbo J, Keltz H, Stone DJ. A prospective study of closed pleural biopsies. JAMA 1971; 218:377–380.
25. Loddenkemper R, Mai J, Scheffler N, et al. Prospective individual comparison of blind needle biopsy and of thoracoscopy in the diagnosis and differential diagnosis of tuberculous pleurisy. Scand J Respir Dis Suppl 1978; 102:196–198.
26. Colt HG. Thoracoscopic management of pneumothorax. In: Beamis JF, Mathur PN, eds. Interventional Pulmonology. New York: McGraw-Hill, 1999:207–219.
27. Boutin C, Astoul P, Rey F, Mathur PN. Thoracoscopy in the diagnosis and treatment of spontaneous pneumothorax. Clin Chest Med 1995; 16:497–503.
28. Janssen JP, Schramel FM, Sutedja TG, et al. Videothoracoscopic appearance of first and recurrent pneumothorax. Chest 1995; 108:330–334.
29. Boutin C, Viallat JR, Cargnino P, et al. Thoracoscopic lung biopsy. Experimental and clinical preliminary study. Chest 1982; 82:44–48.
30. Dijkman JH, van der Meer JW, Bakker W, et al. Transpleural lung biopsy by the thoracoscopic route in patients with diffuse interstitial pulmonary disease. Chest 1982; 82:76–83.
31. Colt HG, Russack V, Shanks TG, et al. Comparison of wedge to forceps videothoracoscopic lung biopsy. Gross and histologic findings. Chest 1995; 107:546–550.
32. Kennedy L, Sahn SA. Noninvasive evaluation of the patient with a pleural effusion. Chest Surg Clin N Am 1994; 4:451–465.
33. Collins TR, Sahn SA. Thoracocentesis. Clinical value, complications, technical problems, and patient experience. Chest 1987; 91:817–822.
34. Villanueva AG, Beamis JF. Medical thoracoscopy: diagnosis of pleural pulmonary disorders. In: Beamis JF, Mathur PN, Mehta AC, eds. Interventional Pulmonary Medicine. New York: Marcel Dekker, 2004:431–449.
35. Chang SC, Perng RP. The role of fiberoptic bronchoscopy in evaluating the causes of pleural effusions. Arch Intern Med 1989; 149:855–857.
36. Feinsilver SH, Barrows AA, Braman SS. Fiberoptic bronchoscopy and pleural effusion of unknown origin. Chest 1986; 90:516–519.
37. Baumann MH. Closed needle pleural biopsy: a necessary tool? Pulm Perspect 2000; 17:1–3.
38. Accreditation Council for Graduate Medical Education. Internal Medicine Program Requirements. Available at: http://www.acgme.org/acWebsite/RRC_140/140_prIndex.asp. Accessed June 12, 2009.,)
39. Baumann MH. Closed pleural biopsy: not dead yet! Chest 2006; 129:1398–1400.
40. Enk B, Viskum K. Diagnostic thoracoscopy. Eur J Respir Dis 1981; 62:344–351.
41. Martensson G, Pettersson K, Thiringer G. Differentiation between malignant and non-malignant pleural effusion. Eur J Respir Dis 1985; 67:326–334.
42. Blanc FX, Atassi K, Bignon J, et al. Diagnostic value of medical thoracoscopy in pleural disease: a 6-year retrospective study. Chest 2002; 121:1677–1683.
43. Munavvar M, Khan MA, Edwards J, et al. The autoclavable semirigid thoracoscope: the way forward in pleural disease? Eur Respir J 2007; 29:571–574.
44. Lee P, Hsu A, Lo C, et al. Prospective evaluation of flex-rigid pleuroscopy for indeterminate pleural effusion: accuracy, safety and outcome. Respirology 2007; 12:881–886.
45. Canto A, Rivas J, Saumench J, et al. Points to consider when choosing a biopsy method in cases of pleurisy of unknown origin. Chest 1983; 84:176–179.
46. Canto-Armengod A. Macroscopic characteristics of pleural metastases arising from the breast and observed by diagnostic thoracoscopy. Am Rev Respir Dis 1990; 142:616–618.
47. Canto A, Ferrer G, Romagosa V, et al. Lung cancer and pleural effusion. Clinical significance and study of pleural metastatic locations. Chest 1985; 87:649–652.
48. Meyer PC. Metastatic carcinoma of the pleura. Thorax 1966; 21:437–443.

49. Rodriguez-Panadero F, Borderas Naranjo F, Lopez Mejias J. Pleural metastatic tumours and effusions. Frequency and pathogenic mechanisms in a post-mortem series. Eur Respir J 1989; 2:366–369.
50. Anderson CB, Philpott GW, Ferguson TB. The treatment of malignant pleural effusions. Cancer 1974; 33:916–922.
51. Oldenburg FA Jr., Newhouse MT. Thoracoscopy. A safe, accurate diagnostic procedure using the rigid thoracoscope and local anesthesia. Chest 1979; 75:45–50.
52. Hansen M, Faurschou P, Clementsen P. Medical thoracoscopy, results and complications in 146 patients: a retrospective study. Respir Med 1998; 92:228–232.
53. Boutin C, Viallat JR, Aelony Y. Practical Thoracoscopy. New York: Springer Verlag, 1991.
54. Astoul P, Boutin C. The role of thoracoscopy for the diagnosis and treatment of pleural cancers. In: Beamis JF, Mathur PN, eds. Interventional Pulmonology. New York: McGraw-Hill, 1999:185–205.
55. Faurschou P, Francis D, Faarup P. Thoracoscopic, histological, and clinical findings in nine case of rheumatoid pleural effusion. Thorax 1985; 40:371–375.
56. Ferrer JS, Munoz XG, Orriols RM, et al. Evolution of idiopathic pleural effusion: a prospective, long-term follow-up study. Chest 1996; 109:1508–1513.
57. Mouchantaf FG, Villanueva AG. The long-term prognosis of patients with the diagnosis of nonmalignant pleural effusions after pleuroscopy. J Bronchol Intervent Pulmonol 2009; 16:25–27.
58. Colt HG. Thoracoscopy. A prospective study of safety and outcome. Chest 1995; 108:324–329.
59. Harris RJ, Kavuru MS, Mehta AC, et al. The impact of thoracoscopy on the management of pleural disease. Chest 1995; 107:845–852.
60. Noppen M, Dekeukeleire T, Hanon S, et al. Fluorescein-enhanced autofluorescence thoracoscopy in patients with primary spontaneous pneumothorax and normal subjects. Am J Respir Crit Care Med 2006; 174:26–30.
61. Bonniot JP, Homasson JP, Roden SL, et al. Pleural and lung cryobiopsies during thoracoscopy. Chest 1989; 95:492–493.
62. Mathur PN, Astoul P, Boutin C. Medical thoracoscopy. Technical details. Clin Chest Med 1995; 16:479–486.
63. Wohlrab JL, Read CA. Medical thoracoscopy: therapy for malignant conditions. In: Beamis JF, Mathur PN, Mehta AC, eds. Interventional Pulmonary Medicine. New York: Marcel Dekker, 2004:451–468.
64. Robinson GR 2nd, Gleeson K. Diagnostic flexible fiberoptic pleuroscopy in suspected malignant pleural effusions. Chest 1995; 107:424–429.
65. Ernst A, Hersh CP, Herth F, et al. A novel instrument for the evaluation of the pleural space: an experience in 34 patients. Chest 2002; 122:1530–1534.
66. Lee P, Colt HG. Rigid and semirigid pleuroscopy: the future is bright. Respirology 2005; 10:418–425.
67. Lee P, Colt HG. Flex-Rigid Pleuroscopy: Step by Step. Singapore: CMP Medica Asia, 2005.
68. Viskum K, Enk B. Complications of thoracoscopy. Poumon Coeur 1981; 37:25–28.
69. Rodriguez-Panadero F, Antony VB. Pleurodesis: state of the art. Eur Respir J 1997; 10:1648–1654.
70. Ronson RS, Miller JI Jr. Video-assisted thoracoscopy for pleural disease. Chest Surg Clin N Am 1998; 8:919–932, x.
71. Walker-Renard PB, Vaughan LM, Sahn SA. Chemical pleurodesis for malignant pleural effusions. Ann Intern Med 1994; 120:56–64.
72. Haas AR, Sterman DH, Musani AI. Malignant pleural effusions: management options with consideration of coding, billing, and a decision approach. Chest 2007; 132:1036–1041.
73. Kolschmann S, Ballin A, Gillissen A. Clinical efficacy and safety of thoracoscopic talc pleurodesis in malignant pleural effusions. Chest 2005; 128:1431–1435.

74. Shaw PHS, Agarwal R. Pleurodesis for malignant pleural effusions. Cochrane Database Syst Rev 2004; 1:CD002916.
75. American Thoracic Society. Management of malignant pleural effusions. Am J Respir Crit Care Med 2000; 162:1987–2001.
76. Baumann MH. Medical thoracoscopy: therapy for benign conditions. In: Beamis JF, Mathur PN, Mehta AC, eds. Interventional Pulmonary Medicine. New York: Marcel Dekker, 2004:469–482.
77. Baumann MH, Strange C, Heffner JE, et al. Management of spontaneous pneumothorax: an American College of Chest Physicians Delphi consensus statement. Chest 2001; 119:590–602.
78. Henry M, Arnold T, Harvey J. BTS guidelines for the management of spontaneous pneumothorax. Thorax 2003; 58(suppl 2):ii39–ii52.
79. Vargas FS, Milanez JR, Filomeno LT, et al. Intrapleural talc for the prevention of recurrence in benign or undiagnosed pleural effusions. Chest 1994; 106:1771–1775.
80. Kennedy L, Sahn SA. Talc pleurodesis for the treatment of pneumothorax and pleural effusion. Chest 1994; 106:1215–1222.
81. Ferrer J, Villarino MA, Tura JM, et al. Talc preparations used for pleurodesis vary markedly from one preparation to another. Chest 2001; 119:1901–1905.
82. Jantz MA, Antony VB. Pathophysiology of the pleura. Respiration 2008; 75:121–133.
83. Marchi E, Vargas FS, Acencio MM, et al. Evidence that mesothelial cells regulate the acute inflammatory response in talc pleurodesis. Eur Respir J 2006; 28:929–932.
84. van den Heuvel MM, Smit HJ, Barbierato SB, et al. Talc-induced inflammation in the pleural cavity. Eur Respir J 1998; 12:1419–1423.
85. Nasreen N, Hartman DL, Mohammed KA, et al. Talc-induced expression of C-C and C-X-C chemokines and intercellular adhesion molecule-1 in mesothelial cells. Am J Respir Crit Care Med 1998; 158:971–978.
86. Light RW, Cheng DS, Lee YC, et al. A single intrapleural injection of transforming growth factor-beta(2) produces an excellent pleurodesis in rabbits. Am J Respir Crit Care Med 2000; 162:98–104.
87. Lee YC, Lane KB, Parker RE, et al. Transforming growth factor beta(2) (TGF beta(2)) produces effective pleurodesis in sheep with no systemic complications. Thorax 2000; 55:1058–1062.
88. Colt HG, Davoudi M. The ideal pleurodesis agent: still searching after all these years. Lancet Oncol 2008; 9:912–913.
89. Aelony Y, King R, Boutin C. Thoracoscopic talc poudrage pleurodesis for chronic recurrent pleural effusions. Ann Intern Med 1991; 115:778–782.
90. Aelony Y, King RR, Boutin C. Thoracoscopic talc poudrage in malignant pleural effusions: effective pleurodesis despite low pleural pH. Chest 1998; 113:1007–1012.
91. Dresler CM, Olak J, Herndon JE II, et al. Phase III intergroup study of talc poudrage vs talc slurry sclerosis for malignant pleural effusion. Chest 2005; 127:909–915.
92. Fentiman IS, Rubens RD, Hayward JL. A comparison of intracavitary talc and tetracycline for the control of pleural effusions secondary to breast cancer. Eur J Cancer Clin Oncol 1986; 22:1079–1081.
93. Hamed H, Fentiman IS, Chaudary MA, et al. Comparison of intracavitary bleomycin and talc for control of pleural effusions secondary to carcinoma of the breast. Br J Surg 1989; 76:1266–1267.
94. Hartman DL, Gaither JM, Kesler KA, et al. Comparison of insufflated talc under thoracoscopic guidance with standard tetracycline and bleomycin pleurodesis for control of malignant pleural effusions. J Thorac Cardiovasc Surg 1993; 105:743–747; discussion 7–8.
95. Steger V, Mika U, Toomes H, et al. Who gains most? A 10-year experience with 611 thoracoscopic talc pleurodeses. Ann Thorac Surg 2007; 83:1940–1945.
96. Tschopp JM, Schnyder JM, Astoul P, et al. Pleurodesis by talc poudrage under simple medical thoracoscopy: an international opinion. Thorax 2009; 64:273–274; author reply 4.

97. Viallat JR, Rey F, Astoul P, et al. Thoracoscopic talc poudrage pleurodesis for malignant effusions. A review of 360 cases. Chest 1996; 110:1387–1393.
98. Mager HJ, Maesen B, Verzijlbergen F, et al. Distribution of talc suspension during treatment of malignant pleural effusion with talc pleurodesis. Lung Cancer 2002; 36:77–81.
99. Tschopp JM, Boutin C, Astoul P, et al. Talcage by medical thoracoscopy for primary spontaneous pneumothorax is more cost-effective than drainage: a randomised study. Eur Respir J 2002; 20:1003–1009.
100. Sudduth CD, Sahn SA. Pleurodesis for nonmalignant pleural effusions. Recommendations. Chest 1992; 102:1855–1860.
101. Gyorik S, Erni S, Studler U, et al. Long-term follow-up of thoracoscopic talc pleurodesis for primary spontaneous pneumothorax. Eur Respir J 2007; 29:757–760.
102. Froudarakis ME, Klimathianaki M, Pougounias M. Systemic inflammatory reaction after thoracoscopic talc poudrage. Chest 2006; 129:356–361.
103. Janssen JP, Collier G, Astoul P, et al. Safety of pleurodesis with talc poudrage in malignant pleural effusion: a prospective cohort study. Lancet 2007; 369:1535–1539.
104. Rinaldo JE, Owens GR, Rogers RM. Adult respiratory distress syndrome following intrapleural instillation of talc. J Thorac Cardiovasc Surg 1983; 85:523–526.
105. Bouchama A, Chastre J, Gaudichet A, et al. Acute pneumonitis with bilateral pleural effusion after talc pleurodesis. Chest 1984; 86:795–797.
106. Nandi P. Recurrent spontaneous pneumothorax: an effective method of talc poudrage. Chest 1980; 77:493–495.
107. Todd TRJ, Delarue NC, Ilves R, et al. Talc poudrage for malignant pleural effusion. Chest 1980; 78:542–543.
108. Kennedy L, Rusch VW, Strange C, et al. Pleurodesis using talc slurry. Chest 1994; 106:342–346.
109. Campos JR, Werebe EC, Vargas FS, et al. Respiratory failure due to insufflated talc. Lancet 1997; 349:251–252.
110. de Campos JR, Vargas FS, de Campos Werebe E, et al. Thoracoscopy talc poudrage: a 15-year experience. Chest 2001; 119:801–806.
111. Rehse DH, Aye RW, Florence MG. Respiratory failure following talc pleurodesis. Am J Surg 1999; 177:437–440.
112. Weissberg D, Ben-Zeev I. Talc pleurodesis. Experience with 360 patients. J Thorac Cardiovasc Surg 1993; 106:689–695.
113. Montes JF, Ferrer J, Villarino MA, et al. Influence of talc dose on extrapleural talc dissemination after talc pleurodesis. Am J Respir Crit Care Med 2003; 168:348–355.
114. Ferrer J, Montes JF, Villarino MA, et al. Influence of particle size on extrapleural talc dissemination after talc slurry pleurodesis. Chest 2002; 122:1018–1027.
115. Maskell NA, Lee YC, Gleeson FV, et al. Randomized trials describing lung inflammation after pleurodesis with talc of varying particle size. Am J Respir Crit Care Med 2004; 170:377–382.
116. Li J. Ultrastructural study on the pleural stomata in human. Funct Dev Morphol 1993; 3:277–280.
117. Lange P, Mortensen J, Groth S. Lung function 22–35 years after treatment of idiopathic spontaneous pneumothorax with talc poudrage or simple drainage. Thorax 1988; 43:559–561.
118. Milanez de Campos JR, Filho LO, de Campos Werebe E, et al. Thoracoscopy and talc poudrage in the management of hepatic hydrothorax. Chest 2000; 118:13–17.
119. Burrows CM, Mathews WC, Colt HG. Predicting survival in patients with recurrent symptomatic malignant pleural effusions: an assessment of the prognostic values of physiologic, morphologic, and quality of life measures of extent of disease. Chest 2000; 117:73–78.

8
Tunneled Pleural Catheters

PAUL MACEACHERN, DAVID STATHER, and ALAIN TREMBLAY
University of Calgary, Calgary, Alberta, Canada

I. Overview

Malignant disease is a frequent cause of exudative pleural effusion, accounting for 42% to 77% of cases (1,2). Bronchogenic carcinoma is the most frequent cause of malignant pleural effusion (MPE) accounting for 24% to 52% of cases (2–5), and with 8% to 15% of all lung cancer patients presenting with malignant effusion and pleural metastasis (1,6). Breast cancer and lymphoma are the next most common cause of MPE, responsible for 13% to 26% and 7% to 26% of cases, respectively (2–5). Ovarian, gastrointestinal, and mesothelial malignancies are additional common causes of MPE. Almost all other cancers have occasionally been documented to cause MPE and, as a group, may be responsible for up to 14% of cases (3).

Patients with MPE usually present with dyspnea. This is the primary complaint in more than half of the cases (1). They may also present with chest pain or cough while some patients may be asymptomatic. Chest pain is a particularly common complaint in patients with mesothelioma.

A malignant effusion usually portends a poor prognosis. In lung cancer, MPE eliminates the possibility of surgical or other aggressive oncologic curative intent treatment modalities. For most other cancers, a malignant effusion indicates metastatic disease and incurability, with the exception of lymphoma where the presence of an effusion has not been shown to affect prognosis (7). The focus of intervention must then become symptom palliation and quality of life rather than oncological cure.

II. Standard Treatments

Multiple options exist for the management of MPE including therapeutic thoracentesis, pleurodesis with a sclerosing agent (via chest tube or thoracoscopy), pleurectomy, and long-term drainage with tunneled pleural catheters (TPCs). Because of the multiple options, professional societies have produced guidelines for MPE management (1,8). Which management strategy will ultimately be chosen depends on the clinical scenario, patient preference, and locally available expertise.

In some cases, such as initial presentations of lymphoma and small cell lung cancer, consideration should be given to treating the underlying malignancy as the primary modality for MPE treatment, as a rapid response to systemic chemotherapy is common. These patients can usually avoid complex pleural interventions other than one or two therapeutic thoracentesis for symptom relief. For symptomatic patients whose effusion is not expected to respond rapidly to systemic therapy, more definitive management of the effusion is usually required. We recommend that symptomatic patients undergo a therapeutic thoracentesis as part of their initial management, as on occasion, removal of large volumes of fluid will not result in relief of dyspnea. This usually indicates additional underlying pathologies such as lymphangitic carcinomatosis, malignant airway obstruction, trapped lung, pulmonary embolus, coexistent cardiac or pericardial disease, COPD, or interstitial lung disease. Patients who do get relief of symptoms are candidates for more definitive management of their pleural fluid.

In general, it is accepted that repeated thoracentesis, pleuroperitoneal shunting, and pleurectomy are less than ideal treatment options for MPE and only useful in well-selected patients (1,8–13). Therapeutic thoracentesis in the treatment of MPE is usually only a temporary solution, as pleural fluid usually recurs quickly. Because of the significant morbidity and mortality associated with pleurectomy, this procedure is rarely used in MPE management (14). Pleuroperitoneal shunting has been reported but is often limited by cost and shunt malfunction (15,16).

A. Pleurodesis

Pleurodesis procedures remain common therapeutic modalities in the management of MPE and have generally been accepted as the gold standard for its treatment (1,8–13), although not an ideal approach for all patients and not without potential complications. Side effects can include pain (17–24), fever (24–28), and prolonged drainage (25–27), and over 40 cases of talc-induced respiratory failure have been reported in the literature (13,21,25,29,30). These procedures typically require hospitalizations of approximately seven days (27,31,32). Despite its widespread application, few randomized controlled trials have addressed the optimal way to create a pleurodesis, with many studies often lacking clear definitions of success or failure and rarely describing the effects on patient symptoms or long-term outcomes. Intention to treat analyses are uncommon, with many studies excluding patients that did not achieve full lung reexpansion following chest drain insertion or at thoracoscopy and those not surviving to 30 days, accounting for as many as 40% of patients studied in some reports (28,33). High success rates reported with talc pleurodesis (28,32,34–36) have not been reproduced in large prospective trials, and recurrences later than 30 days post treatment are not uncommon (28).

III. Outpatient Drainage of Pleural Effusions

An alternative treatment approach to MPE has emerged in the past 10 to 15 years. The use of various catheters to chronically drain MPE without specific attempts at pleurodesis is a relatively simple way to achieve symptom control while avoiding potential toxicity of sclerosing agents or the need for hospitalization or surgical intervention. The focus of this approach is on relieving and preventing dyspnea by maintaining lung reexpansion with repeated drainage although, as described below, many patients will achieve "spontaneous pleurodesis" over time. While initial attempts with these techniques often focused on patients with failed pleurodesis, poor performance status, or trapped lung, chronic pleural drainage has now been validated as a first-line treatment for MPE.

While initial reports of chronic pleural drainage utilized general-use catheters (37–39), a majority of published studies have utilized a specially designed TPC system (PleurX® Catheter, Cardinal Health Systems, McGaw Park, Illinois, U.S.) (31,40–56).

More recently, other similar catheters have been marketed for this purpose with minor variations in design, but we are unaware of any published data using these alternative devices. Subcutaneous implantable access devices have been used in similar fashion in a total of 31 patients (57,58).

The PleurX® catheter system consists of a 15.5 French silicone catheter with a 24-cm distal end with multiple side holes, a tissue cuff that is positioned subcutaneously and a proximal end tipped with a needleless access valve. Dedicated plastic disposable vacuum drainage bottles of 550 or 1000 mL capacity with dressing kits are used to drain the catheter. Details regarding our clinical approach have previously been published (59).

A. Patient Selection

A significant advantage of this treatment approach is the liberal patient selection criteria. The primary indication for tunneled catheters has been malignant pleural disease. Patients ineligible for thoracoscopy or chest tube pleurodesis procedures such as those with trapped lungs and poor performance status and short life expectancy can be successfully treated with this approach. We have also demonstrated excellent results in patients with good lung reexpansion and reasonable life expectancy, suggesting that this approach can be used as first-line treatment in a majority of patients with MPEs (52). Placement of catheters should be limited to patients who experience at least partial symptomatic relief following therapeutic thoracentesis. This will ensure that other explanations for the patient's dyspnea are not neglected and that procedures unlikely to benefit the patient are avoided. In the absence of alternative explanations for the effusion, proof of positive pleural fluid cytology is not required prior to placement in patients with previously confirmed advanced cancer. The use of this technique in nonmalignant disease has been much more limited and is described below.

Contraindications to placement include benign disease, very short life expectancy, uncontrolled coagulopathy, extensive skin involvement with malignancy (inflammatory breast cancer) or infection over the planned insertion site, and multiloculated pleural effusion. Chylothorax and benign disease have previously been considered as contra-indications, but this has been challenged in recent publications. Anticoagulated patients can restart treatment post procedure, but short-term interruption is required for insertion. Bilateral catheters can also be inserted if required and have been well tolerated by our patients.

B. Insertion Technique

Catheter placement can be performed in any adequately equipped procedure room. In our center, a procedure room in the outpatient clinic is utilized for most insertions, or the bronchoscopy suite if patients are already admitted to hospital. Sterile technique with full barrier precautions is utilized. No IV access is established and we have not required the use of sedation (Fig. 1).

We most commonly place the catheters at the anterior axillary line and tunnel the catheter inferiorly over the upper abdomen. In patients with large breasts or diseased skin, a posterior approach is preferred. Bedside ultrasound guidance is used for all of our procedures and allows the selection of an optimal placement location and may avoid failed insertions. This may be especially important if the fluid is partially loculated, in obese patients, if diseased skin is present and in patients with ascites or other reasons for an elevated diaphragm position. Nevertheless, catheters can be inserted safely without

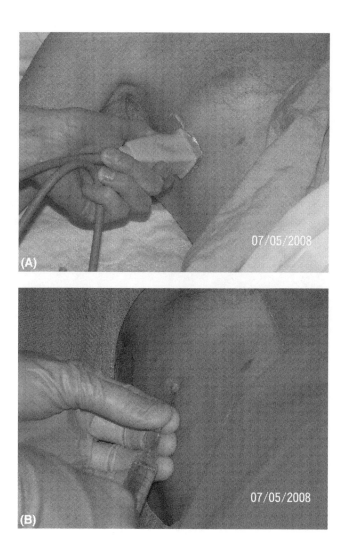

Figure 1 (**A**) Ultrasound localization of optimal insertion site. (**B**) Local anesthesia at insertion site (*Continued on pages 126–130*).

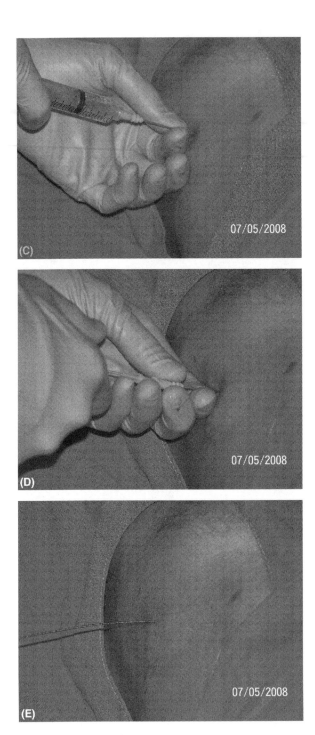

Figure 1 (*Continued*) (**C**) Pleural space is accessed with 18-gauge introducer needle. (**D**) Guidewire insertion. (**E**) Guidewire in situ.

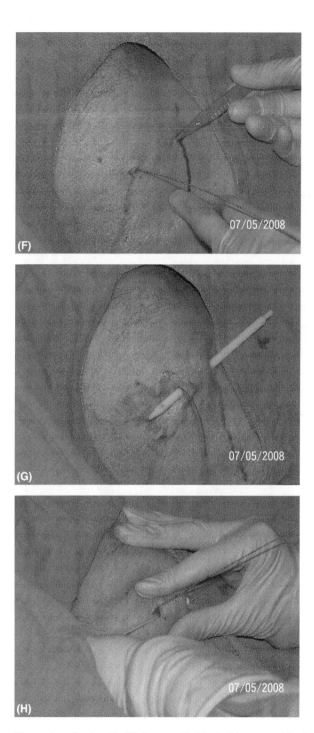

Figure 1 (*Continued*) (**F**) Two small skin incisions at guidewire site and tunnel insertion site. (**G**) Tunneler device advanced subcutaneously. (**H**) TPC advanced through tunnel.

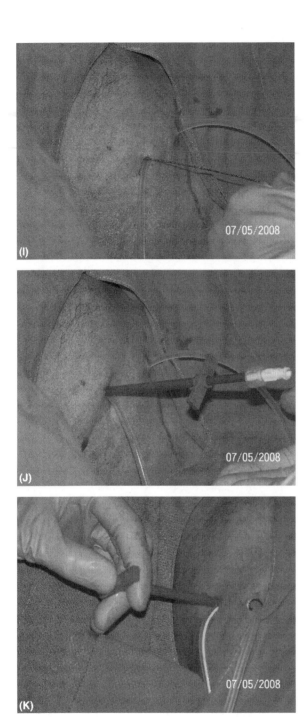

Figure 1 (*Continued*) (**I**) TPC advanced until tissue cuff in subcutaneous position. (**J**) Dilator and peel-away introducer sheath advanced over the guidewire and into the pleural space. (**K**) Dilator is removed, leaving sheath in the pleural space.

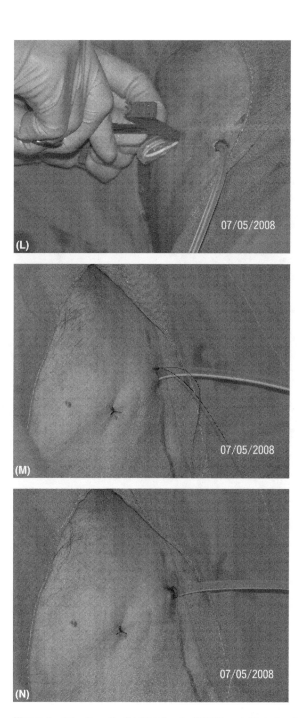

Figure 1 (*Continued*) (**L**) Distal end of TPC inserted into the sheath, which is then pulled apart and removed. A small curved forceps is occasionally required to advance the catheter. (**M**) Two interrupted sutures are placed at the insertion site and one interrupted suture is placed at the tunnel exit site and wrapped around the catheter. (**N**) TPC post insertion.

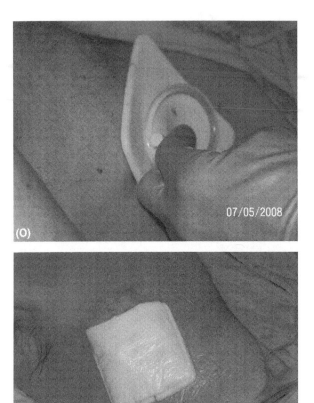

Figure 1 (*Continued*) (**O**) Catheter is coiled over a foam pad. (**P**) Gauze padding under a clear occlusive dressing.

ultrasound guidance in the majority of patients given that the most will have fairly large pleural effusions.

Patients are placed in a supine position with the head of the bed up elevated between 30° and 45° when an anterior axillary approach is chosen. If a posterior approach is anticipated, the patient is placed in a sitting position leaning forward onto a table as is commonly done for thoracentesis. Chest X ray is performed prior to the procedure and previous chest imaging is reviewed if available. Once the patient is in position, ultrasound examination is performed and a skin mark is made to identify planned insertion site.

The skin is prepped with chlorhexidine or proviodine and covered with sterile towels or a fenestrated drape. Local anesthesia with approximately 10 mL of 1% lidocaine is used to anesthetize the skin and access the pleural space. An introducer needle is then advanced into the pleural space through which a guidewire is inserted.

A second syringe of lidocaine is used to anesthetize the skin and subcutaneous tissues for a 5- to 10-cm tunnel. Two small incisions are made with a number 11 scalpel at the site of guidewire insertion (~1 cm) and tunnel insertion site (~6 mm). A plastic tunneler device is inserted through the distal incision toward the guidewire and the catheter pulled through until the tissue cuff is in a subcutaneous position. A peel-away introducer sheath over a dilator is advanced over the guidewire into the pleural space. The dilator is then removed with the guidewire and the distal end of the catheter advanced through the sheath into the pleural space followed by removal of the peel-away introducer sheath. Occasionally, a small curved forceps may be used to assist advancement of the catheter into the pleural space. Two simple interrupted sutures are placed at the pleural insertion site, and one suture at the tunnel insertion site is placed with the ends of the suture wrapped around the catheter. The catheter is then drained until symptoms occur or 1.5 to 2 L of fluid has been removed. A valve cap is placed on the device and sterile dressing applied. A chest X ray is done routinely post procedure and the patient discharged home if no complications are noted. Sutures are removed 10 to 14 days post insertion.

C. Removal Technique

Once a decision has been made to remove the catheter, the patient is brought back to the outpatient clinic. The area around the catheter is cleansed with chlorhexidine and 5 mL of lidocaine 1% is infiltrated with a 25-gauge needle around the tissue cuff. The catheter is then pulled with a firm and constant pressure as well as rotating motion until the cuff is dislodged. Once the cuff is dislodged, the rest of the silicone tube slides out easily. Occasionally, a small curved forceps is used to dislodge the cuff. Small Steri-Strips are applied to the incision, which is then covered with a sterile dressing for 48 hours. Occasionally, pleural fluid leaks out from the insertion site post removal. This is especially common if there is residual loculated effusion on X ray. This is easily managed by applying an ileostomy drainage bag system over the incision that can usually be removed within 48 hours once no further fluid leak is noted.

D. Care Delivery Model

In our center, an outpatient clinic dedicated to management of MPE has been established in a regional cancer center. It is staffed by a dedicated nurse as well as interventional pulmonary physicians. Any patient with suspected MPE can be referred to the clinic for assessment and treatment. Procedures performed in the clinic in addition to TPC placement and removal include thoracentesis, closed pleural biopsy, and intrapleural thrombolytics. All patients are seen two weeks following placement of a TPC and every three months thereafter, with easy access to the clinic if there are difficulties or if spontaneous pleurodesis occurs. All patients are referred to a palliative home care program to assist with catheter drainage and other palliative issues commonly encountered by these patients. Catheter drainage is typically performed three times per week utilizing the 550-mL bottles. A second bottle can be used for each drainage session if the first bottle fills completely and the patient does not have any resulting side effects. Patients and family frequently learn to perform the drainage procedure independently, which allows more freedom and convenience. At the two-week follow-up visits, frequency and amount of drainage is reassessed on the basis of symptoms and any residual fluid on X ray. For patients draining larger amounts of fluid, 1-L bottles are utilized or daily drainage is performed. The interventional pulmonary medicine service remains available to assess patients with TPC on an on-call basis should any problems arise. While other care models can certainly be applied, it is worthwhile pointing out that the actual catheter insertion is but a minor component of the overall care of these patients.

E. Results

To date there have been numerous reports demonstrating that TPC use for treatment of MPE can be achieved on an outpatient basis with minimal morbidity and no reported treatment related mortality (31,40,41,47–50,54,56).

Symptoms and Effusion Control

A large prospective series demonstrating that TPCs are an effective method of treating MPEs was published by our group in 2006 (49). This single-center study described 250 sequential TPC insertions. Symptom control as assessed in 222 of 231 successfully inserted TPCs (96.1%) seen at a two-week follow-up visit demonstrated that 89% of patients experienced partial or complete symptom relief following TPC insertion. One randomized study has directly compared TPCs to doxycycline pleurodesis (40), demonstrating that TPCs were equally efficacious in the management of dyspnea and quality of life in patients with MPE (40). In fact, patients treated with TPC demonstrated a trend toward greater improvement in Borg dyspnea scores although this was not statistically significant. No survival difference was noted between the two groups.

The control achieved using TPCs seems to be durable as well with 90.1% of patients not requiring any further ipsilateral procedures following TPC treatment (49). In those who otherwise would appear to be reasonable candidates for pleurodesis procedures, as determined by good lung reexpansion and survival, there was no need for a repeat procedure in 87% of cases overall and in 92% of patients experiencing spontaneous pleurodesis (52). In the above-mentioned randomized study, 21% of patients who received doxycycline had a late recurrence of pleural effusion, whereas only 13% of patients who had an indwelling catheter had a late recurrence of their effusions or a blockage of their catheter after the initially successful treatment (40). While some would cite prolonged drainage as a downside of TPCs, this appears to be well tolerated by patients. Catheters stayed in place for a median of 56 days in our experience (49) with prolonged drainage, defined as greater than 100 days, reported in 5.2% of patients in another series (54). Longer periods of TPC use is most commonly seen in patients with incomplete lung reexpansion.

Spontaneous Pleurodesis

Spontaneous pleurodesis rates of 42.0% to 70% have been reported following use of TPC for the treatment of MPE, depending on the selected patient population (31,49,52,56). It appears that in patients in whom pleural apposition is achieved, the local inflammatory changes induced by the tumor and/or the catheter is sufficient to create pleurodesis without the administration (and possible related complications) of a sclerosing agent. When only patients who would also be reasonable candidates for pleurodesis procedures were analyzed (as determined by good lung reexpansion and short-term survival), spontaneous pleurodesis rates of 70% were found (52). The time to achieve spontaneous pleurodesis has been variably reported between a median of 26.5 days in one study and a mean of 90 days in another (40,52). When spontaneous pleurodesis was achieved with TPC insertion, the effect was long lasting, with clinically significant reaccumulation of fluid in 2.9% (56) or need for repeat ipsilateral pleural procedures in 8.7% of cases (49). In both these series, catheters were removed once less than 50 cc was drained on three successive drainage attempts. It is difficult to compare symptom control rates and pleurodesis rates between different case series, but it would appear that rates of symptom control, and even eventual pleurodesis and long-term control of pleural fluid, achieved with TPC use can be compared favorably with results achieved with pleurodesis using thoracoscopic or chest tube instillation of sclerosing agents.

Clinical parameters that could influence spontaneous pleurodesis were studied in a retrospective series of 263 patients who underwent insertion of 295 TPCs for MPE (56). The incidence of spontaneous symphysis and catheter removal in the breast (69.6%) and gynecologic cancer (72.5%) groups was significantly higher than in the lung (43.9%) and other cancer (23.9%) groups. Spontaneous pleurodesis and catheter removal was more likely with cytologic positivity, complete expansion of the underlying lung, and in the absence of a history of chest wall irradiation. Another study found no significant impact of tumor cell type on the incidence of spontaneous pleurodesis but did note that patients with good lung expansion (i.e., absence of trapped lung and adequate volume/ frequency of drainages) at the two-week follow-up appointment (post TPC insertion) were more likely to achieve spontaneous pleurodesis (57% vs. 25%) (49). The data from these studies suggest that the likelihood of spontaneous pleurodesis and catheter removal is potentially affected by a number of patient-, tumor-, and treatment-related factors, with complete reexpansion of the underlying lung seeming to be particularly important.

Costs and Hospitalization

In addition to excellent symptom control, TPCs have been shown to reduce, and in most cases, eliminate the need for hospitalization. In the randomized study by Putnam, the median hospitalization time was 1.0 day for the indwelling catheter group compared to 6.5 days for the group receiving doxycycline pleurodesis via a chest tube (40). The overnight admission performed in this initial study is no longer felt to be necessary. Locally, patients are never admitted to hospital post TPC placement, although these are often placed in previously admitted patients to facilitate discharge, and in a recent study, over 90% of 231 catheters where safely inserted on an outpatient basis (54). This approach has not surprisingly been demonstrated to be associated with significantly lower costs during the initial seven days after treatment compared to inpatient pleu- rodesis with doxycycline or talc via a chest tube (41). On the other hand, costs associated with TPC use relate in large part to drainage supplies and support that would not be captured in a short-term study, and no long-term cost analysis has yet been published.

Specific Patient Populations
Debilitated Patients and Trapped Lung

For many patients with MPE, chest tube pleurodesis or thoracoscopy is not considered a viable option because they are too debilitated or have a trapped lung (28). TPCs, however, have been demonstrated in a number of studies to be effective in patients too debilitated to be considered for thoracoscopy or chest tube pleurodesis (43,49,54). TPCs have also been demonstrated in a number of studies to be effective in palliating dyspnea in patients with trapped lung (43,49,53,54). A retrospective study describes 13 catheters placements in 11 consecutive patients who specifically underwent pleural catheter placement for MPE in the setting of a trapped lung syndrome. Malignancies treated included malignant mesothelioma, 6; lymphoma, 3; adenocarcinoma, 1; and multiple myeloma, 1. All but one patient reported improvement in symptoms, as defined by improved dyspnea and exercise tolerance. In 10 patients, the TPC remained in place until death, for a period of 15 to 234 days and one patient required revision after catheter occlusion (53). Two larger retrospective studies (49,54) also reported effective symptomatic relief in the trapped lung subgroups. In a larger study of 127 consecutive patients who underwent thoracoscopy for MPE, 52 (41%) were found to have trapped lung at time of surgery and were managed by insertion of a TPC (53) with symptomatic relief achieved in 49 (94%).

Given the available data, TPC seems to be effective in patients with MPE and trapped lung syndrome although we typically would advocate placing the catheters only in patients who demonstrate at least partial symptomatic improvement following an initial therapeutic thoracentesis.

Pleurodesis Candidates

It is difficult to compare results from large case series of TPC placement for MPE to published data on pleurodesis techniques because of the frequent inclusion of more debilitated patients including those with trapped lung syndrome usually excluded from pleurodesis research. In an attempt to address this issue, patients with survival of three months and absence of trapped lung following two weeks of TPC drainage were selected from a large database (52). Not surprisingly, the authors found higher rates of spontaneous pleurodesis (70%) and symptom control (improvement 100%, complete 67%). This pleurodesis rate is in the range of those reported in a recent large prospective randomized trial of pleurodesis via talc slurry versus thoracoscopic talc insufflation that showed success rates of 71% and 78%, respectively, in patients without trapped lung and alive at 30 days (28).

Mesothelioma

It has been reported that conventional MPE treatments may be less effective in patients with mesothelioma (26,60), and concerns regarding use of TPC in these patients have also been raised (56). Nevertheless, a retrospective analysis in our institution identified 31 TPC procedures in patients with malignant mesothelioma (50). When compared to a control group of 218 TPCs in 195 patients with other tumors causing MPE from the same database, similar efficacy was demonstrated in both groups (50). Dyspnea control in the malignant mesothelioma group was found to be complete or partial after 12 (38.7%) and 17 (54.8%) procedures, respectively, not significantly different than for the control group. The rates of spontaneous pleurodesis, the need for repeat procedures, and complications were no different in the malignant mesothelioma group versus the control group. The TPCs did remain in place longer in patients with malignant mesothelioma than in the control group (83 vs. 52 days), likely as a result of longer survival.

In the above-mentioned study of 11 patients with trapped lung syndrome who underwent TPC insertion for MPE (43), 6 patients had malignant mesothelioma. While results for these patients were not reported separately, all but one patient reported symptomatic benefit, further supporting the use of TPC in this population.

Chylothorax

Chylothorax related to malignancy is usually best treated by addressing the underlying malignancy itself. Recurrent, symptomatic chylothorax in patients with cancer relapse or progressive disease despite adequate treatment is a debilitating condition that is often difficult to manage. Because of concerns regarding chronic drainage of the lymphocyte and lipid-rich liquid, chylothorax has traditionally been considered a contraindication to TPC insertion. The use of TPCs in this patient population has been recently described retrospectively by the MD Anderson Cancer Centre group. They identified 130 patients with chylothorax over a 10-year period (55), 19 of which had recurrent symptomatic chylothorax in association with cancer relapse. TPCs were used in 10 patients while 9 others had other palliative interventions. The authors found no significant difference in the number of patients reporting symptomatic improvement between the groups, yet there were significantly fewer subsequent interventions required during the following 500 days after the index procedure in the TPC group compared to the controls. Serum albumin levels decreased in the TPC group, but the decline was no worse than the decline observed in the control group. Given these results, TPC may be considered in the treatment armamentarium in patients who have recurrent, symptomatic malignant chylothorax, especially if no further oncologic treatment is offered and/or pleurodesis procedures have failed or are contraindicated.

Tunneled Pleural Catheters for Nonmalignant Disease

Pleural space infection is generally considered a contraindication to TPC insertion and the product literature advises against using the product in this situation. Two cases of TPC being used for chronic empyema have recently been reported: in one patient with a bronchopleural fistula and another with an esophagopleural fistula. Both were treated with indwelling pleural catheters, drainage, and long-term antibiotics (61). Both patients had successful resolution of their infection, avoided a surgical intervention, and eventually had the catheters removed. While interesting, the role of TPC in patients with pleural infection would still be considered unproven and experimental.

While we have anecdotal success in a very small number of carefully selected patients with benign pleural disease (infection, postcardiotomy syndrome, anthracycline cardiotoxicity, heart failure in the peritransplant period), there currently exists no evidence to support the use of TPC in nonmalignant conditions and these should still be considered a contraindication to placement of one of these devices.

F. Complications

Both short-term and long-term risks of TPCs have been reported and include infection, loculation of fluid and catheter blockage, pneumothorax, tumor seeding of the tunnel tract, and bleeding. Overall risks are quite low and compare favorably to the previously described complications of standard treatments.

Infection

A common concern is the possibility of infection when a catheter is left in for a prolonged period. While there is a theoretical risk that the tunnel tract will be a conduit for the entrance of microbes, the cuff on the catheter that sits just beneath the exit site is intended to be a barrier to this. Actual rates of infection related to the catheters are quite low. Cellulitis, which usually occurs within a couple of weeks of placement, has been reported to occur following 1.3% to 1.6% of TPC insertions in the two largest case series (49,56). These infections can almost always be treated with oral antibiotics targeted toward normal skin flora such as cloxacillin or cefazolin and without catheter removal. Empyema, which usually occurs after prolonged draining, has been reported to occur between 0.3% and 3.2% of cases (49,56). Our approach to this complication is to admit the patient to hospital, connect the pleural catheter to straight drainage, initiate broad-spectrum antibiotic insuring good coverage for *Staphylococcus aureus* (the most commonly isolated organism in our experience), consider the intrapleural administration of thrombolytic agents, and use CT imaging liberally to ensure appropriate drainage of the pleural cavity. We have rarely needed to insert additional chest drains and have not had to perform surgical decortication in this patient population as yet. Once drainage through the catheter is minimal, this is removed preferably prior to completing the antibiotic course. Interestingly, none of our infections have been associated with neutropenia despite the frequent use of chemotherapeutic agents in this patient population. As such, we do not hesitate to place a TPC in a patient imminently embarking on chemotherapy treatments. Rates of empyema following TPC placement are comparable to those seen after talc pleurodesis with reported rates of 0.7% to 2.5% (24–28).

Loculation of Fluid and Catheter Blockage

Catheter blockage has been reported to occur between 2% and 3.7% of cases (40,56). This can be addressed by replacing the catheter or flushing it with normal saline or even thrombolytics. In our experience, symptomatic loculated collections of fluid can occur in approximately 8% of patients (49). We do also address these with intrapleural thrombolytics as well and occasionally will perform thoracentesis if there is one dominant loculated pocket of fluid and rarely insert a new catheter.

Pneumothorax

Rates of pneumothorax following TPC insertion are 2.4% (49). Most of these are felt to represent entrained air through the large introducer sheath at time of insertion or occasional pleural disruption during reexpansion in the setting of a partially trapped lung. Persistent bronchopleural fistula or subcutaneous emphysema is much less common. In the majority of cases this can be managed by drainage of the air via the usual drainage bottles. For the rare patient with more persistent air leak, admission to hospital and connection of the PleurX to a pleural waterseal device is required. This complication rate is similar to a reported rate of pneumothorax during a large series of 941 ultrasound-guided thoracenteses by radiologists of 2.5% (62) as well as those following pleurodesis (28).

Tumor Seeding

Tumor seeding of tract of the catheter tract is a potential complication given that catheters are often left in place for prolonged periods. The incidence of this complication has been reported to be anywhere from less than 1% to 6.7% (49,56,63). Local irradiation to the catheter tract has been described (63) if this causes discomfort, but tubes do not require removal and can continue to function normally. Of course, tumor seeding can occur following any pleural procedure including thoracoscopy (25,26).

Bleeding and Management of Anticoagulation

Bleeding complications were reported in 2 of 250 patients (0.8%) although the severity of bleeding was not described (49). There are no reports of hemothorax or bleeding requiring surgical intervention or transfusion after TPC insertion. Care should be taken in elderly patients, however, as intercostals artery tortuosity has been shown to increase with advancing age, decreasing the amount of "safe" intercostal space (64). We routinely discontinue anticoagulation prior to tunneled catheter placement, but have not experienced difficulties reinitiating anticoagulation in these patients. Even in patients with a bloody-appearing effusion, measuring the hematocrit of the pleural fluid rarely results in values above 0.03.

Additional Issues

We occasionally have had patients present to other medical centers in need of pleural drainage through their TPC, not being equipped to do so. In these cases, the catheter can be accessed with the plastic portion of a 16- or 14-gauge intravenous cannula, with the needle removed, connected to a standard drainage line to a vacuum bottles, wall suction, or standard pleural drainage unit. Similarly, in bedridden patients, we often connect the pleural catheter to straight drainage on a leg bag to simplify the patient's care and minimize costs.

Occasionally, leakage of pleural fluid occurs around the TPC. This usually occurs in the few days post placement in patients with very large effusions under some degree of positive pressure. It is important to increase the frequency of drainage in these patients and apply frequent dressing changes. This will reduce the risk of infection at the catheter site and favor healing and scarring around the catheter and cuff, resolving the issue.

Dislodged catheters have occasionally occurred, usually within two weeks of placement because the cuff has not healed into place and the patients are still unfamiliar with a device. Once the cuff is out of the subcutaneous tunnel, the catheter should be removed and a new one inserted. The site should be carefully inspected for cellulitis or infection as occasionally this may have led to the dislodgment or occurred as a consequence.

Patients without good lung reexpansion on follow-up should be assessed for insufficient drainage volume, blocked catheter, loculated fluid, trapped lung syndrome, and/or endobronchial obstruction. According to the clinical setting pleural ultrasonography, chest CT scan imaging and bronchoscopy could be considered.

IV. Conclusion

Patients with malignant pleural disease require a management approach that minimizes complications, hospitalizations, and discomfort. Their life expectancy is usually quite short and in our opinion is better spent outside our medical centers. The advent of TPC treatment for MPE has allowed a simple minimally invasive method to palliate patients' symptoms on an outpatient basis with minimal complications. It has been our experience and that of others (54) that once presented with this treatment option, very few patients elect to undergo more invasive inpatient pleurodesis–type procedures. The successful application of this technique to a variety of patient populations attests that TPC can be considered as a primary treatment option for most patients with MPE.

References

1. American Thoracic Society. Management of malignant pleural effusions. Am J Respir Crit Care Med 2000; 162(5):1987–2001.
2. Light RW. Pleural effusions related to metastatic malignancies. In: Light RW, ed. Pleural Diseases. Philadelphia: Lippincott Williams & Wilkins, 2007:133–161.
3. Sahn SA. Pleural diseases related to metastatic malignancies. Eur Respir J 1997; 10(8):1907–1913.
4. Johnston WW. The malignant pleural effusion. A review of cytopathologic diagnoses of 584 specimens from 472 consecutive patients. Cancer 1985; 56(4):905–909.
5. Hsu C. Cytologic detection of malignancy in pleural effusion: a review of 5,255 samples from 3,811 patients. Diagn Cytopathol 1987; 3(1):8–12.
6. Spiro SG, Gould MK, Colice GL. Initial evaluation of the patient with lung cancer: symptoms, signs, laboratory tests, and paraneoplastic syndromes: ACCP evidenced-based clinical practice guidelines (2nd edition). Chest 2007; 132(suppl 3):149S–160S.
7. Elis A, Blickstein D, Mulchanov I, et al. Pleural effusion in patients with non-Hodgkin's lymphoma: a case-controlled study. Cancer 1998; 83(8):1607–1611.
8. Antunes G, Neville E, Duffy J, et al. BTS guidelines for the management of malignant pleural effusions. Thorax 2003; 58(suppl 2):ii29–ii38.
9. Neragi-Miandoab S. Malignant pleural effusion, current and evolving approaches for its diagnosis and management. Lung Cancer 2006; 54(1):1–9.
10. Tan C, Sedrakyan A, Browne J, et al. The evidence on the effectiveness of management for malignant pleural effusion: a systematic review. Eur J Cardiothorac Surg 2006; 29(5):829–838.
11. Lee YC, Light RW. Management of malignant pleural effusions. Respirology 2004; 9(2): 148–156.
12. Bennett R, Maskell N. Management of malignant pleural effusions. Curr Opin Pulm Med 2005; 11(4):296–300.
13. West SD, Davies RJ, Lee YC. Pleurodesis for malignant pleural effusions: current controversies and variations in practices. Curr Opin Pulm Med 2004; 10(4):305–310.
14. Bernard A, de Dompsure RB, Hagry O, et al. Early and late mortality after pleurodesis for malignant pleural effusion. Ann Thorac Surg 2002; 74(1):213–217.
15. Genc O, Petrou M, Ladas G, et al. The long-term morbidity of pleuroperitoneal shunts in the management of recurrent malignant effusions. Eur J Cardiothorac Surg 2000; 18(2):143–146.
16. Petrou M, Kaplan D, Goldstraw P. Management of recurrent malignant pleural effusions. The complementary role of talc pleurodesis and pleuroperitoneal shunting. Cancer 1995; 75(3): 801–805.
17. Light RW, O'Hara VS, Moritz TE, et al. Intrapleural tetracycline for the prevention of recurrent spontaneous pneumothorax. Results of a Department of Veterans Affairs cooperative study. JAMA 1990; 264(17):2224–2230.
18. Heffner JE, Unruh LC. Tetracycline pleurodesis. Adios, farewell, adieu. Chest 1992; 101(1): 5–7.
19. Mansson T. Treatment of malignant pleural effusion with doxycycline. Scand J Infect Dis Suppl 1988; 53:29–34.
20. Herrington JD, Gora-Harper ML, Salley RK. Chemical pleurodesis with doxycycline 1 g. Pharmacotherapy 1996; 16(2):280–285.
21. Brant A, Eaton T. Serious complications with talc slurry pleurodesis. Respirology 2001; 6(3): 181–185.
22. Wied U, Andersen K, Schultz A, et al. Silver nitrate pleurodesis in spontaneous pneumothorax. Scand J Thorac Cardiovasc Surg 1981; 15(3):305–307.
23. Marom EM, Patz EF, Jr, Erasmus JJ, et al. Malignant pleural effusions: treatment with small-bore-catheter thoracostomy and talc pleurodesis. Radiology 1999; 210(1):277–281.
24. Stefani A, Natali P, Casali C, et al. Talc poudrage versus talc slurry in the treatment of malignant pleural effusion. A prospective comparative study. Eur J Cardiothorac Surg 2006; 30(6):827–832.

25. de Campos JRM, Vargas FS, de Campos Werebe E, et al. Thoracoscopy talc poudrage: a 15-year experience. Chest 2001; 119(3):801–806.

26. Viallat JR, Rey F, Astoul P, et al. Thoracoscopic talc poudrage pleurodesis for malignant effusions. A review of 360 cases. Chest 1996; 110(6):1387–1393.

27. Arapis K, Caliandro R, Stern JB, et al. Thoracoscopic palliative treatment of malignant pleural effusions: results in 273 patients. Surg Endosc 2006; 20(6):919–923.

28. Dresler CM, Olak J, Herndon JE, et al. Phase III intergroup study of talc poudrage vs talc slurry sclerosis for malignant pleural effusion. Chest 2005; 127(3):909–915.

29. Rehse DH, Aye RW, Florence MG. Respiratory failure following talc pleurodesis. Am J Surg 1999; 177(5):437–440.

30. Bondoc AY, Bach PB, Sklarin NT, et al. Arterial desaturation syndrome following pleurodesis with talc slurry: incidence, clinical features, and outcome. Cancer Invest 2003; 21(6): 848–854.

31. Pollak JSM. Treatment of malignant pleural effusions with tunneled long-term drainage catheters. J Vasc Interv Radiol 2001; 12(2):201–208.

32. Diacon AH, Wyser C, Bolliger CT, et al. Prospective randomized comparison of thoracoscopic talc poudrage under local anesthesia versus bleomycin instillation for pleurodesis in malignant pleural effusions. Am J Respir Crit Care Med 2000; 162(4 pt 1):1445–1449.

33. Steger V, Mika U, Toomes H, et al. Who gains most? A 10-year experience with 611 thoracoscopic talc pleurodeses. Ann Thorac Surg 2007; 83(6):1940–1945.

34. Zimmer PW, Hill M, Casey K, et al. Prospective randomized trial of talc slurry vs bleomycin in pleurodesis for symptomatic malignant pleural effusions. Chest 1997; 112(2):430–434.

35. Walker-Renard PB, Vaughan LM, Sahn SA. Chemical pleurodesis for malignant pleural effusions. Ann Intern Med 1994; 120(1):56–64.

36. Kennedy L, Sahn SA. Talc pleurodesis for the treatment of pneumothorax and pleural effusion. Chest 1994; 106(4):1215–1222.

37. Robinson RD, Fullerton DA, Albert JD, et al. Use of pleural Tenckhoff catheter to palliate malignant pleural effusion. Ann Thorac Surg 1994; 57(2):286–288.

38. Hussain SA, Burton GM, Yuce M. Symptomatic loculated malignant pleural effusion treatment with indwelling Tenckhoff catheter. Chest 1990; 97(3):766–767.

39. Vázquez-Pelillo JC, Gonzalez EP, Atance PL, et al. Malignant pleural effusions: a description of an alternative method of external drainage with a fine-caliber catheter. Arch Bronconeumol 1997; 33(9):450–452.

40. Putnam JB Jr., Light RW, Rodriguez RM, et al. A randomized comparison of indwelling pleural catheter and doxycycline pleurodesis in the management of malignant pleural effusions. Cancer 1999; 86(10):1992–1999.

41. Putnam JB Jr., Walsh GL, Swisher SG, et al. Outpatient management of malignant pleural effusion by a chronic indwelling pleural catheter. The Ann Thorac Surg 2000; 69(2):369–375.

42. Smart JM, Tung KT. Initial experiences with a long-term indwelling tunnelled pleural catheter for the management of malignant pleural effusion. Clin Radiol 2000; 55(11):882–884.

43. Pien GW, Gant MJ, Washam CL, et al. Use of an implantable pleural catheter for trapped lung syndrome in patients with malignant pleural effusion. Chest 2001; 119(6):1641–1646.

44. Pollak JSM. Malignant pleural effusions: treatment with tunneled long-term drainage catheters. Curr Opin Pulm Med 2002; 8:302–307.

45. Brubacher S, Gobel BH. Use of the Pleurx Pleural Catheter for the management of malignant pleural effusions. Clin J Oncol Nurs 2003; 7(1):35–38.

46. Ohm C, Park D, Vogen M, et al. Use of an indwelling pleural catheter compared with thoroscopic talc pleurodesis in the management of malignant pleural effusions. Am Surg 2003; 69(3):198–202.

47. Musani AI, Haas AR, Seijo L, et al. Outpatient management of malignant pleural effusions with small-bore, tunneled pleural catheters. Respiration 2004; 71(6):559–566.

48. van den Toorn LM, Schaap E, Surmont VF, et al. Management of recurrent malignant pleural effusions with a chronic indwelling pleural catheter. Lung Cancer 2005; 50(1):123–127.

49. Tremblay A, Michaud G. Single-center experience with 250 tunnelled pleural catheter insertions for malignant pleural effusion. Chest 2006; 129(2):362–368.

50. Tremblay A, Patel M, Michaud G. Use of tunneled pleural catheters in malignant mesothelioma. J Bronchol 2006; 12(4):203–206.

51. Burgers JA, Olijve A, Baas P. Chronic indwelling pleural catheter for malignant pleural effusion in 25 patients. Ned Tijdschr Geneeskd 2006; 150(29):1618–1623.

52. Tremblay A, Mason C, Michaud G. Use of tunnelled catheters for malignant pleural effusions in patients fit for pleurodesis. Eur Respir J 2007; 30(4):759–762.

53. Qureshi RA, Collinson SL, Powell RJ, et al. Management of malignant pleural effusion associated with trapped lung syndrome. Asian Cardiovasc Thorac Ann 2008; 16(2):120–123.

54. Warren WH, Kalimi R, Khodadadian LM, et al. Management of malignant pleural effusions using the Pleur(x) catheter. Ann Thorac Surg 2008; 85(3):1049–1055.

55. Jimenez CA, Mhatre AD, Martinez CH, et al. Use of an indwelling pleural catheter for the management of recurrent chylothorax in patients with cancer. Chest 2007; 132(5):1584–1590.

56. Warren WH, Kim AW, Liptay MJ. Identification of clinical factors predicting Pleurx catheter removal in patients treated for malignant pleural effusion. Eur J Cardiothorac Surg 2008; 33(1):89–94.

57. Daniel C, Kriegel I, Di MS, et al. Use of a pleural implantable access system for the management of malignant pleural effusion: the Institut Curie experience. Ann Thorac Surg 2007; 84(4):1367–1370.

58. Verfaillie G, Herreweghe RV, Lamote J, et al. Use of a Port-a-Cath system in the home setting for the treatment of symptomatic recurrent malignant pleural effusion. Eur J Cancer Care (Engl) 2005; 14(2):182–184.

59. Michaud G, Barclay P, Tremblay A. Tunneled pleural catheters for palliation of malignant pleural effusions. J Bronchol 2006; 12(4):245–248.

60. Sterman DH, Kaiser LR, Albelda SM. Advances in the treatment of malignant pleural mesothelioma. Chest 1999; 116(2):504–520.

61. Davies HE, Rahman NM, Parker RJ, et al. Use of indwelling pleural catheters for chronic pleural infection. Chest 2008; 133(2):546–549.

62. Jones PW, Moyers JP, Rogers JT, et al. Ultrasound-guided thoracentesis: is it a safer method? Chest 2003; 123(2):418–423.

63. Janes SM, Rahman NM, Davies RJ, et al. Catheter-tract metastases associated with chronic indwelling pleural catheters. Chest 2007; 131(4):1232–1234.

64. Carney M, Ravin CE. Intercostal artery laceration during thoracocentesis: increased risk in elderly patients. Chest 1979; 75(4):520–522.

9

Bronchoscopic Lung Volume Reduction in COPD

ENRIQUE DIAZ-GUZMAN
University of Kentucky, Lexington, Kentucky, U.S.A.

ATUL C. MEHTA
Sheikh Khalifa Medical City, managed by Cleveland Clinic, Abu Dhabi, UAE

I. Introduction

Chronic obstructive pulmonary disease (COPD) represents a leading cause of disease morbidity and mortality worldwide, with estimates affecting >10% of the world's adult population (1). The term COPD is nonspecific and most commonly refers to patients with chronic bronchitis or emphysema and a subset of patients with asthma (2). The disease is characterized by destruction of the lung parenchyma (emphysema), airway inflammation, and increase in mucus-producing cells (3).

Emphysema consists in permanent and anatomically irreversible enlargement of distal airspaces caused by destruction of the alveolar walls (3). These anatomical changes result in irreversible airflow obstruction with variable degrees of air trapping and lung hyperinflation. Importantly, the development of significant lung hyperinflation at rest reduces the patients' ventilatory capacity during exertion, increases airway conductance at rest, and induces several cellular molecular alterations in the diaphragm, leading to inspiratory muscle weakness (4,5). These mechanical and pathologic changes affect exercise capacity and contribute to dyspnea and exercise intolerance in patients with COPD.

Reduction in lung volume is associated with an improvement in respiratory mechanics: normalization of diaphragmatic and chest wall size, shortening of the respiratory muscle length, increase in vital capacity, and restoration of normal trans-pulmonary recoil pressures. The use of pharmacologic agents such as bronchodilators is aimed at improving airflow obstruction and reducing lung hyperinflation. Nevertheless, pharmacologic lung volume reduction (LVR) is less effective in patients with irreversible airway obstruction, in whom surgical or endoscopic approaches are often considered.

Several surgical procedures, including bullectomy, the Monaldi–Brompton technique (6), lung volume reduction surgery (LVRS), and lung transplantation, have shown success in improving quality of life in patients with COPD. Among these, LVRS has gained popularity, particularly since a recent national trial demonstrated improvements in survival and exercise capacity in a subgroup of patients with upper lobe predominant emphysema and limited exercise capacity (7). Nevertheless, LVRS is associated with significant morbidity, carries a mortality risk even at centers with large experience (8), and is associated with high cost and prolonged hospitalization (9).

Because of poor cost-effectiveness of LVRS, endoscopic alternatives are being developed in an attempt to provide less invasive, safer, and cost-effective methods to perform LVR. Bronchoscopic lung volume reduction (BLVR) comprises a variety of techniques and designs to achieve the beneficial physiologic effects observed after LVRS. The basic principle of BLVR consists in creating an area of atelectasis, which simulates the volume loss obtained through surgical resection. A description of the different approaches, technology, experience, and outcomes is presented here. Table 1 summarizes technologies that have been used for BLVR.

The principles of currently available BLVR techniques are the following: (a) closure of anatomical airway passages to emphysematous areas of the lung to induce a

Table 1 Summary of Available Technologies for BLVR.

Device	Affiliated company	Available data	Disadvantages
Silicone balloons	None	Anectodic reports. Minimal number of patients	Potential for postobstructive pneumonia. Questionable efficacy
Watanabe spigot	None	Used for other purposes (pneumothorax treatment, fistula treatment). Only one report with small number or patients	Questionable efficacy to achieve lung volume loss in all patients
Endobronchial valves	Emphasys Medical Inc.	Several studies available, including one multicentric trial	Questionable maintenance of lung volume reduction at long term because of collateral airways
	Spiration Inc.	Several studies available, including multicentric trial	Questionable maintenance of lung volume reduction at long term because of collateral airways
Endobronchial coils	PneumRx Inc.	Pilot study with five patients demonstrated safety of technology	The effects should be independent of collateral ventilation
Artificial accessory airways	Bronchus Technologies Inc.	Only preliminary reports available	Occlusion of artificial airways may develop, reducing efficacy and increasing risk for infection
Biologic therapy	Aeris Therapeutics Inc.	Phase 2 clinical studies underway	Irreversible damage to the lung. Risk for abscess formation and V/Q mismatch
Vapor therapy	Uptake Medical Corp.	Pilot study	Irreversible damage induced by water vapors. May need several treatments (20–30 min). Side effects appear to be common

collapse and reduce volume; these techniques include use of balloons, spigots, and one-way valves; (b) opening of extra-anatomical airway passages to improve collateral flow from hyperinflated lung regions; and (c) restructuring of emphysematous lung by applying biologic agents.

II. Blockade of Airway Passages

A. Mechanical Endobronchial Occluders

Silicone Balloons

This technique consists in blocking airflow into the emphysematous segment(s) of the lung. Sabanathan et al. reported eight patients who underwent BLVR in targeted areas of upper lobes segments using silicone balloons filled with contrast medium. Five patients had migration of endobronchial occluders and required to be replaced by stainless steel Gianturco-type stents blocked with biocompatible sponge (10). Although the majority of the patients subjectively improved, there were no changes in pulmonary function tests, and four developed late infectious complications.

Endobronchial Spigots

Watanabe et al. described the use of endobronchial spigots constructed with biocompatible materials designed to obstruct airways (11). In their report, the authors presented the use of spigots in the management of persistent bronchopleural fistulas in 12 patients with emphysema (12). The spigots were deployed using a rigid bronchoscope in a conventional way similar to the deployment of a Dumont stent. The authors reported two patients who developed segmental atelectasis after the procedure, providing evidence that this technique could be used for BLVR. Similarly, Toma et al. reported the use of spigots in the management of patients with persistent pneumothorax. Two out of 23 patients developed an upper lobe collapse (13). Miyazawa et al. subsequently modified the original technique and employed a guidewire placed under fluoroscopy to target the segmental bronchus. Using a push-and-slide method with the guide-catheter into the bronchus, they applied spigots in six patients with severe emphysema (14). Although the authors reported improvement in dyspnea in four patients and an increase in 10% in vital capacity, CT scans after the bronchial occlusion did not show regional volume loss.

Endobronchial Valves

This method consists in applying a device that functions as a one-way valve allowing air to exit the airways and impeding air re-entry into the targeted lung segments. Compared with the other mechanical occluders, endobronchial valves (EBVs) have the theoretical advantage of allowing the exit of air from the blocked segment. This results in a reduced risk of hyperinflation of the lung distal to the occlusion caused by collateral ventilation pathways.

Two different EBVs are currently under clinical evaluations: Spiration® umbrella and the Emphasys one-way valve. Emphasys Inc. (Emphasys, Redwood City, California, U.S.) developed its first EBV consisting of a silicone duckbill, one-way valve attached to a nitinol (nickel-titanium) self-expanding stent retainer with silicone seals to occlude the airway around the valve. The device is deployed using a guidewire placed by flexible bronchoscopy. The company released a second generation of valves, Zephyr®, currently manufactured in two sizes with overlapping diameter ranges (4.0–7.0 mm and 5.5–8.5 mm). A recent prospective, randomized, multicentric trial using Zephyr EBV (VENT

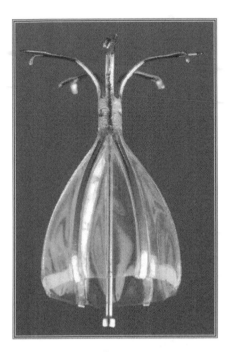

Figure 1 Spiration® intrabronchial valve.

trial) evaluated the safety and efficacy in 321 patients. The study showed that it met both its primary efficacy endpoints, showing statistically significant improvements in lung function and exercise tolerance. Additionally, the study suggested that the Zephyr EBV had a favorable safety profile in comparing major complications between the treatment and control groups.

The Spiration Umbrella implantable intrabronchial valve (IBV) (Spiration Inc., Redmond, Washington, U.S.) consists of an umbrella-shaped device made of a polyurethane membrane on a nitinol framework with five anchors that attach to the airway for providing stability (Fig. 1). The proximal part of the IBV conforms to the airway wall functioning like an umbrella, expanding during inspiration to prevent air entry, and retracting during expiration allowing escape of air. The IBV is deployed via a delivery catheter that is inserted through the instrument channel of a bronchoscope. The IBV also includes a proximal central knob that allows removal, if required with the help of a bronchoscopic forceps (Fig. 2). Both valve systems offer the possibility of being removed if complications arise during placement or over time (Fig. 3). A multicentric clinical trial evaluating the efficacy of the IBV will be completed in 2009. The study will compare IBV versus sham procedures and will evaluate effects of the EBVs on quality of life [disease-related health status (St. George's Respiratory Questionnaire, SGRQ)] and will assess regional lung volume changes as measured by quantitative CT scan.

A summary of the available EBV studies published in the literature is presented in Table 2 (Fig. 4). Most of the current available studies show that EBV placement is

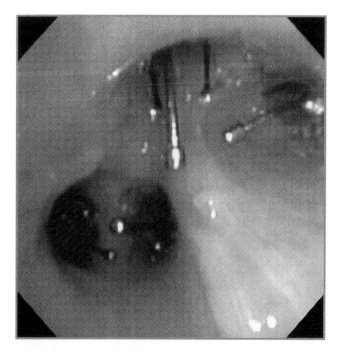

Figure 2 Note intrabronchial valves in place, in the subsegments of the right upper lobe bronchus. Proximal central knob facilitates removal of the valve if required.

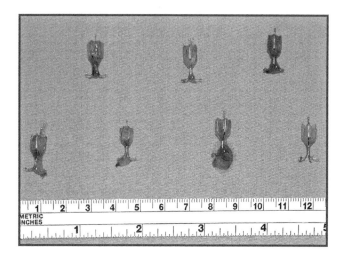

Figure 3 If required intrabronchial valves can be easily removed.

Table 2 Summary of Available Studies with Endobronchial Valves

Device	Study design	Results	Complications	Comments	Reference
Spiration IBV	Multicentric, prospective. 30 patients with upper lobe disease	No improvement in FEV_1 or exercise capacity, but improvement in QOL (SGRQ)	No migration or bleed; 2 patients developed pneumonia	Average of 6.1 valves/patient;.average procedure time 41 min	(15)
Emphasys EBV	Single center, 8 patients	Follow-up at 4 wk showed improvement in FEV_1 and DLCO, particularly in patients with radiographic evidence of volume reduction	2 pneumothorax; 3 COPD exacerbation	25 valves unilaterally Objective: improvement in lung function decreased with time	(16)
Emphasys EBV	Single center, 10 patients	Improvement in DLCO but no improvement in FEV_1 or dyspnea scores	2 COPD exacerbation; 1 pneumonia; 1 pneumothorax	Average 4–11 valves. No radiographic evidence of volume reduction	(17)
Emphasys EBV	Single center, 20 patients	Improvement in FEV_1, FVC, 6MWT, and QOL after 90 days	4 pneumonthorax; 1 severe bronchospasm	Average 2–8 valves. Follow-up CT showed 10/23 lobes with significant volume loss	(18)
Emphasys EBV	Single center, 13 patients	Improvement in FEV_1 and 6MWT. 43% patient able to discontinue O_2	Six complications in 3 patients, including 2 bilateral pneumothorax	Unilateral procedures in 11 patients	(19)
Emphasys EBV	Multicentric, 98 patients	Improvement in FEV_1, FVC, RV, and exercise capacity	8 complications including 1 death	Mean 4 ± 1.6 valves, predominantly RUL	(20)

Abbreviations: IBV, intrabronchial valve; FEV_1, forced expiratory volume in one second; SGRQ, St. George's Respiratory Questionnaire; QOL, quality of life; EBV, endobronchial valve; FVC, forced vital capacity; 6MWT, six-minute walk test; DLCO, diffusion lung capacity; RUL, right upper lobe; COPD, chronic obstructive pulmonary disease.

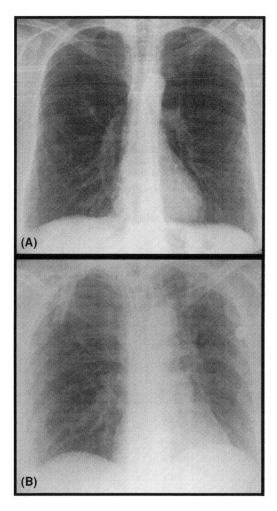

Figure 4 Posteroanterior view of the chest before (**A**) and immediately after (**B**) the intrabronchial valve placement in a patient with severe upper lobe emphysema. Note the position of the diaphragm before and after.

feasible and safe. Moreover, studies have demonstrated beneficial physiologic effects despite absence of significant radiographic LVR. The explanation for the later may be related to a decrease in physiologic dead space and reduction of dynamic hyperinflation (21). Although the studies with different EBV devices demonstrate that the procedure is safe, several potential limitations exist.

1. The majority of patients with advanced emphysema fail to develop evidence of complete atelectasis and significant LVR on CT scans.

2. Extensive collateral ventilation may exist around the targeted segments, allowing significant gas flow around the valves.
3. Theoretically, the high closing volume in the emphysema lung may result in obstruction of conducting airways distal to an EBV, thus reducing efficacy of the device.
4. Few studies have demonstrated sustained long-term beneficial effects.
5. Perioperative complications are common.

Endobronchial Coils

Nitinol self-actuating coils have been manufactured (PneumRx, Inc., Mountain View, California, U.S.) to induce LVR independent of collateral ventilation. Initial data on five patients showed that the coils may be placed safely and without complications. Short-term follow-up showed that all the patients tolerated the devices and showed improvement in lung function (22). Further studies to establish long-term efficacy and safety of these devices are needed.

III. Opening of Extra-Anatomical Pathways

The concept of opening extra-anatomical pathways to alleviate hyperinflation and improve respiratory mechanics in patients with emphysema was postulated in 1978 (23). In emphysema, airways resistance may exceed collateral resistance, redirecting airflow preferentially through collateral pathways. Therefore, when peripheral airways become obstructed or obliterated, collateral channels may provide for more even distribution of ventilation (24).

Lausberg et al. studied collateral airflow in 12 explanted emphysematous lungs placed in an airtight ventilation chamber. The authors created bronchoscopic airway bypasses by puncturing the wall of segmental bronchi with a radiofrequency catheter and inserting a small stent to keep the accessory channels patent (25). The authors found that the forced expiratory volume in one second (FEV_1) increased from 245 ± 107 mL at baseline to 447 ± 199 mL after the placement of three stents, and to 666 ± 284 after placement of five stents ($p < 0.001$). When attempted in normal lungs, the procedure was not associated with a significant change in FEV_1.

On the basis of this principle, Bronchus Technologies Inc. (Mountain View, Washington, U.S.) developed the Exhale Emphysema Treatment System. This system uses a radiofrequency probe to create bronchial fenestrations, and includes an endo-bronchial Doppler device to avoid injury to the surrounding blood vessels. Rendina et al. evaluated this technique in 10 patients who underwent lobe resection for malignancy, and in 5 patients who underwent lung transplantation. Only two episodes of minor hemorrhage were reported, and the procedure was considered to be feasible and safe (26). A modification of the original technique was described in an animal model using a #22-gauge transbronchial needle aspirate (TBNA) needle to create a fenestration, fol-lowed by an angioplasty catheter with an expandable balloon to place an expandable metallic stent. Nevertheless, after three-weeks follow-up, the majority of the new channels were occluded, and the authors had to apply topical mitomycin C to delay occlusion of these passages. In another animal model with dogs, paclitaxel-eluting stents were used to prevent stent occlusion. Compared with complete occlusion in all controls,

65% of the drug-eluting stents were patent after three months of follow-up. Up to date, no clinical studies in humans have evaluated the use of drug-eluting stents to maintain patency of extra-anatomical pathways.

IV. Lung Volume Reduction Using Biologic Agents

Reduction in lung volume can be achieved without the use of an implantable device, by applying biologic reagents that induce inflammation and scarring in areas of the lung. Ingenito et al. described the use of a fibrin-based alveolar lavage in an animal model with sheeps. The technique consisted in a first phase of surfactant wash-out solution, followed by application of a fibrin glue. Although the procedure was associated with radiographic evidence of volume reduction by CT and a significant reduction in total lung capacity (TLC) and residual volume (RV), when compared with the surgical approach, the biologic method was associated with a 45% failure rate and a 15% rate of abscess formation (27).

The method was subsequently modified (Aeris Therapeutics, Woburn, Massachusetts, U.S.). The authors developed a three-step system, which uses a series of biologically active agents delivered through a flexible bronchoscope. Two small aliquots of 10 mL are applied to each segment of the lung. The first aliquot contains a trypsin-based solution used to inactivate surfactant and cause epithelial cell disruption. The second contains a buffered isotonic salt solution to rinse detached epithelial cells, surfactant, and residual trypsin. Subsequently, a dual-lumen catheter is placed into the target site and used to deliver solutions that contain fibrinogen, thrombin, and polymer that form a hydrogel in situ. Once stabilized, this solution will promote local release of fibroblast growth factor-1, transforming growth factor $\beta 1$, and platelet-derived growth factor, causing fibroblast attachment, myofibroblast proliferation, and collagen expression (28). In comparison to previously described BLVR techniques, the volume loss caused by scar formation is not affected by collateral ventilation; nevertheless, the affected area of the lung suffers irreversible damage. As compared to the original method, the three-step technique was associated with a 91% success rate and there were no reports of lung abscess formation (29). Aeris Therapeutics has recently completed a prospective, open-label, noncontrolled, multicenter phase 2 study evaluating the efficacy and safety of this system in patients with advanced upper lobe predominant emphysema involving 50 patients treating 8 subsegmental sites. The conclusion was that biologic LVR improves pulmonary physiology and the functional status of the patients with upper lobe predominant emphysema for up to at least six months. Overall improvement was greater and longer lasting if 20 mL/site dosage was used compared with 10 cc/site. Further long-term studies are required (30).

Although the biologic LVR appears to be superior to other techniques because of a reduced chance of collateral ventilation, no studies have compared the efficacy of these different methods. Additionally, the main disadvantages of the biologic method consist in the irreversibility nature of the procedure, the risk of postobstructive infections because of the inability to drain secretions, and the potential to cause V/Q mismatch because of spillage of the agent to "healthier" areas of the lungs.

V. Lung Volume Reduction Using Thermal Ablation

Bronchoscopic thermal vapor ablation (BTVA) (Uptake Medical Corp., Seattle, Washington, U.S.) consists of delivering heated water vapor into the bronchial tree of targeted lung regions. BTVA utilizes a vapor generator and a metal balloon vapor catheter, with target dosing at 3 to 7.5 cal/g according to a prior CT-based tissue-air algorithm resulting in permanent parenchymal damage and resulting in loss of lung volume. Initial data in 11 patients with heterogeneous emphysema demonstrated that the procedure is safe, although side effects (COPD exacerbation, pneumonia, and hemoptysis) were common (31). Currently studies are underway to establish if BTVA is safe and effective to achieve LVR in patients with COPD.

VI. Conclusions

There are several endoscopic alternatives to achieve successful LVR in patients with COPD. Current evidence suggests that LVR can be safely achieved using different types of EBV, and that these are associated with improvements in lung function in carefully selected patients with severe COPD. The role of newer endoscopic technologies such as thermal vapor application or endobronchial coils is still under investigation.

References

1. Buist AS, McBurnie MA, Vollmer WM, et al. International variation in the prevalence of COPD (the BOLD study): a population-based prevalence study. Lancet 2007; 370:741–750.
2. Mannino DM. COPD: epidemiology, prevalence, morbidity and mortality, and disease heterogeneity. Chest 2002; 121:121S–126S.
3. American Thoracic Society. Standards for the diagnosis and care of patients with chronic obstructive pulmonary disease. Am J Respir Crit Care Med 1995; 152:S77–S121.
4. Ottenheijm CA, Heunks LM, Dekhuijzen RP. Diaphragm adaptations in patients with COPD. Respir Res 2008; 9:12.
5. O'Donnell DE, Webb KA. The major limitation to exercise performance in COPD is dynamic hyperinflation. J Appl Physiol 2008; 105:753–755; discussion 755–757.
6. Shah SS, Goldstraw P. Surgical treatment of bullous emphysema: experience with the Brompton technique. Ann Thorac Surg 1994; 58:1452–1456.
7. Fishman A, Martinez F, Naunheim K, et al. A randomized trial comparing lung-volume-reduction surgery with medical therapy for severe emphysema. N Engl J Med 2003; 348:2059–2073.
8. Patients at high risk of death after lung-volume-reduction surgery. N Engl J Med 2001; 345:1075–1083.
9. Ramsey SD, Sullivan SD, Kaplan RM, et al. Economic analysis of lung volume reduction surgery as part of the National Emphysema Treatment Trial. NETT Research Group. Ann Thorac Surg 2001; 71:995–1002.
10. Sabanathan S, Richardson J, Pieri-Davies S. Bronchoscopic lung volume reduction. J Cardiovasc Surg (Torino) 2003; 44:101–108.
11. Watanabe Y. LVRS with WBA. World Bronchology Conference, Boston, MA, 2002.
12. Watanabe Y, Matsuo K, Tamaoki A, et al. Bronchial occlusion with endobronchial Watanabe spigot. J Bronchol 2003; 10:264–267.
13. Toma T, Matsuo K, Tamaoki A. Endoscopic bronchial occlusion with spigots in patients with emphysema. Am J Respir Crit Care Med 2002; 165(suppl): B9 (abstr).
14. Miyazawa H, Shinno H, Noto H, et al. Bronchial occlusion using EWS by push and slide method and a pilot study of bronchoscopic lung volume reduction using EWS for severe emphysema. J Japan Soc Bronch 2003; 25:695–703.
15. Wood DE, McKenna RJ Jr., Yusen RD, et al. A multicenter trial of an intrabronchial valve for treatment of severe emphysema. J Thorac Cardiovasc Surg 2007; 133:65–73.

16. Toma TP, Hopkinson NS, Hillier J, et al. Bronchoscopic volume reduction with valve implants in patients with severe emphysema. Lancet 2003; 361:931–933.
17. Snell GI, Holsworth L, Borrill ZL, et al. The potential for bronchoscopic lung volume reduction using bronchial prostheses: a pilot study. Chest 2003; 124:1073–1080.
18. Yim AP, Hwong TM, Lee TW, et al. Early results of endoscopic lung volume reduction for emphysema. J Thorac Cardiovasc Surg 2004; 127:1564–1573.
19. Venuta F, de Giacomo T, Rendina EA, et al. Bronchoscopic lung-volume reduction with one-way valves in patients with heterogenous emphysema. Ann Thorac Surg 2005; 79:411–416; discussion 416–417.
20. Wan IY, Toma TP, Geddes DM, et al. Bronchoscopic lung volume reduction for end-stage emphysema: report on the first 98 patients. Chest 2006; 129:518–526.
21. Hopkinson NS, Toma TP, Hansell DM, et al. Effect of bronchoscopic lung volume reduction on dynamic hyperinflation and exercise in emphysema. Am J Respir Crit Care Med 2005; 171:453–460.
22. Ernst A, Herth F. Clinical Experience Using a Non-Valve Minimally Invasive Implantable Device for the Treatment of Late Stage Homogeneous and Heterogeneous Emphysema. Philadelphia: American College of Chest Physicians, 2008.
23. Macklem PT. Collateral ventilation. N Engl J Med 1978; 298:49–50.
24. Terry PB, Traystman RJ, Newball HH, et al. Collateral ventilation in man. N Engl J Med 1978; 298:10–15.
25. Lausberg HF, Chino K, Patterson GA, et al. Bronchial fenestration improves expiratory flow in emphysematous human lungs. Ann Thorac Surg 2003; 75:393–397; discussion 398.
26. Rendina EA, De Giacomo T, Venuta F, et al. Feasibility and safety of the airway bypass procedure for patients with emphysema. J Thorac Cardiovasc Surg 2003; 125:1294–1299.
27. Ingenito EP, Reilly JJ, Mentzer SJ, et al. Bronchoscopic volume reduction: a safe and effective alternative to surgical therapy for emphysema. Am J Respir Crit Care Med 2001; 164:295–301.
28. Ingenito EP, Tsai LW, Sullivan SD, et al. Fibroblast growth factor-1 therapy for advanced emphysema—a new tissue engineering approach for achieving lung volume reduction. J Bronchol 2006; 13:114–123.
29. Ingenito EP, Berger RL, Henderson AC, et al. Bronchoscopic lung volume reduction using tissue engineering principles. Am J Respir Crit Care Med 2003; 167:771–778.
30. Criner GJ, Pinto-Plata V, Strange C, et al. Biologic lung volume reduction in advanced upper lobe emphysema: phase 2 results. Am J Respir Crit Care Med 2009; 179:791–798.
31. Snell GI, Hopkins G, Westall G, et al. The Feasibility and Safety of Bronchoscopic Thermal Vapour Ablation Therapy: A Novel Treatment of Severe Upper Lobe Heterogenous Emphysema. Philadelphia: American College of Chest Physicians, 2008.

10
Bronchial Thermoplasty

MARTIN L. MAYSE and MARIO CASTRO
Washington University School of Medicine, St. Louis, Missouri, U.S.A.

I. Introduction

Bronchial thermoplasty is an investigational bronchoscopic procedure for the treatment of asthma designed to reduce the amount of airway smooth muscle (ASM) (1) with the goal of decreasing bronchoconstriction and the frequency and severity of asthma symptoms (2). Bronchial thermoplasty is achieved by the controlled delivery of radio-frequency (RF) electrical energy to the airway wall via a special catheter electrode. This heats the airway wall to a specific target temperature, which ultimately leads to a decrease in ASM without airway perforation or stenosis. Energy is systematically applied to the majority of airways between 3 and 10 mm in diameter throughout the tracheobronchial tree.

Bronchial thermoplasty is performed with the investigational Alair® Bronchial Thermoplasty System (Asthmatx, Inc. Sunnyvale, California, U.S.) (3) and has been used safely in animals (2) and both nonasthmatic (4) and asthmatic human subjects (5). Previous unblinded clinical studies comparing bronchial thermoplasty to standard medical therapy in asthmatic subjects have demonstrated an improvement in asthma control (5,6) and quality of life (7). While conceptually straightforward, the bronchial thermoplasty procedure is meticulous and procedural duration is substantially longer than that encountered during routine bronchoscopy. Optimal patient selection, procedural planning, and patient management are critical for success. This chapter describes the theory behind bronchial thermoplasty, reviews the preclinical data, describes the equipment and procedure, discusses patient selection and preparation, outlines special considerations for patient management during the procedure, and finally presents the results of published clinical trials to date.

II. Theory
A. Overview

Asthma is a chronic airway disease in which patients typically present with dyspnea, wheezing, chest tightness, and cough. The pathophysiology of asthma is characterized by airway inflammation and remodeling, variable airflow obstruction, and bronchial hyperresponsiveness. The airway remodeling in asthma refers to structural changes in the airway, including epithelial changes, subepithelial fibrosis, goblet cell metaplasia, blood vessel hyperplasia, and importantly ASM hypertrophy. Contraction of the ASM results in subsequent airway narrowing and airflow obstruction. Current therapy for asthma includes short- and long-term bronchodilators and anti-inflammatory therapy; however, no therapy exists for long-term modulation of ASM.

B. Physiologic Basis

ASM plays a prominent role in the pathophysiology of asthma. During asthma exacerbations, patients respond to drugs that relieve spasm of smooth muscle in the airways, and asthmatics are hyperresponsive to smooth muscle agonists. Examination of airways obtained at postmortem, open lung biopsy, or bronchial biopsy demonstrates smooth muscle hypertrophy and hyperplasia, indicating that ASM may be causally related to the hyperresponsiveness of asthma (8).

The physiologic basis for ASM contraction leading to airway hyperresponsiveness has not been well delineated, but it is felt to be because of geometrical narrowing of the airway because of the hypertrophy of ASM (9), exaggerated narrowing of the ASM (10), limited capacity to relax with inspiration (11), thicker remodeled airways because of altered mucosal folding (12,13), and altered lung mechanics because of altered elastic recoil and airway closure (14,15). Triggers of bronchoconstriction in asthma, for example, allergens and irritants, are associated with ASM contraction. A reduction in the amount of functioning ASM should reduce the bronchoconstriction characteristic of asthma.

Bronchial thermoplasty is a new procedure that may reduce ASM. Bronchial thermoplasty is achieved by the controlled heating of the airway wall to decrease the amount of ASM. In its current embodiment, an electrode array is placed within the airway, expanded to contact the airway walls, and RF electrical energy is passed from this electrode into the tissues of the airway wall. As electrical energy passes from the electrode to the tissue, resistance at the electrode-tissue interface and within the tissue itself causes the electrical energy to be converted to heat. While similar in basic principles to conventional RF ablation, the delivery of RF electrical energy during bronchial thermoplasty utilizes continuous feedback to tightly control the degree of tissue heating, thereby decreasing ASM without leading to airway perforation or stenosis.

C. Preclinical Data

Preclinical studies of bronchial thermoplasty have been performed in a canine model (2). In this model, airway responsiveness to methacholine was significantly reduced following bronchial thermoplasty for up to 3 years. Furthermore, airway responsiveness to methacholine was inversely correlated to the extent of ASM by histologic examination. Treatment effects were limited to the airway wall and the immediate peribronchial region. A separate study in a canine model using computed tomography demonstrated a significant reduction in methacholine responsiveness two to four weeks post treatment (16).

A feasibility study of bronchial thermoplasty has also been performed in patients who have been scheduled for lung resection for a suspected lung cancer (4). Bronchial thermoplasty was performed during preoperative bronchoscopy in the segmental airways within the lobe that was to be removed up to three weeks prior to the scheduled lung resection. There were no adverse effects from the procedure or bronchoscopic evidence of scarring. Histologic examination of the resected specimens demonstrated reduction in

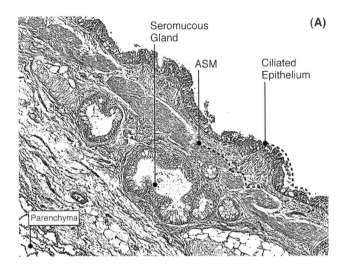

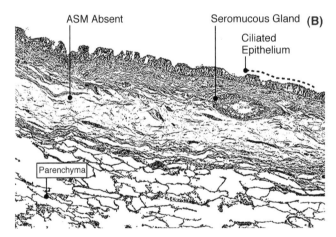

Figure 1 Histopatholology before and after bronchial thermoplasty. Histopathologic features of untreated control airway (**A**) and an airway 12 weeks after treatment with RF bronchial thermoplasty (**B**) (trichrome stain, original magnification 100×). ASM in the untreated airway is normal, and ASM in the airway treated with bronchial thermoplasty is essentially absent. The parenchyma, epithelium, and mucous glands in the treated airway are unaffected. *Abbreviation*: ASM, airway smooth muscle. *Source*: Modified from Ref. 2.

ASM and the treatment was confined to the airway wall and immediate peribronchial region (Fig. 1).

These preclinical studies in dogs and humans lend support to the safety and feasibility of performing bronchial thermoplasty to reduce smooth muscle in asthma patients.

III. Procedure

A. Overview

Bronchial thermoplasty is performed during bronchoscopy with the patient under moderate (formerly called conscious) sedation. All accessible airways distal to the main stem bronchi and between 3 and 10 mm in diameter, with the exception of the right middle lobe, are treated under bronchoscopic direct visualization. To treat the entire target airway, contiguous and nonoverlapping activations of the device are used, moving from distal to proximal along the length of the airway, and systematically from airway to airway as described previously (1,2,5). The entirety of both lungs are treated in three bronchoscopy sessions, each lasting approximately one hour and each separated by about three weeks.

B. Equipment

Bronchial thermoplasty is currently performed using the investigational Alair Bronchial Thermoplasty System composed of the Alair catheter and the Alair RF controller (Fig. 2). The Alair catheter is a single-use, flexible device with an expandable 4-wire electrode array at one end and a deployment handle at the other. This device is designed to be delivered into the airways under direct visualization through the working channel of an RF or high-frequency (HF) compatible bronchoscope; ideally the smallest diameter bronchoscope possible. Larger bronchoscopes (>5.2 mm OD) are not recommended since they limit access and thereby the treatment of smaller airways. Once in place, the electrode array is expanded by an actuator on the deployment handle to contact the airway walls. The Alair RF controller is an RF electrical generator with a foot pedal activator switch. It continuously monitors temperature at the electrode-tissue interface and adjusts the rate of energy delivery into the tissue in a manner appropriate for the asthma treatment application. The Controller also monitors the system to ensure proper setup. For instance, energy cannot be delivered until all accessories are properly connected, and if the electrode array is not in proper contact with the airway wall, the front panel notifies the bronchoscopist to reposition the electrode array to make proper contact. A standard gel-type patient return electrode is affixed to the patient and connected to the controller to provide a complete circuit.

C. Technique

The following is based on the described procedure used in the previous human clinical studies and the current ongoing pivotal trial of bronchial thermoplasty. The bronchial thermoplasty treatment for the entirety of both lungs is performed during three separate bronchoscopy sessions, each session separated by about three weeks. This divided treatment is done to minimize the risk of an asthma exacerbation or diffuse airways edema that might occur if the entire tracheobronchial tree were accessed and treated in one session, and to avoid excessive procedural length. The right lower lobe is treated in the first bronchoscopy. The left lower lobe is treated in the second bronchoscopy. Both the right and left upper lobes are treated in the third and final bronchoscopy (5). The right middle lobe is not treated because of theoretical concerns that circumferential heating of the bronchus may lead to right middle lobe syndrome (1,17), although no experience in treating the right middle lobe with bronchial thermoplasty currently exists.

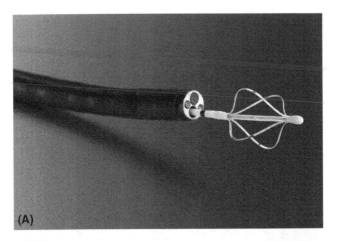

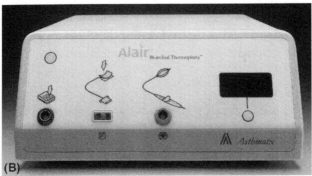

Figure 2 Alair catheter and controller. (**A**) The Alair catheter with expandable electrode array passed through the working channel of a flexible bronchoscope. (**B**) The front panel of the Alair RF controller.

For an individual bronchoscopy session, the patient is prepared in the manner outlined in the patient management section below. The bronchoscope is then introduced and any previously treated airways are inspected to evaluate for possible mucous impaction or scarring and to ensure adequate healing. If previously treated areas have not healed, consideration should be given to postponing treatment. Following inspection, the bronchoscope is navigated to the region of the lung to be treated, and the order in which the airway segments are to be accessed and treated is planned. Treatment planning is crucial to the success of bronchial thermoplasty. If the airways are approached in a random fashion, some airways may be treated twice while other airways may be skipped entirely. We recommend a systematic approach from distal to proximal, working methodically from airway to airway across the region of lung being treated to ensure that all accessible airways are carefully identified and treated once and only once. As an example, treatment planning for the right lower lobe might allow initial treatment of the anterior segment followed by the lateral and posterior segments. The medial segment is then treated followed by the distal portion of the right lower lobe bronchus up to the level of the superior segment, and finally the superior segment is treated. Within each segment, the subsegmental airways should also be treated in a similar systematic manner, moving from superior airways to those that are more inferior, or moving from airways to the right of the field of view to those that are more to the left.

Following treatment planning, the bronchoscope is navigated to the most distal region of the first airway to be treated. The catheter is then passed through the working channel of the bronchoscope and advanced to the targeted region under continuous bronchoscopic visualization. The electrode array is expanded by depressing the activator on the deployment handle until the four electrode wires firmly contact the airway wall. Care should be taken not to overexpand the electrodes as this may distort the electrode array. Energy delivery is then initiated by pressing and releasing the controller footswitch. The controller will deliver RF energy automatically for approximately 10 seconds, adjusting the rate of energy delivery according to preprogrammed parameters. Following each activation, the electrode array is partially collapsed and repositioned proximally the length of the exposed electrode wire, about 5 mm. This positions the exposed portion of the electrode adjacent to, but not overlapping, the previous activation site. This process is repeated along the entire length of each targeted airway as shown in Figure 3, and progresses from airway to airway as determined during treatment planning. The electrode array position should be referenced to anatomical landmarks because of the potential for relative motion between the bronchoscope, catheter, and airways that may occur with breathing, coughing, or during repositioning. The use of a "map" of the airways to plan and track the progression of the treatment has been used with success and is recommended (18).

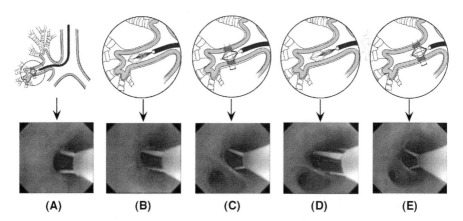

| (A) | (B) | (C) | (D) | (E) |

Figure 3 Contiguous activations with the Alair catheter in an airway. The two images in each panel are a graphic representation of the Alair catheter in the airway with a matched bronchoscopic photograph of the catheter in the airway. (**A**) The catheter placed distally in airway, with the electrode array expanded and controller activated. (**B**) Following completion of the activation, the electrode array partially collapsed and moved 5 mm proximal to previous activation site. (**C**) The electrode array reexpanded in position adjacent but not overlapping previous activation site. The controller is again activated. (**D**) After completion of the activation, the electrode array partially collapsed and moved 5 mm proximal to previous activation. (**E**) The electrode array reexpanded in a position adjacent but not overlapping previous activation site. The controller is activated once again.

On occasion, mucus may build up in the airways and obscures bronchoscopic visualization. When this occurs, the electrode array can be completely retracted and the catheter removed from the bronchoscope, allowing irrigation and suctioning. Advantage can be taken of this to gently clean the electrode array with sterile saline and to apply more topical anesthesia to the airways if needed.

IV. Patient Selection

Before considering a patient for bronchial thermoplasty the physician should obtain a detailed medical history and perform appropriate medical evaluations to determine the patient's suitability to undergo this procedure. It should be assured that the patient is appropriate for bronchial thermoplasty, on the basis of patient populations that have been studied in clinical trials, and is safe to undergo bronchoscopy. Table 1 outlines considerations for patient selection and safety.

Table 1 Patient Selection

Patients may be considered for bronchial thermoplasty if they meet the following minimal criteria[a]

Appropriate for bronchial thermoplasty

- Adults with documented diagnosis of asthma:
  - documented reversible decrease in FEV_1 or
  - airway responsiveness by methacholine challenge
- Nonsmoker for 1 year or greater (and, if former smoker, <10 pack years)
- Symptomatic despite treatment with stable maintenance medication [such as fluticasone (or equivalent) >500 μg per day ± long-acting β_2-agonist (LABA)]
- Prebronchodilator $FEV_1 \geq 60\%$ predicted
- Stable with respect to asthma status
  - no current respiratory tract infection
  - no severe asthma exacerbation within the last 2 weeks
  - forced expiratory volume in one second (FEV_1) within 10% of the best value

Safe to undergo bronchoscopy

- Able to undergo bronchoscopy as per hospital guidelines
- No known sensitivity to medications required to perform bronchoscopy (such as lidocaine, atropine, opiates such as fentanyl, and benzodiazepines such as midazolam)
- No known unstable comorbid conditions that would present a risk for bronchoscopy, such as untreated obstructive sleep apnea or clinically significant cardiovascular disease, epilepsy, diabetes, or cancer
- No internal pacemaker or neurostimulator

---

[a]Based on inclusion and exclusion criteria that were used in prior clinical trials of bronchial thermoplasty and accepted guidelines for treatment of asthma. For complete information on inclusion and exclusion criteria, see http://www.clinicaltrial.gov.

V. Patient Management

The success of bronchial thermoplasty depends not only on an appropriately selected patient and the technique of the bronchoscopist, but also on adequate patient management before, during, and after the procedure. While patient management for bronchial thermoplasty is similar to that of any bronchoscopic procedure, there are special considerations for the management of patients undergoing bronchial thermoplasty. These considerations arise for several reasons: patients undergoing bronchial thermoplasty have moderate persistent asthma, patients must undergo a total of three bronchoscopic sessions to complete treatment, and the individual bronchoscopy sessions tend to be relatively long when done properly. To overcome these issues, asthma stability is reassessed on the day of each bronchoscopy, steroids are given to decrease postprocedure inflammation, inhaled bronchodilators are administered, drying agents are given to decrease mucus production, good topical anesthesia of the airway and an appropriate level anesthesia are provide to facilitate the procedure and increase patient willingness to undergo repeat bronchoscopies, and lastly the administration of topical anesthesia, anxiolytics, and analgesics are repeated as needed during the longer procedure.

A. Patient Preparation and Premedication

To minimize postprocedure inflammation of the airways, patients are given prophylactic prednisone at a dosage of 50 mg/day (or equivalent) for five days: the three days prior to the procedure, the day of procedure, and the day after the procedure (3).

On the day of each procedure, patients should be reevaluated to ensure they remain a good candidate for bronchial thermoplasty (Table 2) and bronchoscopy should be postponed if they no longer meet recommended criteria. If the patient has not taken their prescribed oral prednisone on the day of the procedure, premedication should include intravenous (IV) administration of 40 mg methylprednisolone or its equivalent. An albuterol nebulizer of 2.5 to 5.0 mg or 4 to 8 puffs of albuterol with a metered dose inhaler and an antisialogogue agent such as glycopyrrolate at a dosage of 0.2 to 0.4 mg IV or intramuscular (IM) (a minimum of 30 minutes prior to the procedure) should be administered. Caution should be exercised while using this agent because of its chronotropic risk. Glycopyrrolate is preferred over atropine because it is a superior drying agent with fewer propensities for adverse central nervous system effects or tachyarrhythmias. While perhaps not clinically proven to have a meaningful impact in other bronchoscopic procedures (19), the benefits of treating with an effective drying agent to reduce the amount of airway secretions and improve visibility through the bronchoscope have been experienced during bronchial thermoplasty (7,18).

B. Topical Anesthesia

Judicious application of topical anesthesia is very important to the success of bronchial thermoplasty. Any standard approach to the application of topical anesthesia to the upper airway can be used, so long as the nasal and/or oral passages are anesthetized and lubricated and the posterior pharynx is sufficiently anesthetized so as to significantly diminish or eliminate the patient's gag reflex. The patient's sedation level is reassessed and considerations are made for supplementing with more anxiolytic or antitussive medications (see Sedation section) as needed.

Table 2 Considerations on the Day of Bronchoscopy

Immediately prior to bronchoscopy, postpone the procedure for any of the following reasons:

- Prescribed prednisone or prednisolone was not taken on the 3 days prior to bronchoscopy
- SpO$_2$ less than 90% on room air
- Increase in asthma symptoms in last 48 hours requiring more than 4 puffs/day on average of rescue bronchodilator over pretreatment usage
- Less than 14 days from completion of a course of oral corticosteroid use for an exacerbation of asthma
- Postbronchodilator FEV$_1$ is less than 85% of pretreatment value
- Active respiratory infection, active allergic sinusitis, or other clinical instability
- Physician feels for any reason the treatment should be postponed

During bronchoscopy, terminate the procedure if any of the following observations are made:

- Airways are unusually edematous or inflamed
- Extensive and/or prolonged bronchoconstriction
- Airways accessed in previous bronchoscopy session do not appear to be sufficiently healed
- Presence of purulent or abnormally tenacious sputum or mucus plugging
- Inability to access airways because of excessive secretions, excessive coughing, or tortuous anatomy
- Physician feels for any reason that the treatment should be terminated

Once the patient's upper airway has been sufficiently anesthetized, anesthetizing the vocal cords and bronchial tree can proceed. Although different concentrations of lidocaine may be used, 1% lidocaine is recommended to limit the potential for lidocaine toxicity. At the vocal cord level, 1% lidocaine can be applied in small (2 mL) aliquots through the working channel of the bronchus until the patient appears comfortable with minimal coughing. As the bronchoscope is advanced down the airway, 1% lidocaine should be used in small (2 mL) aliquots down the bronchial tree. Application of local anesthetic should focus more on the airway segments being targeted for treatment. After 30 to 40 minutes into the procedure, additional topical anesthesia should be considered if necessary.

The maximum dose of lidocaine is often institution specific; however, 600 mg of lidocaine or 8.2 mg/kg or less has been used safely in asthmatics undergoing bronchoscopy (20). The patient should be continuously monitored for signs and symptoms of lidocaine toxicity. Toxic reactions to local anesthetics most frequently involve the central nervous system and may include lightheadedness, tongue numbness, visual changes, auditory disturbances, seizures, or loss of consciousness (21). If doses exceed the maximum limits, consider monitoring lidocaine levels post procedure.

C. Sedation

Simultaneous with achieving adequate anesthesia in the patient's airway, it is critically important to achieve and maintain an optimal level of sedation. Most patients can undergo bronchial thermoplasty under moderate sedation. Moderate sedation, as defined by the American Society of Anesthesiologists (ASA) (22), is when a patient responds purposefully to either verbal commands alone or with light tactile stimulation. The choice of medications necessary for good patient management will ultimately be the choice of the physician performing the procedure and may vary on the basis of country- or institution-specific guidelines and practices. However, the combination of a short-acting benzodiazepine and a narcotic, namely midazolam and fentanyl, are excellent choices because of their familiarity and ability to be carefully titrated and, if necessary, to be rapidly reversed.

Midazolam is a fast-acting benzodiazepine with a short half-life, and it can be easily titrated to effect. It is often initially given in a 1 to 2 mg loading dose followed by incremental doses of 0.5 to 1 mg as needed. The onset of the effect is within one to three minutes, with a maximum duration of about two hours. Midazolam also produces antegrade amnesia or anxiolysis, and has an anticonvulsant effect. The objective is patient anxiolysis and patient comfort while still maintaining adequate spontaneous ventilation during the procedure. Supplemental doses should be given if the patient is anxious or has minimal sedation assuming adequate oxygenation and ventilation. The precise timing of sedation will vary between patients and largely depends on the clinical judgment of the physician.

Fentanyl is also an effective sedating agent used during bronchial thermoplasty and it is beneficial because it has both potent analgesic and antitussive properties. An effective loading dose is 50 to 100 μg IV with additional doses of 25 to 50 μg IV as needed. Onset of action is 2 to 4 minutes with a peak effect at 10 to 15 minutes and duration ranging from 30 to 60 minutes. Supplemental doses should be administered if the patient has minimal sedation, is having pain, or is coughing excessively. The ultimate objective is to provide the patient with adequate analgesia and sedation with minimal coughing.

It is important to note that benzodiazepines and opiates have different mechanisms of action, but potentiate each other's actions including respiratory depression and hypotension. Therefore, frequent smaller supplemental sedative/analgesic doses allow for more effective titration. The main advantage of using midazolam and fentanyl to induce moderate sedation is their fast onset times, which make them more easily titratable. In addition, both medications have reversal agents (naloxone and flumazenil, respectively) that can be used to antagonize their effects if necessary. Sedation can be produced while avoiding side effects.

D. Postprocedure Care

In addition to standard milestones used during post–bronchoscopy recovery milestones, patients should be discharged only after the patient's postbronchodilator FEV_1 is within 80% value and the patient is feeling well. It should also be verified that patients have their prophylactic steroid to be taken the day following each bronchoscopy.

As with any bronchoscopic procedure, there is an expected increase and worsening of respiratory-related symptoms in the period immediately following bronchial thermoplasty, such as breathlessness, wheeze, cough, chest discomfort, night awakenings, and productive cough (5,7). These symptoms typically present within one week of bronchoscopy and resolve with standard medical care on average within one week. Therefore, it is very important to contact the patient 24, 48 hours, and 7 days post procedure to assess their status following bronchoscopy. In particular, there is a potential for excess mucus production in response to bronchoscopy and bronchial thermoplasty in asthma patients. It is expected that coughing will clear any excess mucus; however, it is possible that the mucus may become thickened and occlude the airway. In the event thickened mucus is suspected, a chest radiograph should be obtained, and if mucus plugging is confirmed, patients should be treated with chest physiotherapy and/or therapeutic bronchoscopy as indicated. They should also be monitored carefully until resolution occurs.

E. Clinical Data

Preliminary studies have demonstrated the safety and efficacy of bronchial thermoplasty. In a feasibility study, Cox et al. evaluated the safety of bronchial thermoplasty in 16 subjects with mild to moderate persistent stable asthma at two different sites (5). At baseline lung function testing, including methacholine bronchoprovocation, peak flow measurements, symptoms, and medications were recorded. Evaluations were performed at 12 weeks, 1, and 2 years post treatment. All treatments were completed within 30 minutes. Acutely blanching of the airways was noted but there were no subsequent changes in structure of the airways. There were 312 adverse events: 74% mild, 25% moderate, and 1% severe. The severe adverse events involved hospitalization for an unrelated event. The most frequent procedure-related adverse events were increased cough, dyspnea, wheeze, and bronchospasm, and all resolved within one week of the procedure. Most of these procedure-related events required bronchodilators, though 3% required systemic corticosteroids.

In this feasibility study (5), subjects following bronchial thermoplasty demonstrated a significant improvement in airway responsiveness. The mean PC20 increased by 2.4 ± 1.7 ($p < 0.001$), 2.8 ± 1.5 ($p = 0.007$), and 2.6 ± 1.5 doublings ($p < 0.001$) at 12 weeks, and 1 and 2 years post treatment, respectively. There was no significant change in FEV_1 at two years though there were significant improvements at 12 weeks and 1 year. There were significant improvements in symptom-free days ($p = 0.015$) and morning ($p = 0.01$) and evening peak flows ($p = 0.007$). Therefore, this feasibility study of bronchial thermoplasty demonstrated a significant improvement in airway hyperresponsiveness for up to two years in a small group of mild to moderate asthma patients.

A follow-up study focused on quality of life and satisfaction with bronchial thermoplasty performed on 16 subjects (6). Approximately one year post thermoplasty, patients reported an increased ability to carry out activities, tolerate allergens, and perform physical activity. All patients indicated they would probably or definitely undergo the procedure again and would recommend it to others.

In the largest study published to date of bronchial thermoplasty, Asthma Intervention Research (AIR) trial, Cox et al. randomized 112 subjects with moderate to severe persistent asthma requiring inhaled corticosteroids and long-acting β-agonists (LABA) and in whom asthma control worsened when the LABA was withdrawn to either bronchial thermoplasty or usual care control group (7). The primary end point in this study was mild exacerbations during LABA withdrawal at 3, 6, and 12 months. The mean rate of mild exacerbations was significantly reduced following bronchial thermoplasty but unchanged in the control group: -0.16 ± 0.37 versus $+0.04 \pm 0.29$ exacerbations per subject per week, $p = 0.005$ (Fig. 4). This translates to approximately 10 fewer mild exacerbations per subject per year. There was not a significant difference in severe exacerbations between the groups.

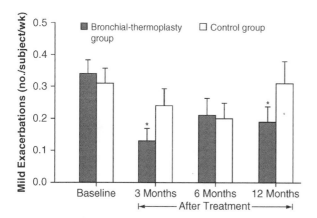

Figure 4 Rates of mild exacerbations per subject per week. Mean values are shown for all subjects receiving inhaled corticosteroids alone for whom data were available at the given time points. Asterisks indicate a statistically significant difference in the mean change from baseline between the two groups, and I-bars represent the standard errors. $p = 0.03$ for the comparison between subjects in the two groups treated with inhaled corticosteroids alone at 3 and 12 months. *Source*: Modified from Ref. 7.

In the AIR study, there was a significant improvement in morning peak flows (39 $\pm$ 49 L/min, $p = 0.003$) and reduction in β-agonist use (approximately 9 puffs per week, $p = 0.04$) although there was no significant difference in FEV_1 or PC_{20} at 12 months (Fig. 5) (7). Asthma quality of life (1.3 ± 1.0 vs. 0.6 ± 1.1, $p = 0.003$) and asthma control (-1.2 ± 1.0 vs. -0.5 ± 1.0, $p = 0.001$) significantly improved following thermoplasty. Furthermore, there was a 2.6-fold increase in symptom-free days (-41 ± 40 vs. 17 ± 38, $p = 0.005$) and improvement in symptom scores (-1.9 ± 2.1 vs. 0.7 ± 2.5, $p = 0.01$). This translates to approximately three additional symptom-free months per subject per year. Interestingly, in a post hoc analysis these benefits were even greater in a subgroup of subjects requiring high maintenance doses of inhaled corticosteroids (>1000 μg of beclomethasone or the equivalent).

Finally, in the AIR study, adverse events were more common immediately following thermoplasty but similar after 6 weeks and 12 months after treatment (7). During the treatment period, there were 407 adverse respiratory events: 69% mild, 30% moderate, and 1% severe. The majority of these adverse events occurred within one day of the procedure and resolved an average of seven days after the onset. Four subjects required six hospitalizations in the bronchial thermoplasty group compared with only two hospitalizations in the control group. These hospitalizations post thermoplasty included asthma exacerbation, pleurisy, and partial collapse of the left lower lobe two days following treatment. There was no relationship noted between these adverse events and the experience of the bronchoscopist with thermoplasty.

A recent controlled study in subjects with severe asthma complements the previous findings from the AIR trial. In the Research in Severe Asthma (RISA) trial, the primary objective was to determine the safety of bronchial thermoplasty in 32 subjects with severe symptomatic asthma (23). These subjects required high doses of inhaled or oral corticosteroids (>750 μg of inhaled fluticasone and/or ≤30 mg of oral pre-dnisolone/day) and were symptomatic on at least 10 out of 14 days. In this study, bronchial thermoplasty did result in transient worsening of asthma symptoms that resolved within one week after the onset similar to the AIR trial. However, there were

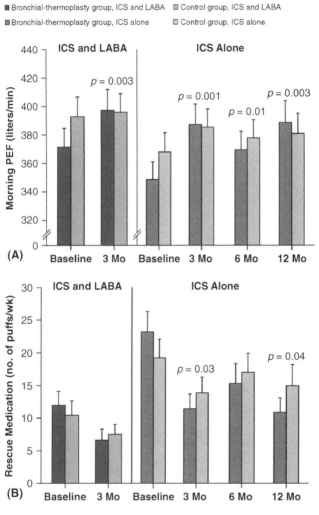

Figure 5 Measures of asthma control at baseline and during follow-up. Mean values are shown for all subjects for whom data were available at the given time points. *p* values are for comparisons of the mean change from baseline between the two groups. I-bars represent standard errors. (**A**) Morning peak expiratory flow rates in liters per minute. (**B**) Use of rescue medications over the study period. (**C**) The percentage of symptom-free days. (**D**) Responses to the Asthma Quality of Life Questionnaire (AQLQ), which are scored on a scale of 1 to 7, with higher numbers indicating a better quality of life. The minimal important difference is thought to be 0.5. Modified from Ref. 7.

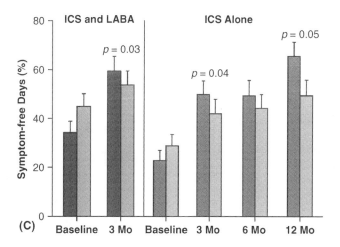

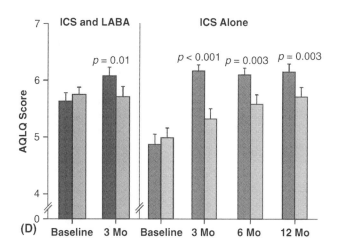

Figure 5 (*Continued*)

seven hospitalizations that occurred in 4 of the 15 bronchial thermoplasty including two subjects with segmental lobar collapse requiring treatment. After six weeks, there was no significant difference in adverse events between the two groups.

Interestingly, the RISA study had beneficial response in improving asthma control in this small study of severe asthma. Subjects following thermoplasty were able to reduce their rescue medication use (-27 ± 40 vs. -2 ± 12 puffs per week, $p < 0.05$, treated vs. control, respectively) and improve their asthma control score -1.0 ± 1.0 vs. -0.1 ± 1.0, $p = 0.02$). Unlike the AIR trial, these subjects experienced a significant improvement in lung function (15 ± 17 vs. -0.9 ± 22 FEV_1 percent predicted, $p = 0.04$). These improvements in asthma control and rescue medication use persisted one year after thermoplasty treatment. These studies suggest that bronchial thermoplasty can result in lasting improvements in asthma control with less rescue medication use though with an associated short-term increase in asthma morbidity.

Additional studies are under way to evaluate the safety and efficacy of bronchial thermoplasty in a double-blind, sham-controlled trial in 297 subjects with moderate-persistent asthma (3).

VI. Summary

Bronchial thermoplasty is an investigational procedure using RF energy to heat airway tissue in a way designed to reduce the amount of ASM (1) and hence the potential for bronchospasm and asthma symptoms. In an unblinded, multicenter, randomized clinical trial involving patients with asthma, bronchial thermoplasty was shown to improve asthma control and quality of life (7). While the potential for a strong placebo effect exists in this unblinded study, the magnitude and persistence of the effects observed were likely greater than what could be attributed to placebo alone.

Successful bronchial thermoplasty requires that all accessible airways distal to the main stem bronchi between 3 and 10 mm in diameter, with the exception of the right middle lobe, be treated once and only once. To achieve this goal, a systematic approach moving from distal to proximal within an airway and working methodically from airway to airway across the region of lung being treated is recommended. This systematic approach results in a bronchoscopy that is generally longer in duration than bronchoscopies performed for bronchoalveolar lavage or tissue biopsy. Patient management during bronchial thermoplasty must be emphasized because optimal administration of the treatment requires minimal patient movement during the procedure. Thus, adequate and effective administration of sedatives and analgesics to achieve and maintain moderate sedation is critically important. Because the full treatment of the entire lung requires more than one bronchoscopy session, it is important that patient comfort is maximized so that the patient's anxiety for future bronchoscopies is minimized.

Preliminary clinical results of bronchial thermoplasty appear encouraging (5,7), although these findings should be interpreted with caution, as these were unblinded studies of a procedure with a high potential for placebo effect. An appropriately powered, blinded, sham-controlled study is currently under way to assess the ultimate risk to benefit ratio of this procedure.

Acknowledgments

We are indebted to Michael D. Laufer, MD, who pioneered the method of treating airway smooth muscle physically to ameliorate asthma, to Gerard Cox, MB and John Miller, MD (McMaster University, Hamilton, Ontario) for the first use and development of this technique in the clinical setting, and The AIR, RISA and AIR2 Trial Study Groups for their important contributions to the advancement of bronchial thermoplasty.

The Alair Bronchial Thermoplasty System has received a CE mark to sell the device in the European Union and it is currently under investigation in an FDA-approved IDE pivotal clinical trial in the United States (3). This trial is supported by Asthmatx, Inc., Sunnyvale, California, United States.

Alair and Asthmatx are registered trademarks of Asthmatx, Inc.

References

1. Cox PG, Miller J, Mitzner W, et al. Radiofrequency ablation of airway smooth muscle for sustained treatment of asthma: preliminary investigations. Eur Respir J 2004; 24:659–663.
2. Danek CJ, Lombard CM, Dungworth DL, et al. Reduction in airway hyperresponsiveness to methacholine by the application of RF energy in dogs. J Appl Physiol 2004; 97:1946–1953.
3. AIR2 Trial. Available at: http://www.clinicaltrials.gov/ct/show/NCT00231114?order=1.
4. Miller JD, Cox G, Vincic L, et al. A prospective feasibility study of bronchial thermoplasty in the human airway. Chest 2005; 127:1999–2006.
5. Cox G, Miller JD, McWilliams A, et al. Bronchial thermoplasty for asthma. Am J Respir Crit Care Med 2006; 173:965–969.
6. Wilson S, Cox G, Miller J, et al. Global assessment after bronchial thermoplasty: the patient's perspective. J Outcomes Res 2006; 10:37–46.
7. Cox G, Thomson NC, Rubin AS, et al. Asthma control in the year following bronchial thermoplasty. N Engl J Med 2007; 356:1327–1337.
8. Heard B, Hossain S. Hyperplasia of bronchial muscle in asthma. J Pathol 1971; 110:319–331.
9. James A, Paré P, Hogg J. The mechanics of airway narrowing in asthma. Am Rev Respir Dis 1989; 139:242–246.
10. Fredberg JJ, Inouye D, Miller B, et al. Airway smooth muscle, tidal stretches, and dynamically determined contractile states. Am J Respir Crit Care Med 1997; 156:1752–1759.
11. Skloot G, Permutt S, Togias A. Airway hyperresponsiveness in asthma: a problem of limited smooth muscle relaxation with inspiration. J Clin Invest 1995; 96:2393–2403.
12. Lambert R, Wiggs B, Kuwano K, et al. Functional significance of increased airway smooth muscle in asthma and COPD. J Appl Physiol 1993; 74:2771–2781.
13. Wiggs B, Bosken C, Paré P, et al. A model of airway narrowing in asthma and in chronic obstructive pulmonary disease. Am Rev Respir Dis 1992; 145:1251–1258.
14. Ding D, Martin J, Macklem P. Effects of lung on maximal methacholine-induced bronchoconstriction in normal humans. J Appl Physiol 1987; 62:1324–1330.
15. Macklem P. A theoretical analysis of the effect of airway smooth muscle load on airway narrowing. Am J Respir Crit Care Med 1996; 153:83–89.
16. Brown R, Wizeman W, Danek C, et al. In vivo evaluation of the effectiveness of bronchial thermoplasty with computed tomography. J Appl Physiol 2005; 98:1606.
17. Gudmundsson G, Gross TJ. Middle lobe syndrome. Am Fam Physician 1996; 53(8): 2547–2550.
18. Mayse ML, Laviolette M, Rubin AS, et al. Clinical pearls for bronchial thermoplasty. J Bronchol 2007; 14:115–123.
19. Triller N, Debeljak A, Kecelj P, et al. Topical anesthesia with lidocaine and the role of atropine in flexible bronchoscopy. J Bronchol 2004; 11:242–245.
20. Langmack EL, Martin RJ, Pak J, et al. Serum lidocaine concentrations in asthmatics undergoing research bronchoscopy. Chest 2000; 117:1055–1060.
21. Moore DC, Green J. Systemic toxic reactions to local anesthetics. Calif Med 1956; 85:70–74.
22. Continuum of depth of sedation definition of general anesthesia and levels of sedation/analgesia. Approved by ASA House of Delegates on October 13, 1999 and amended on October 27, 2004.
23. Pavord ID, Cox G, Thomson NC, et al. Safety and efficacy of bronchial thermoplasty in symptomatic, severe asthma. Am J Respir Crit Care Med 2007; 176:1185–1191.

11

Sedation, Analgesia, and Anesthesia for Airway Procedures

PERRY NYSTROM and PRAVEEN MATHUR
Indiana University School of Medicine, Indianapolis, Indiana, U.S.A.

I. Introduction

Interventional pulmonology is a new field within pulmonary medicine that focuses on the use of sophisticated bronchoscopic and pleuroscopic techniques for the treatment of a spectrum of thoracic disorders ranging from tracheobronchial stenosis to pleural effusions. These efforts are facilitated by sedative-hypnotics and analgesics, resulting in greater patient comfort, cooperation, and satisfaction. Newer drugs expand the opportunities for minimally invasive procedures in medically complex patients. In recognition of the growing number of personnel utilizing potent sedating and anesthetizing drugs, specialty societies have promulgated guidelines for the safe conduct of sedation, monitoring, and reanimation by qualified healthcare providers (1–3).

The success of interventional pulmonary medicine depends on patient safety and comfort. To achieve these objectives, the interventionalist must always be cognizant of the potential for airway and respiratory compromise. If an airway will be shared between the anesthesiologist and bronchoscopist, for example, rigid bronchoscopy under general anesthesia, communication must start preoperatively and continue until the patient's full recovery. When interventions become urgent or emergent, the clinician must resist the tendency toward a cursory review of medical details and physical features that may contribute to adverse events and suboptimal outcomes.

II. Procedural Sedation and Analgesia

Drugs used for anxiolysis, amnesia, and comfort should be easy to titrate to the desired effect with a low incidence of adverse cardiorespiratory effects, while providing for a rapid return to baseline cognitive function. To date, an ideal drug does not exist, and drug combinations are common. Adequate sedation requires patience; thus small doses, titrated to effect, decreases the risk for deep sedation while promoting patient comfort and acceptance. After bronchoscopy, a minority of adults report poor pain control despite the use of sedation, analgesics, and topical anesthesia (4). Operative conditions and stimulation can change rapidly, and the clinical objectives of sedation are dynamic as well, but the principles of safe drug administration remain applicable. Specific drug selection and route of administration are determined by a therapeutic goal, the pharmacologic properties, and anticipated effect of the drug. Intravenous drug administration avoids any delay caused by absorption, and drug response is more predictable.

Table 1 Sedation Continuum and Physiologic Function

Function	Sedation			General anesthesia
	Minimal	Moderate	Deep	
Response to stimulus	Appropriate to verbal stimulus	Purposeful to verbal or tactile stimulation	Painful stimulation elicits response	No response to painful stimuli
Airway	Patent	Patent	Assistance likely	Assistance necessary
Spontaneous ventilation	Adequate	Adequate	Potentially inadequate	Inadequate
Cardiovascular	Maintained	Usually maintained	Usually maintained	Impaired (?)

"Conscious" sedation is considered moderate sedation.

Levels of drug-induced sedation-analgesia are a continuum characterized by patient response and physiologic functions (Table 1). During "minimal sedation," or anxiolysis, patients respond normally to verbal commands. Although cognitive function and coordination may be impaired, cardiorespiratory function is not. In "moderate sedation," that is, conscious sedation, patients respond purposefully to verbal commands or light tactile stimulation. Airway patency and cardiorespiratory function are unaffected. In contrast, patients who experience "deep sedation" cannot be easily aroused but respond purposefully following repeated or noxious stimulation. Airway patency and ventilatory function may be compromised. Heart rate and blood pressure are usually maintained. When drugs cause a loss of consciousness accompanied by an inability to arouse the patient even by noxious stimulation, a state of "general anesthesia" has been achieved. Airway management and positive pressure ventilation may be required because of depressed spontaneous ventilation and neuromuscular function.

III. Patient Evaluation and Preparation

Prior to any intervention, the clinician should review the patient's medical history with emphasis on cardiopulmonary problems, exercise tolerance, and prior experiences with procedural sedation or general anesthesia. The history may suggest a sensitivity or intolerance to agents commonly used for sedation, analgesia, and anesthesia. Experiences that portend difficulty are delayed emergence, unanticipated admission or observation, and airway problems. Patients are risk-stratified by physical status (Table 2).

The preoperative review of systems and physical exam focuses on the airway and the cardiopulmonary system. The Mallampati airway classification I to IV describes the progressively poor visualization of the oropharynx, uvula, and soft palate as the size of the tongue increases. Mallampati classes III and IV are suggestive of airway difficulty during sedation and intubation. The clinician should inquire about arthritic conditions affecting cervical spine mobility and body positioning, temperomandibular joint dysfunction, symptoms of untreated or treated gastroesophageal reflux, esophageal pathology, and gastric or small bowel dysmotility. Vital signs are reviewed and documented.

Table 2 American Society of Anesthesiologists Physical Status Classification

Physical status	Description of disease status
I	Healthy
II	Mild systemic disease, e.g., controlled asthma or COPD, hypertension, diabetes, prior MI, smoker, and age > 70
III	Severe systemic disease that impacts daily activity but is not incapacitating, e.g., moderate COPD, CAD with angina
IV	Severe systemic disease that may be incapacitating and is a constant threat to life, e.g., chronic CHF, arrhythmia, unstable angina
V	Moribund patient, not expected to survive 24 hours
VI	Brain death organ donor
E	Emergency procedure (e.g., removal of foreign body, III-E)

The risk of aspiration is ever-present during moderate sedation, especially when airway reflexes are attenuated or abolished by topical or nerve block anesthesia. Accepted fasting guidelines are "nothing per os" (NPO) two to three hours for clear liquids and at least six hours for solids. Longer periods may be necessary for patients with upper intestinal delayed transit time, for example, gastroparesis (1). Prescribed antireflux medications should be taken on the day of the procedure. Patients should be counseled as to when cardioactive, antiplatelet, and glycemic control medications are to be taken.

Preoperative laboratory testing is influenced by the history, physical exam, recent evaluations, and the likelihood that the results will impact perioperative management. Cardiac risk assessment by clinical predictors and reported exercise capacity may prompt a comprehensive evaluation in accordance with good medical practice, not because it will significantly influence management for a minimally invasive pulmonary procedure. Bacterial endocarditis prophylaxis should be considered if there is a history of endocarditis, prosthetic heart valve, or asplenia (3).

The sedation and anesthetic plan should be discussed with the patient, questions answered, and incorporated into the written informed consent for the pulmonary intervention. An anesthesia provider should be included in the perioperative care team when

- a prolonged or therapeutic endoscopic procedure may require more than moderate sedation, that is, deep sedation;
- there is anticipated intolerance, documented intolerance, or paradoxical response, to standard sedatives during an unsuccessful or aborted procedure;
- there is risk of complication related to severe comorbidity (ASA III or greater); and
- airway problems are anticipated by history or anatomic variation.

Otherwise, the routine assistance of an anesthesia provider in the care of low-risk patients for routine pulmonary interventions is not warranted (5).

IV. Equipment and Personnel
The endoscopy center of an institution is an ideal site for interventional pulmonology because the equipment, personnel, and protocols are in place to prepare and recover patients for minimally invasive procedures. Personnel are cross-trained, and a select

Table 3 Recommended Equipment for Pulmonary Procedures

Oxygen source
Nasal cannula
Oxygen mask capable of delivering $FiO_2 > 90\%$
Oropharyngeal and nasopharyngeal airways in various sizes
Laryngeal mask airways (LMA 4 and 5 for most adults)
Endotracheal tubes in various sizes
Laryngoscope with Macintosh and Miller blades, various sizes
Ambu bag with appropriate size masks; consider PEEP valve
Suction device and canister capable of continuous suction at -150 mmHg
Yankauer suction catheter

group of nurses will have sedation training and advanced life support skills. Staff responsible for procedural sedation will likely participate in a program to maintain sedation skills through experience, continuing education in pharmacology, and opportunities for simulator training.

Table 3 lists the recommended equipment for pulmonary procedures. In addition to frequent clinical assessment, standard monitoring consists of cardiac telemetry, noninvasive blood pressure, and pulse oximetry. Carbon dioxide (CO_2) monitoring should be considered in patients with moderate to severe pulmonary disease or baseline hypercapnia. Capnography, or end-tidal CO_2, would be appropriate when an endotracheal tube or laryngeal mask airway have been placed. Without an artificial airway, transcutaneous CO_2 is an accurate estimate of the arterial partial pressure of CO_2 when compared with end-tidal CO_2 during thoracic surgery and one-lung ventilation (6).

V. Physiology: The Lateral Decubitus Position and Medical Thoracoscopy

Patient positioning for medical thoracoscopy will be determined by the patient's body habitus and the operator's experience. A lateral decubitus position is common. This allows the operator ease of access to the lateral chest and improved thoracoscopic visualization of anterior and posterior aspects of the pleural space and lung surface.

A. Normal Physiology

In the upright position, the traditional concept of gravity-dependent pulmonary blood flow characterizes four zones relating perfusion to ventilation. Normally, the distribution of blood flow is 55% in the right lung and 45% in the left lung. In the lung apices (zone 1), alveolar pressure dominates and no gas exchange occurs, but in the lung bases, perfusion may be influenced by the arterial to interstitial fluid pressure difference (zone 4). In the mid to lower lungs, the ventilation-perfusion relationship is improved as arterial and venous pressures increase. Normally, very little of zone 1 exists.

B. Lateral Decubitus Position Physiology

Ventilation and perfusion physiology changes little in the lateral decubitus position. Gravity decreases blood flow to the nondependent lung by at least 10%, resulting in 60% blood flow to the dependent lung and 40% to the nondependent lung, regardless of the side down. The dependent lung ventilation is greater than the nondependent lung because the dependent hemidiaphragm rests at a higher position in the chest. A more forceful hemidiaphragm contraction produces greater negative pleural pressure. Perfusion increases more than ventilation in the dependent lung compared to the nondependent lung. Overall, the lateral decubitus ventilation-perfusion relationship (V/Q) remains similar to the upright position. During spontaneous breathing and moderate sedation, the V/Q relationship should not change. In contrast, a state of deep sedation or general anesthesia decreases functional residual capacity. Now, the nondependent lung becomes more compliant relative to the dependent lung, and the distribution of ventilation favors the nondependent lung. Blood flow distribution is not affected, and dependent lung perfusion is greater than the nondependent lung.

While sedated and breathing spontaneously, if the chest is open to atmospheric pressure, there should not be any significant V/Q alterations. However, the mechanics of the chest will change somewhat. With inspiration, the mediastinum shifts toward the dependent pleural space because of the negative pleural pressure relative to the atmospheric pressure of the nondependent pleural space. The tidal volume of the dependent lung will be decreased an amount equal to the mediastinal shift. The mediastinum shifts back to the nondependent side during exhalation. Paradoxical respirations of the nondependent lung may be observed. It will appear to collapse during inspiration when residual air flows to the dependent lung caused by negative pleural pressures, and partial lung expansion occurs during exhalation as air flows into the trachea and nondependent lung because of the dependent pleural pressure increase relative to the nondependent atmospheric pleural pressure (7).

If the operative nondependent lung collapses during the procedure, one-lung ventilation physiology will ensue. Right to left perfusion shunting occurs by a gravitational effect as well as hypoxic pulmonary vasoconstriction (HPV), which protects the patient from a significant drop in arterial partial pressure of oxygen (PaO_2). For HPV to be most effective, it is important to maintain adequate FiO_2, normocapnia, and normothermia. HPV is maximal when pulmonary artery pressure is normal. Sedative-hypnotics and opioid analgesics studied to date have no significant effect on HPV. Nitrous oxide may reduce HPV.

VI. Anesthetic Techniques

In many parts of the world, bronchoscopy is performed on cooperative patients with topical anesthesia only, albeit most patients prefer some sedation for procedures. Indeed, adequate topical anesthesia of the tracheobronchial tree is critical to successful bronchoscopy, and local anesthetic infiltration of soft tissue and periosteum at pleural insertion sites facilitates thoracic procedures.

A. Local Anesthetics

Local anesthetics prevent or relieve pain by impairing permeability of neuronal membranes to sodium, preventing depolarization of the membrane and interrupting nerve conduction. They interact directly with one or more sites within the voltage-gated sodium channels to raise the threshold necessary for depolarization, leading to failure of impulse generation and propagation (8). The duration of action is proportional to the time of contact with the neuronal membrane. Vasoconstrictors, for example, epinephrine,

Table 4 Manifestations of Lidocaine Toxicity

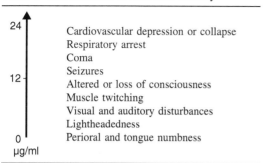

increase contact time by delaying vascular absorption; local anesthetic effect is prolonged and peak blood concentrations are lower.

Serious toxicity is related to effects on the central nervous system (CNS) and cardiovascular system (Table 4). Adverse reactions are attributed to dose, absorption, vascular injections, and rate of rise to peak plasma concentration. Initial signs of local anesthetic toxicity are excitatory because of blockade of inhibitory pathways in the CNS. Patients may be drowsy, dysphoric, confused, or agitated. Higher levels produce muscle twitching, tremors, and generalized convulsions. Still higher levels will lead to coma, respiratory depression, and cardiovascular collapse. Rarely, cardiovascular collapse with cardiac arrhythmias and death may occur before signs of CNS excitation. The convulsive threshold for local anesthetics is decreased in the presence of hypercapnia. Elevated PCO_2 increases cerebral blood flow, causes respiratory acidosis, and results in less protein binding and more free drug. Rapid action to administer antiseizure drugs and respiratory support is essential to avoid respiratory acidosis. Convulsions are treated with small doses of benzodiazepines (BZD), barbiturates (thiopental), or propofol. The lethal dose of bupivacaine was increased in a rat model (9) and survival was increased in dogs given cardiotoxic doses of bupivacaine (10).

Amide-type local anesthetics are extensively bound to proteins, particularly $\alpha 1$-acid glycoprotein and albumin. Hypoproteinemia will alter the amount of free drug available for hepatic metabolism and influence the potential for systemic toxicity. Solutions of local anesthetics may contain preservatives, or epinephrine, which may cause true allergic reactions or hemodynamic changes, respectively.

Lidocaine, the prototypical amide local anesthetic, is used routinely for tracheobronchial anesthesia. Lidocaine is rapidly absorbed and possesses antitussive properties. Clinically significant cardiovascular depression usually occurs at serum lidocaine levels that produce marked CNS effects. The amount of lidocaine used during bronchoscopy has traditionally been limited to 4 mg/kg total dose in gel, aerosolized, nerve block, and dilute topical solution (Fig. 1). Absorption from alveoli is rapid. The British Thoracic Society guidelines recommend using the smallest dose necessary with a limit of 8.2 mg/kg in adults (3). Frey et al. demonstrated the safety of high-dose lidocaine (> 12 mg/kg) during routine bronchoscopy with moderate sedation by midazolam and fentanyl. Serum lidocaine levels and methemoglobin levels remained very low (11). For infiltration anesthesia, the lidocaine limit is approximately 7 mg/kg.

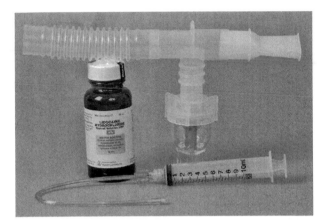

Figure 1 Lidocaine 4% can be nebulized to anesthetize the oropharnyx, glottis, and proximal trachea. Transtracheal injection of lidocaine 4% (3–4 mL; 120–160 mg) will anesthetize the proximal trachea and glottic structures. Atomizer tubing can be attached to a syringe to apply lidocaine 4% to the base of the tongue, oropharynx, epiglottis, and hypopharynx.

Bupivacaine is not used as a topical anesthetic but rather for subcutaneous infiltration at the superior aspect of the rib for prolonged anesthesia and analgesia after pleuroscopy or chest tube insertion. Bupivacaine infiltration for the placement of an indwelling pleural catheter will provide up to 24 hours of postprocedural analgesia. It can be combined with lidocaine for a rapid onset. The total dose should not exceed 3.5 mg/kg, especially when administered in anatomic sites with rapid absorption, for example, intercostal nerve block. Except for less cardiotoxicity, *ropivacaine* pharmacology is similar to bupivacaine. *Mepivacaine* is not effective as a topical anesthetic. It is similar to lidocaine except for greater protein and tissue binding that increases the duration up to four hours. Addition of vasoconstrictor will prolong the anesthetic action (8).

Infiltration Technique Field Block Anesthesia
The following conditions are necessary for this technique: Use an alcohol swab or chlorhexidine sponge to clean the skin at the planned site(s) of pleural instrumentation. After adequate sedation, local anesthetic is injected liberally into subcutaneous tissues with a 25-gauge, 1.5 inch needle. By the time the patient is prepped, draped, and the operator has sterile attire, the operative site will be anesthetized. If anesthesia is inadequate, take time to inject additional local anesthetic so that patient comfort by deep sedation can be avoided.

B. Airway Anesthesia
Superior Laryngeal Nerve Block
The superior laryngeal nerve is easily anesthetized where it penetrates the thyrohyoid membrane between the greater cornu of the hyoid bone and the superior cornu of the thyroid cartilage (Fig. 2). The hyoid bone can be identified as the small mobile bone in the crease of the neck just superior to the thyroid cartilage. In the semirecumbent

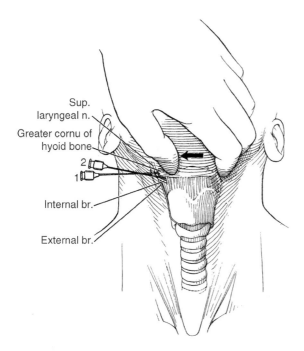

Sup. laryngeal n.

Greater cornu of hyoid bone

2

1

Internal br.

External br.

Figure 2 Superior laryngeal nerve block. (1) Needle contact on the greater cornu, (2) needle directed inferiorly. From Ref. 12.

position with the head extended, the hyoid bone is displaced toward the side to be blocked with the index finger while the greater cornu is palpated with the thumb of the same hand. A 25-gauge needle is advanced until it makes contact with this structure, then walked off the bone inferiorly and advanced 2 to 3 mm so that the tip of the needle rests between the thyrohyoid membrane laterally and the laryngeal mucosa medially. If careful aspiration for blood and air is negative, 2 to 3 mL of lidocaine 1% is injected. An additional 1 mL can be injected as the needle is withdrawn. Alternatively, the needle can be walked cephalad off the superior cornu of the thyroid cartilage. The injection is repeated on the opposite side.

Transtracheal/Translaryngeal Injection
Transtracheal injection is a rapid, simple, and effective method of applying topical local anesthetic to the infraglottic larynx and upper trachea (Fig. 3). Knowledge of neck anatomy is critical to avoid needle injury to neck structures or intravascular injection. Coughing is reduced if the injection is preceded by aerosolized lidocaine and/or light sedation with a sedative and opioid. In the semirecumbent position with the neck extended, the cricothyroid membrane is located in the space between the thyroid and cricoid cartilages. The midline of the membrane is then located and held in place by the index and middle finger of the nondominant hand. After a skin wheal is placed, a 20-gauge needle connected to a 5-mL syringe containing 3 to 4 mL of lidocaine 4% is then advanced perpendicular to the skin while being aspirated. Penetration of the

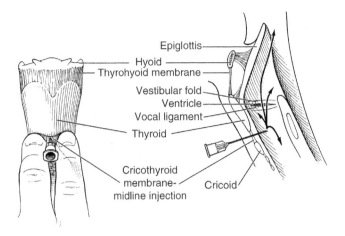

Figure 3 Transtracheal lidocaine injection. From Ref. 12.

membrane and entry into the trachea are confirmed by free aspiration of air. The needle should not be advanced any further; inject lidocaine quickly and immediately remove the needle from the airway. Alternatively, a 20-gauge IV catheter-over-needle and fluid-filled syringe are inserted until air is aspirated. The needle is removed, and after confirming the catheter position within the trachea by air aspiration, lidocaine is injected. Local anesthetic injection at the end of inspiration will deliver more solution to the proximal trachea and subglottic mucosa. After injection, the catheter is removed.

VII. Sedation and Analgesia Pharmacology
A. Benzodiazepines

Four BZD are commonly used for procedural sedation. Three drugs are BZD receptor agonists: midazolam, diazepam, and lorazepam. They produce anxiolysis, sedation, antegrade amnesia, and centrally mediated muscle relaxation, but they lack any analgesic properties. One drug, flumazenil, is a BZD receptor antagonist.

Benzodiazepines enhance gamma-aminobutyric acid (GABA) neuroinhibitory effects mediated by GABA receptor, subtype A, in the brain and spinal cord. Receptor activation by benzodiazepines alters the receptor-associated chloride ionophores, resulting in a prolonged, intense neuronal hyperpolarization resistant to excitation. Enhanced receptor affinity for GABA may play a role (13,14).

Individual BZD lipophilicity and protein binding differ, which influences their varied pharmacokinetics. Diazepam and midazolam are metabolized through oxidation by the cytochrome P450 (CYP) enzymes, CYP2C19 and CYP3A4. Hepatic enzyme induction by ethanol abuse or antiepileptic drugs, and drug interactions, specifically CYP3A4 inhibition (antiretroviral drugs, macrolide antibiotics, calcium channel antagonists), may influence the dose response. Lorazepam undergoes glucuronide conjugation, and drug effect is influenced less by drug-drug interactions or coexisting liver disease. Individuals older than age 65 more frequently exhibit paradoxical agitation, not sedation.

Cardiorespiratory effects are minimal to moderate even at large doses. In general, midazolam causes a slightly greater decrease in blood pressure. Central respiratory depression, even apnea, can occur, but in general, the therapeutic margin is wide for this adverse effect (15). When BZD are combined with opioids, greater hemodynamic alterations, respiratory depression or apnea, may be seen with relatively small doses (16).

Midazolam is commonly used for procedural sedation. Its popularity is related to water solubility, lack of venous irritation, rapid onset, and a brief duration of action. Rapid redistribution from the brain and metabolism account for the short duration of action. The elimination half-life of midazolam is one to four hours (13,14).

Midazolam can increase heart rate and decrease blood pressure. The hemodynamic effects are dose related, and midazolam with an opioid may be supra-additive for hypotension. Adequate sedation with midazolam and alfentanil will attenuate the cardiovascular response to diagnostic or interventional bronchoscopy as effectively as labetolol (17). Central respiratory drive can be depressed by as little as 2 mg, especially in patients with COPD. The peak effect is seen in five minutes and may last for two hours. Transient apnea may occur when midazolam is combined with opioids (18).

Incremental doses of 0.5 to 2 mg IV are appropriate to induce sedation. The total dose required for sedation ranges from 0.05 to 0.15 mg/kg. Rapid hypnosis occurs when a single dose of 0.1 to 0.15 mg/kg is given IV. In general, the elderly require less drug and far less drug is required for sedation when administered with an opioid. Stem cell transplant recipients and HIV patients who abuse drugs require higher doses of midazolam for bronchoscopy, even when combined with opioids. Increased drug requirement might be related to CYP3A4 enzyme induction (19).

The highly lipid soluble BZD, *diazepam*, is useful for the treatment of seizures, alcohol withdrawal syndrome, anxiety, and skeletal muscle spasm. It may cause pain and venous inflammation when injected intravenously. Metabolism creates two active metabolites, desmethyldiazepam and oxazepam. Desmethyldiazepam is slightly less potent than diazepam; metabolism is slow, contributing to sustained effects lasting two to four days in the elderly and patients with advanced liver disease (13); thus, a disadvantage for use in procedural sedation.

One of the most potent BZD, *lorazepam* is intermediate to long acting with a profound amnestic effect compared with diazepam or midazolam. It is seldom used for procedural sedation in the outpatient setting because of the slow onset of peak effect and a potential for prolonged psychomotor impairment.

Flumazenil antagonizes the central effects of agents acting at the BZD receptor. BZD-induced sedation and psychomotor impairment are rapidly reversed by flumazenil administered IV, but less consistent effect occurs for neurocognitive dysfunction and respiratory depression. Flumazenil has been used after bronchoscopy to improve breathing and oxygen saturation (15). Side effects associated with rapid reversal of BZD-induced sedation include nausea, emesis, tachycardia, hypertension, headache, and rarely seizures. Sedation reversal is evident within 1 to 3 minutes and peaks in 10 minutes. The usual dose is between 0.2 and 0.6 mg. A dose of 0.2 mg is associated with partial antagonism, and doses as high as 1.0 mg usually produce complete competitive antagonism of sedation-hypnosis. Repeated doses of 0.2 mg can be given at one-minute intervals to a maximum of 3 mg in one hour (13). Respiratory depression after an opioid and a BZD should be reversed with the opioid antagonist naloxone before flumazenil.

The half-life of flumazenil, approximately one hour, is the maximal duration of clinical benefit from a single intravenous dose unless the patient has severely impaired liver function (13). Sedation may reappear gradually within one to two hours after flumazenil. The patient should remain closely monitored until all possible central BZD effects have subsided. If sedation recurs, repeated doses can be given or a continuous infusion started at a dose of 0.1 to 0.4 mg/hr.

B. Propofol

Propofol is a rapid and short-acting intravenous anesthetic that has been evaluated extensively and used for sedation. If administered by continuous infusion, different levels of sedation can be achieved rapidly by changing the dose. Recovery is rapid and not accompanied by a hangover effect, even after prolonged infusions. Amnesia is not a consistent feature of propofol use, but the addition of a small dose of midazolam does not delay recovery or interfere with "euphorigenic" mood alteration and antinausea properties (20). Drug effect cannot be reversed because propofol does not have a specific antagonist.

In the present formulation, the drug is highly lipid soluble, resulting in an onset of action within 60 seconds. After a single bolus, the rapid decline in drug level is explained by redistribution and elimination. Biotransformation of propofol is exceptionally high. Cirrhosis does not alter the pharmacokinetic properties. Extrahepatic clearance of propofol exists because propofol's clearance exceeds hepatic blood flow, and metabolism has been confirmed during the anhepatic phase of liver transplantation. The drug may impair its own clearance by decreasing hepatic blood flow (21). The lung is an important extrahepatic site for metabolism of propofol, responsible for approximately 30% uptake and first-pass elimination after a bolus dose (22). The initial distribution half-life is two to eight minutes with an elimination half-life of one to three hours.

The mechanism and site of action probably involves interactions with the GABA subtype A receptor complex, causing changes in chloride ion conductance. Sedation and hypnosis are dose dependent (13,20). Doses of 2 to 2.5 mg/kg induce rapid loss of consciousness not associated with any significant excitatory effects. Sedation loading doses of 0.25 to 0.75 mg/kg are followed by a continuous infusion of 25 to 75 μg/kg/min. Lower infusion rates are possible when propofol is used with BZD and opioids. Alternatively, sedation can be accomplished by titrating small doses of 10 to 40 mg IV.

Alternatively, sedation can be accomplished by titrating small doses of 10 to 40 mg IV.

The effects on different organ systems are dose dependent and predictable. Propofol decreases systemic vascular resistance and myocardial contractility, but heart rate is unchanged. Upper airway reflex inhibition frequently causes airway obstruction. The ventilatory response to hypoxia and hypercapnia can be depressed, necessitating oxygen therapy, but with small doses, there are no significant changes in tidal volume, minute ventilation, end-tidal CO_2, or arterial blood gas values. Low concentrations of propofol can attenuate vagally mediated bronchoconstriction; higher doses attenuate methacholine-induced bronchoconstriction. In sedation doses, there is less blood pressure change, respiratory depression, or apnea (20). Adverse events are related to the dose, speed of injection, and concomitant use of opioids. Dosage reductions are recommended in hypovolemia, low cardiac output states, and the elderly.

The lipid emulsion formulation causes pain on injection, especially in the small veins on the dorsum of the hand. This may be mistaken as an excitatory reaction during the induction of sedation or general anesthesia. To minimize injection pain, a venous catheter should be placed in the larger veins of the arm, and lidocaine 20 to 40 mg injected prior to propofol or added to the propofol syringe. The clinician should follow strict aseptic technique and discard any unused drug within six hours to avoid bacterial growth in the lipid emulsion.

Fospropofol Disodium

A water soluble prodrug of propofol, fospropofol disodium (LUSEDRA™ Eisai Corporation of North America) was approved as an intravenous sedative-hypnotic by the Food and Drug Administration (FDA) in December 2008. Fospropofol biotransformation to propofol delays the peak concentration of propofol by four to six minutes, and consequently, the peak concentration is lower and more sustained compared to propofol emulsion (23). Study patients reported a minor adverse effect of inguinal and perineal parasthesias. The drug manufacturer is seeking FDA approval of fospropofol disodium use by nonanesthesia personnel, and additional clinical studies are planned for cohorts consisting of adolescents, patients at the extremes of age, and patients who are ASA class III or IV.

C. Dexmedetomidine

Dexmedetomidine (DEX) was approved by the FDA in 1999 for short-term sedation of critically ill adults. Since then, off-label use as an anesthetic adjunct and in other clinical settings has grown steadily (24). DEX is an imidazole derivative that is highly selective for the α-2 adrenergic receptor. Activation of the alpha-2A (α-2A) adrenergic receptor produces both sedation and analgesia but does not reliably produce general anesthesia even at maximal doses. Sedation occurs by α-2A receptor activation in the locus ceruleus and spinal cord and acts through the endogenous sleep-promoting pathways to exert the sedative effect (13,25), which has been described as similar to natural sleep. Patients are relatively easy to arouse during and after DEX infusion. Adequate sedation is characterized by anxiolysis, comfort, cooperation, and communication. However, amnesia is not a reliable feature of DEX sedation. When used for dental procedures, DEX sedation was comparable to midazolam except for decreased hemodynamic variables and less amnesia (26). The recommended loading dose is 1 µg/kg given over 10 minutes, followed by continuous infusion at a rate of 0.2 to 0.7 µg/kg/hr (13). The distribution and terminal half-lives are six minutes and two hours, respectively. The drug has not been studied in pregnancy and may be harmful to the fetus (C rating, potential risk). A combination of opioid and DEX is synergistic for analgesia but not for respiratory depression, an apparent opioid-sparing effect for analgesia. Activation of the α-2A adrenergic receptor is sympatholytic. Reduced dosing, even forgoing the loading dose, should be considered in patients with risk factors for severe hypotension or bradycardia.

Sedation and analgesia are achieved without significant respiratory depression. Minute ventilation may decrease slightly, but PCO_2 and PaO_2 remain stable, even during deep sedation. The slope of the ventilatory response to increasing CO_2 is unchanged. Respiratory parameters are similar to those induced during natural sleep, a distinct advantage in patients who are not intubated and mechanically ventilated. Reports of

DEX use for pulmonary procedures are emerging. The Cleveland Clinic reported a case of uneventful endobronchial valve deployment for lung volume reduction in an elderly patient with severe COPD (27). In a pilot study of 10 patients with moderate-to-severe COPD undergoing bronchoscopy, patients received small amounts of midazolam and fentanyl followed by an infusion of DEX at 1 µg/kg/hr. Hemodynamics remained stable, and no respiratory complications occurred (28).

D. Ketamine

Ketamine is the only IV anesthetic with potent analgesic, hypnotic, and anterograde amnestic effects. A phencyclidine derivative, it induces a state of dissociative anesthesia from electrophysiologic dissociation between limbic system excitation and cortical inhibition. Patients appear to be in a cataleptic state with open eyes, slow gaze, maintenance of spontaneous respiration, and occasional reflex movements. Therefore, the usual signs of sedation depth may not apply. There is no specific antagonist of ketamine. Although the drug is versatile, it has not gained popularity for procedural sedation because of a lack of experience with the drug and potential psychomimetic effects (29). The mechanism of action appears to involve competitive antagonism at N-methyl-D-aspartate (NMDA) receptors throughout the central nervous system. Hepatic metabolism generates a less active metabolite, norketamine. The elimination half-life is two hours (13). The onset of action is rapid after usual doses of 0.5 to 2 mg/kg IV. Lower doses, titrated to effect, are appropriate for moderate sedation when combined with BZD, propofol, or both. The combination decreases emergence reactions. Airway patency, oropharyngeal muscle tone, and spontaneous respirations are maintained during ketamine sedation-anesthesia, especially when the drug is given slowly. Cardiovascular stimulation and cerebral vasodilation are dose dependent (29). A ketamine-propofol combination may be superior to other drug combinations for sedation during bronchoscopy, but a large comparison trial has not been conducted (30).

E. Opioids

Opioids are a structurally related class of natural or synthetic agents that have morphine-like properties. Opioids are classified by pharmacodynamic activity: agonists, antagonists (naloxone), mixed agonist-antagonists (butorphanol, nalbuphine). The clinical effects depend on opioid-specific receptor binding: mu, kappa, sigma, and delta. Sedation and respiratory depression are mediated by mu, kappa, and delta receptors. Analgesia results from opioid interaction with peripheral receptors on sensory nerves and central receptors in the dorsal horn of the spinal cord, brainstem medulla, and cerebral cortex (31).

Central Nervous System Effects

High doses of opioids may cause deep sedation or hypnosis; they do not reliably produce amnesia. Opioids can reduce cerebral metabolic oxygen requirements, cerebral blood flow, and intracranial pressure if ventilation is unchanged. Stimulation of the chemoreceptor trigger zone located in the area postrema of the brain stem can result in vomiting. Actions within the medullary cough center are antitussive, although fentanyl in moderate doses (2–7 µg/kg) can induce coughing when given rapidly. Normeperidine, an excitatory metabolite of meperidine, can accumulate with repeated dosing or impaired kidney function. Normeperidine may cause seizures.

Respiratory Effects

Opioids activate mu receptors in the respiratory centers of the ventromedial medulla responsible for respiratory rhythm and frequency (32). Minute ventilation decreases primarily by a reduction in respiratory rate. The ventilatory response to CO_2 is depressed; the CO_2 response curve is decreased and shifted to the right. The ventilatory response to hypoxemia is blunted. These opioid-induced alterations depend on the dose, route of administration, comorbidities, genetics, sex, and age (33). Generalized skeletal muscle rigidity can occur with rapid injection of large doses of opioids. Loss of chest wall compliance and contraction of laryngeal and pharyngeal muscles can be severe, resulting in ventilatory difficulty even with positive-pressure ventilation. Muscle rigidity occurs more frequently with the synthetic opioids fentanyl, sufentanil, and remifentanil. Small amounts injected slowly avoid muscle rigidity. Naloxone, a pure narcotic antagonist, will reverse all receptor-mediated effects of opioids, including rigidity (34).

Cardiovascular Effects

At clinically relevant doses, opioids do not cause significant myocardial depression, but stimulation of the medullary vagal nuclei causes bradycardia. One exception, meperidine, which has a chemical structure resembling atropine, may cause tachycardia. Hypotensive effects are most prominent in patients with increased sympathetic tone as seen in congestive heart failure or hypovolemia. Blood pressure changes are less common in isovolemic, supine patients. However, orthostatic hypotension may be seen in patients with autonomic neuropathy. Morphine and meperidine can cause vasodilatation and tachycardia from a non-IgE-mediated release of histamine. Fentanyl and sufentanil tend to decrease heart rate more than morphine. Blood pressure may drop in response to diminished sympathetic tone. Neither has any direct, negative inotropic properties, nor do they trigger histamine release. Nonetheless, hemodynamic disturbances are generally minimal in patients with preserved left ventricular function. Alfentanil does not cause histamine release or direct myocardial depression. As a sedative, remifentanil provides more stable hemodynamics than propofol (34).

Morphine is a poor choice for sedation because of the slow onset and intermediate duration of action. The active metabolite, morphine-6-glucuronide, has mu receptor activity equal to morphine. In some individuals, peak effect for analgesia and respiratory depression may not be seen for 30 to 45 minutes. The once popular analgesic, meperidine, has been implicated in a variety of adverse events.

Fentanyl

A synthetic opioid 100 times more potent than morphine, fentanyl increases pain threshold, alters pain reception, and inhibits ascending pain pathways. If administered IV, the duration of sedation and analgesia is 0.5 to 1 hour, but respiratory depression may last longer. The drug is highly lipophilic with redistribution into muscle and fat. Protein binding is high and metabolism primarily hepatic by CYP3A4. For minor procedures, small doses of 25 to 50 µg are given IV and repeated every three to five minutes until the desired effect is achieved. Total dose decreases when fentanyl is combined with other sedatives.

Other synthetic opioids, such as the fentanyl congeners alfentanil, sufentanil, and remifentanil, may not be as useful as fentanyl for sedation and analgesia. Sufentanil is significantly more potent than fentanyl and must be used in very small amounts to avoid respiratory compromise. Remifentanil is a unique narcotic, equipotent to fentanyl, with a five- to eight-minute duration of action. It is rapidly metabolized by plasma esterases and, therefore, must be administered by continuous infusion (34).

F. Opioid Antagonism: Naloxone

A nonselective, competitive opioid receptor antagonist, naloxone, reverses sedation and respiratory depression caused by opioids. The onset occurs within two minutes; duration of action is 30 to 60 minutes. The depressive effects of mixed agonist-antagonist such as butorphanol tartrate (Stadol), nalbuphine (Nubain), and buprenorphine (Buprenex) can also be reversed by naloxone. Adverse reactions associated with abrupt reversal of opioid effect include tachycardia, hypertension, arrhythmias, pulmonary edema, nausea, and vomiting. Seizures can occur, but no causal relationship has been established. Naloxone may precipitate a withdrawal syndrome in narcotic-dependent patients. Drug effects on the developing fetus are not known.

Initially, airway support is the priority for patients who are hypoventilating and hypoxemic. The usual dose of naloxone given to reverse an oversedated patient with respiratory depression is 0.4 mg given intravenously, intramuscularly, or a larger dose with 10 mL saline by endotracheal tube. To avoid abrupt reversal, low-dose naloxone, 40 µg IV (0.04 mg), can be repeated every few minutes until an increased respiratory rate is observed or the patient wakes up. Naloxone has a short half-life, and individuals must be observed carefully to detect any return of opioid effect. A continuous infusion of 5 µg/kg/hr can be used for the expected duration of narcotic effect. Recovery room personnel should be alerted when naloxone has been given.

G. Alternative Methods

Patient-Controlled Sedation

Patient-controlled sedation (PCS) uses single agents or drug combinations administered by the patient to meet their desired level of sedation and comfort. Theoretically, deep sedation should be avoided (35). Specialized pumps deliver a preset dose of medication and allow time for the peak effect. Procedure efficiency may be compromised by the dosing regimen (36). For colonoscopy, maximal sedation scores, adverse events, and patient satisfaction were equivalent to traditional methods of sedation for similar procedures (37,38). Efficacy of PCS for bronchoscopy was demonstrated in a comparison of propofol combined with alfentanil or ketamine. Amnesia and overall comfort were rated highly by patients (34). More study is required to demonstrate significant advantages of PCS over the simplified techniques utilized in contemporary practice.

Nitrous Oxide Sedation

The use of nitrous oxide (N_2O) outside of the operating room has gained popularity because it is easy to administer by facemask with a predictable short duration. The colorless, odorless gas is insoluble in blood and tissues, undergoes no biotransformation, and is eliminated by the lungs. It is a weak anesthetic agent unable to produce reliable surgical anesthesia, but analgesia is possible at concentrations as low as 20%, and higher concentrations induce moderate sedation. Premixed 50:50 nitrous oxide and oxygen has been used successfully in bronchoscopy. Overall pain and cough were lower in the patients receiving nitrous oxide by facemask, potentially an alternative to general anesthesia (39). A similar study in pediatric patients demonstrated improved sedation-analgesia and minor side effects (40). The use of nitrous oxide during bronchoscopy with an artificial airway (endotracheal tube, laryngeal mask airway) has not been studied. Obvious disadvantages of nitrous oxide use are waste gas scavenging and delivering an adequate FiO_2 during periods of oxygen desaturation.

H. Neuromuscular Blockade

Because adequate operating conditions are achieved routinely with topical anesthesia and moderate sedation, neuromuscular blockade is not used for interventional pulmonary procedures. Patient movement, in most instances, does not necessarily present a threat to life or hinder the successful completion of the procedure. There are exceptions. Patients requiring mechanical ventilation may be paralyzed with neuromuscular blockers and heavily sedated because of lung injury, difficulty oxygenating and ventilating, airway obstruction, and fistulas. Other exceptions may be related to operator preference in patients on mechanical ventilatory support who are adequately sedated and need (*i*) an endotracheal tube changed to accommodate a larger diagnostic or therapeutic broncho-scope, (*ii*) percutaneous tracheostomy, (*iii*) airway procedures but have intracranial pathology or brain injury with an elevated intracranial pressure, or (*iv*) tracheal or bron-chial staged procedures when postprocedural mechanical ventilation is planned. If neu-romuscular blockade is needed, adequate sedation must be ensured and mechanical ventilatory support adjusted to optimize oxygenation and ventilation in the paralyzed patient.

The two intermediate-acting, nondepolarizing, neuromuscular blocking agents, rocuronium and cisatracurium, are the most appropriate choices. *Rocuronium* has a steroid nucleus similar to vecuronium, and a rapid onset at dosages of 0.6 to 0.9 mg/kg. With the lower dose, peak effect may take up to three minutes after intravenous injection. There is no histamine release and no significant hemodynamic changes associated with the use of this drug. *Cisatracurium*, chemically similar to atracurium, undergoes in vivo inactivation by chemical structure rearrangement. Adequate muscle relaxation occurs in two to three minutes with doses of 0.1 to 0.15 mg/kg. The duration of neuromuscular blockade will be 20 to 40 minutes. There is no significant histamine release or cardiovascular change with large doses of cisatracurium.

If neuromuscular blockade is a consideration in any other setting, such as the endoscopy suite or the operating room, it would be prudent to call upon anesthesiology colleagues to provide their expertise in managing the patient during the procedure. This will ensure adequate preparation, equipment, and personnel are available to meet a high standard of safety and comfort for the patient and bronchoscopist.

VIII. Recovery After Procedural Sedation

A patient who has undergone a procedure requiring moderate sedation requires con-tinuous monitoring during the recovery phase. Supplemental oxygen should be admin-istered until the patients return to their baseline oxygen saturation (room air or baseline supplemental oxygen) or they maintain a saturation of greater than 92% to 95% on room air. Vital signs are monitored at 15-minute intervals until the patient is awake, alert, and meets discharge criteria (1). Recovery personnel assess patients' readiness for discharge by scoring systems for physiologic functions (respiration, circulation, consciousness, activity level) and well-being (nausea/emesis, tolerating oral liquids).

References

1. Practice guidelines for sedation and analgesia by nonanesthesiologists: an updated report by the American Society of Anesthesiologists Task Force on sedation and analgesia by non-anesthesiologists. Anesthesiology 2002; 96:1004–1017.
2. European Respiratory Society/American Thoracic Society Task Force. ERS/ATS statement on interventional pulmonology. Eur Respir J 2002; 19:356–373.
3. British Thoracic Society Bronchoscopy Guidelines Committee. British Thoracic Society guidelines on diagnostic flexible bronchoscopy. Thorax 2001; 56(suppl I): i1–i21.
4. Lechtzin N, Rubin HR, Jenckes M, et al. Predictors of pain control in patients undergoing flexible bronchoscopy. Am J Respir Crit Care Med 2000; 162:440–445.
5. Faigel DO, Baron TH, Goldstein JL, et al. Guidelines for the use of deep sedation and anesthesia for GI endoscopy. Gastrointest Endosc 2002; 56:613.
6. Tobias S. Noninvasive carbon dioxide monitoring during one-lung ventilation: end-tidal versus transcutaneous techniques. J Cardioth Vasc Anesth 2003; 17:306–308.
7. Triantacillou AN, Benumoff JL, Lecamwasam HS. Physiology of the lateral decubitus position, the open chest, and one-lung ventilation. In: Kaplan JA, Slinger PD, eds. Thoracic Anesthesia. 3rd ed. Philadelphia: Churchill Livingstone, 2003:71–79.
8. Cotterall WA, Mackie K. Local anesthetics. In: Brunton LL, Lazo JS, Parker KL, eds. Goodman and Gilman's The Pharmacological Basis of Therapeutics. 11th ed. New York: McGraw-Hill, 2006:369–381.
9. Weinber GL, VadeBoncouer T, Ramaraju GA, et al. Pretreatment or resuscitation with a lipid infusion shifts the dose-response to bupivacaine induced asystole in rats. Anesthesiology 1998; 88:1071–1075.
10. Winberg G, Ripper R, Feinstein DL, et al. Lipid emulsion infusion rescues dogs from bupivacaine-induced cardiac toxicity. Reg Anesth Pain Med 2003; 28:198–202.
11. Frey WC, Emmons EE, Morris MJ. Safety of high dose lidocaine in flexible bronchoscopy. J Bronchol 2008; 15:33–37.
12. Brown DL. Regional Anesthesia and Analgesia. Philadelphia: W.B. Saunders, 1996:249, 250.
13. Charney DS, Mihic SJ. Hypnotics and sedatives. In: Brunton LL, Lazo JS, Parker KL, eds. Goodman and Gilman's The Pharmacological Basis of Therapeutics. 11th ed. New York: McGraw-Hill, 2006:401–413.
14. Coleman RL, Temo J. Benzodiazepines. In: White PF, ed. Textbook of Intravenous Anesthesia. Philadelphia: Lippincott Williams and Wilkins, 1997:77–84.
15. Williams TJ, Bowie PE. Midazolam sedation to produce complete amnesia for bronchoscopy: 2 years' experience at a district general hospital. Respir Med 1999; 93:361–365.
16. Bahhady IJ, Ernst A. Risks of and recommendations for flexible bronchoscopy in pregnancy: a review. Chest 2004; 126:1974–1981.
17. Fox BD, Krylov Y, Leon P, et al. Benzodiazepine and opioid sedation attenuate the sympathetic response to fiberoptic bronchoscopy. Prophylactic labetalol gave no additional benefit. Results of a randomized double-blind placebo-controlled study. Respir Med 2008; 102:978–983.
18. Crawford M, Pollock J, Anderson K, et al. Comparison of midazolam with propofol for sedation in outpatient bronchoscopy. Br J Anaesth 1993; 70:419–422.
19. Chhajed PN, Wallner J, Stolz D, et al. Sedative drug requirements during flexible bronchoscopy. Respiration 2005; 72:617–621.
20. White PF, Smith I. Propofol. In: White PF, ed. Textbook of Intravenous Anesthesia. Philadelphia: Lippincott Williams and Wilkins, 1997:111–113, 119–122.

21. Chen TL, Ueng TH, Chen SH, et al. Human cytochrome P450 mono-oxygenase system is suppressed by propofol. Br J Anaesth 1995; 74:558–562.
22. Dawidowicz AL, Fornal E, Mardarowicz M, et al. The role of human lungs in the biotransformation of propofol. Anesthesiology 2000; 83:992–997.
23. Rechner J, Ihnsen H, Hatterscheid D, et al. Pharmacokinetics and clinical pharmacodynamics of the new propofol prodrug GPI 15715 in volunteers. Anesthesiology 2003; 99:303–313.
24. Popat K, Purugganan R. Off-label uses of dexmedetomidine. Adv Anesth 2006; 24:177–192.
25. Nelson LE, Lu J, Guo T, et al. The α2-adrenoceptor agonist dexmedetomidine converges on an endogenous sleep-promoting pathway to exert its sedative effects. Anesthesiology 2003; 98:428–436.
26. Cheung CW, Ying CLA, Chiu WK, et al. A comparison of dexmedetomidine and midazolam for sedation in third molar surgery. Anaesthesia 2007; 62:1132–1138.
27. Castro PE, Abdelmalak B, Gildea T. Dexmedetomidine in bronchoscopic lung volume reduction. Available at: http://www.nysaa-pga/PGA-60-Poster/PGA-60_P-9154.pdf. Accessed April 2008.
28. Abouzgheib W, Littman J, Pratter M, et al. Efficacy and safety of dexmedetomidine during bronchoscopy in patients with moderate to severe COPD or emphysema. J Bronchol 2007; 14:233–236.
29. Craven R. Ketamine. Anaesthesia 2007; 62:48–53.
30. Hwang J, Jeon Y, Park HP, et al. Comparison of alfentanil and ketamine in combination with propofol for patient-controlled sedation during fiberoptic bronchoscopy. Acta Anaesthesiol Scand 2005; 49:1334–1338.
31. Bailey P, Egan TD. Fentanyl and its congeners. In: White PF, ed. Textbook of Intravenous Anesthesia. Philadelphia: Lippincott Williams and Wilkins, 1997:215–220.
32. Gray PA, Reckling JC, Bocchiaro CM, et al. Modulation of respiratory frequency by peptidergic input to rhythmogenic neurons in the pre-Bötzinger complex. Science 1999; 286:1566–1568.
33. Dahan A. Novel data on opioid effect on breathing and analgesia. Semin Anesth 2007; 26: 58–64.
34. Hwang J, Jeon Y, Park HP, et al. Comparison of alfentanil and ketamine in combination with propofol for patient-controlled sedation during fiberoptic bronchoscopy. Acta Anesthesiol Scand 2005; 49:1334–1338.
35. Thorpe SJ, Balakrishnan VR, Cook LB. The safety of patient-controlled sedation. Anaesthesia 1997; 52:1144–1150.
36. Kulling D, Bauerfeind P, Fried M, et al. Patient-controlled analgesia and sedation in gastrointestinal endoscopy. Gastrointest Endosc Clin N Am 2004; 14:353–368.
37. Bright E, Rosereare C, Dalgleish D, et al. Patient-controlled sedation for colonoscopy: a randomized trial comparing patient-controlled administration of propofol and alfentanil with physician-administered midazolam and pethidine. Endoscopy 2003; 35:683–687.
38. Mandel JE, Tanner JW, Lichtenstein GR, et al. A randomized, controlled, double-blind trial of patient-controlled sedation with propofol/remifentanil versus midazolam/fentanyl for colonoscopy. Anesth Analg 2008; 106:434–439.
39. Atassi K, Mangiapan G, Fuhrman C, et al. Prefixed equimolar nitrous oxide and oxygen mixture reduces discomfort during flexible bronchoscopy in adult patients. A randomized, controlled, double-blind trial. Chest 2005; 128:863–868.
40. Fauroux B, Onody P, Gall O, et al. The efficacy of premixed nitrous oxide and oxygen for fiberoptic bronchoscopy in pediatric patients: a randomized, double-blind, controlled study. Chest 2004; 125:315–321.

12

Advanced Bronchoscopic Techniques for Diagnosis of Peripheral Pulmonary Lesions

ROBERT LEE
Lahey Clinic Medical Center, Burlington, Massachusetts, U.S.A.

DAVID OST
The University of Texas M.D. Anderson Cancer Center, Houston, Texas, U.S.A.

I. Introduction

The number of newly diagnosed lung cancers will be greater than 200,000 in 2008 (1). As many as 25% to 30% of these will present as peripheral lesion (2). When a peripheral lesion is initially identified, the pretest probability of lung cancer should be assessed. This estimate of the probability of lung cancer being present should be based on a careful history, physical exam, and review of CT images. Factors to focus on include the lesion's size, morphology, type of opacity, and growth rate (3). However, to confirm a diagnosis, a tissue biopsy will frequently be required.

The site of biopsy will depend on the clinical context. Often, the diagnostic workup answering the question whether a patient has cancer is occurring in parallel with the staging workup, which answers the question of the extent of cancer spread. A concurrent staging evaluation is usually warranted if the pretest probability of malignancy is high. In this way, diagnosis and staging can be provided with the least number of invasive procedures. Often this entails performing a biopsy at a site that would identify the greatest extent of disease. For example, biopsy of an enlarged lymph node may be more desirable than biopsy of a mass, since it may serve the dual purpose of diagnosis and staging. In other instances, biopsy of a peripheral lesion may be the best approach, especially if there is already evidence of metastatic disease elsewhere.

In those instances in which biopsy of a peripheral lesion is warranted, it is useful to be familiar with a wide range of diagnostic techniques, since the best approach will often vary with the clinical context in a given patient. In this chapter, we will review specific techniques that target peripheral lesions, focusing on their diagnostic sensitivity, specificity, and complication rates.

II. Traditional Techniques

Traditional diagnostic techniques for peripheral lesions can be divided into bronchoscopic and percutaneous approaches. Bronchoscopic approaches typically utilize flexible bronchoscopy with a combination of bronchoalveolar lavage (BAL), cytology brushing, transbronchial biopsy (TBBX), and peripheral transbronchial needle aspiration (TBNA). Percutaneous approaches typically use some form of image guidance, such as fluoroscopy, CT imaging, or ultrasound, to guide percutaneous fine needle aspiration.

A. Bronchoscopic Approaches

Conventional flexible bronchoscopy has had limited success when used for small peripheral lesions. A review of 30 studies evaluating the role of flexible bronchoscopy for peripheral bronchogenic carcinoma demonstrated an overall mean sensitivity of 69% that decreased to 33% in peripheral lesions <2 cm (2). Diagnostic sensitivity and yield seem to vary significantly on the basis of size and location of the lesion. For example, in one study of 129 patients with peripheral solitary pulmonary nodules (SPNs), diagnostic yield was 64% for malignant and 35% for benign lesions (4). However, stratification based on size and location demonstrated a diagnostic yield of 14% for SPNs <2 cm in diameter that were located in the outer 1/3 of the lung. For lesions <2 cm in size located in the middle 1/3 of the lung, the yield increased to 31%. If the lesions were greater than 4 cm and in the outer 1/3 of the lung, the yield was still 77%. We can conclude that flexible bronchoscopy using traditional methods had a significantly higher yield when lesions are larger than 4 cm or are centrally located.

One important way to improve the sensitivity of bronchoscopic diagnosis for peripheral lesions than one diagnostic technique. For example, in the study cited above, all patients had BAL, TBBX, and brushing. However, peripheral TBNA was not utilized at that time as part of the standard approach to peripheral nodules. Subsequently, other investigators have demonstrated that using peripheral TBNA in addition to traditional methods (BAL, brushing, and TBBX) increases sensitivity from about 31% to 50% without any significant increase in complication rates (5). In this study, when BAL, brushing, TBBX, and peripheral TBNA were performed, TBNA was the sole method that was diagnostic in 20% of the patients. So the incremental benefit of adding peripheral TBNA to the standard approach for peripheral lesions was quite large. TBNA is still underutilized in clinical practice, so this offers an opportunity to improve diagnostic yield for patients with a minimal increase in cost (6,7).

B. Percutaneous Approach

Transthoracic fine needle aspiration under CT guidance has been studied extensively and is a valuable modality for diagnosing peripheral lesions. The reported mean sensitivity and specificity are 90% and 97%, respectively, for malignant disease (2). However, the complication rate of pneumothorax can be high, ranging from 17% to 33% (8). Also, there is a potential to spread malignant cells into the pleural space, although the exact magnitude of this risk is difficult to estimate and there are relatively few studies reporting this (9,10). In addition, potentially fatal arterial air embolism has been reported, but these are exceptionally rare occurrences (11,12).

III. Advanced Techniques

Recent advances in imaging technology have facilitated the development of advanced diagnostic techniques for biopsies of peripheral lung lesions. The focus has been overcoming two major roadblocks that limit the diagnostic sensitivity of flexible bronchoscopy. The first is how to successfully navigate to small distal lesions; the second is verification that the biopsy site is correct. The remainder of the chapter will focus on these advanced diagnostic techniques, such as ultrathin bronchoscopy, CT-guided bronchoscopy, virtual bronchoscopy, electromagnetic navigation and guidance for bronchoscopy (ENB), and endobronchial ultrasound (EBUS).

A. Ultrathin Bronchoscopy

Bronchoscopes <3 mm in external diameter have been used since the 1980s as a means to observe peripheral lesions (13,14). Ultrathin bronchoscopes are well suited to addressing the issue of how to navigate to small distal lesions. However, given the number of branches, it is easy to become disoriented and it is often not possible to address the issue of how to verify that the ultrathin scope is actually in the correct place. In addition, early models had no working channel, so they had limited clinical utility. With the development of a built-in working channel and improved range of motion for the tip, there may be a role for newer models to be used in the diagnosis of peripheral lesions (15). Current commercially available models have an external diameter of 2.8 mm with a channel diameter of 1.2 mm, allowing BAL, TBBX, and brushing with specially designed forceps and brushes. The entire scope can be passed through the working channel of a large conventional bronchoscope once wedged at the lung segment of interest. Currently, ultrathin bronchoscopy remains an adjunct to conventional bronchoscopy for the diagnosis of peripheral lesions. How much improvement, if any, in diagnostic yield can be obtained by using ultrathin bronchoscopy in addition to routine bronchoscopic techniques remains to be determined. Small series have shown mixed results and the actual techniques used varied (16,17). One promising method of utilizing ultrathin bronchoscopy is to use ultrathin bronchoscopy only when conventional bronchoscopy yields no immediate diagnosis with rapid onsite cytology. When employed in this manner, diagnostic yield increased from 54.3% to 62.8% in a series of 32 patients (17).

B. CT Fluoroscopic Guidance for Bronchoscopy

Real-time CT fluoroscopy is an attractive concept since CT provides three-dimensional verification that the bronchoscope or its instruments are in the right place. CT fluoroscopic guidance is performed with the patient on the CT scanner table with the feet first into the scanner (18–20). Once the bronchoscope is in place, CT fluoroscopy is performed and the location of biopsy tools (forceps, brush, or TBNA) can be determined. Importantly, while CT fluoroscopy can provide image verification of the location of biopsy instruments, it cannot necessarily help steer them to the correct location. Tsushima et al. compared CT fluoroscopy and X-ray fluoroscopy in 160 patients and found a significantly higher diagnostic yield with CT fluoroscopy in lesions ≤15 mm (<10 mm size 42.9% vs. 7.7%, $p = 0.028$; 10–15 mm size = 54.2% vs. 20% $p = 0.039$) (21). Other studies have demonstrated diagnostic yields ranging from 62% to 89% (Table 1). When peripheral TBNA of nodules was added to CT fluoroscopy–guided bronchoscopy for nodules up to 3.0 cm in size, a 67% diagnostic yield was achieved (prevalence of malignancy being 42%) (19). The mean radiation exposure in these studies was approximately twice the amount of X-ray fluoroscopy. The clinical significance of this amount of additional radiation exposure depends in large part on the clinical context. Given that most bronchoscopy patients are older and often have cancer, it is doubtful that the long-term effects of increased radiation exposure will manifest.

Ultrathin bronchoscopes have been used in conjunction with CT fluoroscopy for more controlled maneuverability in the small peripheral airways (20–23). Theoretically, this can increase the diagnostic yield by providing additional steerability in addition to image verification of the biopsy site. However, the studies using ultrathin bronchoscopes in addition to CT fluoroscopic guidance did not have a comparator arm with

Table 1 Real Time CT Fluoroscopy for Peripheral Lung Lesions

Studies	*n*	Mean size (mm) (range)	Ultrathin	VB	Yield (%)
Wagner et al., 1996 (18)	9	26 (10–45)	No	No	89
White et al., 2000 (19)	12	22 (10–30)	No	No	67
Asano et al., 2002 (20)	23	14 (all <20)	Yes	No	78.3
Shinagawa et al., 2004 (22)	26	13.2	Yes	Yes	65
Tsushima et al., 2006 (21)	82	16.7 (5–51)	No	Yes	62.2
Shinagawa et al., 2007 (23)	85	13.6	Yes	Yes	66
Ost et al., 2008 (24)	15	37 ± 16	No	No	71

Abbreviation: VB, virtual bronchoscopy.

conventional bronchoscopy, which makes it difficult to draw any definitive conclusion regarding the incremental benefit of utlrathin bronchoscopy.

CT fluoroscopy–guided bronchoscopy has been used for TBNA in patients who have undergone nondiagnostic TBNA of lymph nodes performed blindly (25). After the needle pass is made, CT fluoroscopy is performed intermittently to verify that the tip of the TBNA needle is in the target lymph node. On the basis of the CT fluoroscopy image, adjustments or additional passes can be made.

One additional interesting role of CT fluoroscopy is bronchoscopic dye marking for peripheral lesions prior to surgical resection (26,27) In this procedure, a catheter is placed via the bronchoscope near the visceral pleura closest to the lesion of interest under CT guidance. Once in place, 0.5 mL of either barium sulfate suspension or other dye such as indigo carmine can be injected. This facilitates locating the nodule for surgical biopsy or resection, especially when it is not palpable or visible.

C. Virtual Bronchoscopy

Virtual bronchoscopy provides a virtual reality, three-dimensional display of the bronchial lumen reconstructed from preprocedure CT data (28). Virtual bronchoscopy has been used to evaluate endobronchial abnormalities such as tumors and obstructing lesions, and to guide TBNA of the lymph nodes (29). Virtual bronchoscopy may have a role as an adjunct in navigation systems to help guide the bronchoscope to the correct bronchus that leads to a peripheral lesion. Virtual bronchoscopy can image up to 6th generation bronchi, depending on the CT technique and algorithms used (30). With faster multidetector scanners and newer programs, imaging to even higher order bronchi may be feasible. However, this is done prior to the actual bronchoscopy, so other imaging methods such as X-ray fluoroscopy, CT fluoroscopy, or EBUS are usually used in real time to verify the location of biopsy tools (22,30–32). Potentially, virtual bronchoscopy can decrease procedure time and limit radiation. Currently, there are only limited data as to whether this technique improves the diagnostic yield, since the results from studies are confounded by the use of other imaging adjuncts, such as EBUS, CT fluoroscopy, or X-ray fluoroscopy. Larger studies comparing virtual imaging against a standard control would be needed to definitively answer this question. To date, there are no randomized trials assessing the efficacy and usefulness of virtual bronchoscopy.

D. Electromagnetic Navigation and Guidance for Bronchoscopy

ENB is a new type of real-time guidance for accessing small peripheral lesions and lymph nodes. ENB was built on the concept of virtual bronchoscopy, but also incorporates novel features such as steerable forceps and a locatable probe. An extended working channel (EWC), which is just a sheath that extends beyond the bronchoscope and allows accessory tools to pass through, is used as a mechanism to maintain the biopsy site while the locatable steerable probe is withdrawn and switched to biopsy tools. ENB allows for improved maneuverability and accuracy beyond the optical limitations of the bronchoscope. The necessary equipment includes an electromagnetic board placed under the patient, which detects and localizes the position of the locatable probe in three dimensions. On the basis of the reconstructed virtual 3D images from a preprocedure CT, simultaneous radiologic and endobronchial mapping is performed using five to seven prominent anatomic landmarks. Typically, these are the main carina and the secondary carinas in the right upper lobe, right middle lobe, right lower lobe, left upper lobe, and left lower lobe. Once these landmarks are registered, real-time guidance of the locatable probe to the target lesion can be performed. The steerable probe allows a 180° turn with an angulation radius of 2.5 cm without kinking of the EWC (33).

The first set of studies that evaluated this type of technology in bronchoscopy was in 1998 using the Biosense® intrabody navigation system (34,35). A 1.5-mm electromagnetic sensor tip was attached to the tip of the bronchoscope with its wire running outside the bronchoscope that had to be covered with a sheath. In addition, 10 metallic skin markers were placed on the chest wall prior to CT scanning that made the procedure cumbersome. Of note, this system did not contain a steerable forceps.

The next generation of ENB systems was introduced shortly thereafter (super-Dimension™), which simplified and improved the technology with the introduction of an extended working channel and steerable electromagnetic probe. A pilot study using this system showed a 69% diagnostic yield in 29 patients with an average navigation accuracy of 6.12 mm (target registration error value) (36). Subsequent studies showed a comparable diagnostic yield of 62.5% to 74% (37–39) (Table 2).

Fluoroscopy was used in all of the above studies during biopsy to verify the biopsy site and the distance from the pleura because of the concern that the EWC might dislodge when biopsy tools are introduced. However, a study comparing ENB with ENB plus peripheral EBUS demonstrated only modest complication rates (up to 8% for pneumothorax), so it is feasible to use ENB without fluoroscopy (40). Total procedure time was reduced when ENB was performed without fluoroscopy (39,40). However, no study has definitively addressed whether or not the addition of fluoroscopy to the ENB procedure impacts either safety or diagnostic yield significantly.

E. Endobronchial Ultrasound

Endoscopic ultrasound was initially used in the field of gastroenterology. The first bronchoscopic application was described in 1992, and has been commercially available since 1999 (41). Current clinical applications of EBUS technology include mediastinal lymph node biopsy and staging, assessment of local tumor tissue invasion, and more recently, evaluation of peripheral lung lesions (42), which will be the focus of this section.

In peripheral lung lesions, a flexible high-frequency 20-MHz ultrasound probe with external diameter ranging from 1.4 mm to 2.5 mm is inserted through the working

Table 2 Electromagnetic Navigation Bronchoscopy

Studies	n	Mean size ± SD (mm) (range)	Yield by size	Other imaging used	Biopsy	Navigation accuracy (mm) (mean ± SD)	Complications
Becker et al., 2005 (36)	29	(12–106)[a]	Overall: 69%	Fluoro and EBUS	Forceps, Brush, or Currette	6.12 (2.85–9.53)	1 pt: PTX 3 pts: Self limit-ing Bleeding
Schwarz et al., 2006 (37)	13	33.5 ± 11 (15–50 mm)	Overall: 69% ≤20mm: 50% >20 to ≤30mm: 66% >30mm: 75%	Fluoro	Forceps, Brush	5.7	None
Gildea et al., 2006 (39)	54	22.8 ± 12.6 (8–78)	Overall: 74% ≤20 mm: 74.1% >20 to ≤40 mm: 66.6% >40 mm: 100%	Fluoro	Forceps, Brush, TBNA	6.6 ± 2.1 (2.9–13.8)	2 pts: PTX (3.5%)
Makris et al., 2007 (38)	40	23.5 ± 9.5 (8–49)[b]	Overall: 62.5% ≤20 mm: 43.7 % >20 to ≤30 mm: 71.4% >30 mm: 76.9 %	None	Forceps (9 attempts for each lesion)	4 ± 0.95[b]	3 pts: PTX
Eberhardt et al., 2007 (40)	92	24 ± 8 (10–58)	Overall: 67% ≤20 mm: 63% >20 mm: 70% ≤30 mm: 67% >30 mm: 75%	None	Forceps, brush, TBNA, washing	9 ± 6	2 pts: PTX 1 pt: Intubation 1 pt: EWC perforation

[a]No mean reported for the entire sample size.
[b]Originally reported as SEM converted to SD for comparison.
Abbreviations: PTX, pneumothorax; pt, patient; EWC, extended working channel.

Table 3 Endobronchial Ultrasound Diagnostic Yield

Studies	n	Technique	Additional imaging	Size in mean ± SD (range)	Yield by size	Complication
Herth et al., 2002 (43)	50	Forceps	Fluoroscopy	33.1 ± 9.2 mm (20–60 mm)	Overall: 80% <3 cm: 80% >3 cm: 79%	None
Kurimoto et al., 2004 (44)	150	GS ± curette Brush/forceps	Fluoroscopy	No range given	Overall: 77% ≤10 mm: 76% >10 to ≤15: 76% >15 to ≤20: 69% >20 to ≤30: 77% >30: 92%	Mod bleeding 1%
Kikuchi et al., 2004 (47)	24	GS + curette Brush/forceps	Fluoroscopy	18.4 ± 6.3 mm (8.0–27.5 mm)	Overall: 58.3% <20 mm: 53.3% 20 to 30 mm: 66.7%	PTX: one pt (4.2%)
Shirakawa et al., 2004 (50)	50	GS ± curette Forceps	Fluoroscopy	No range given	Overall: 70.8%	
Paone et al., 2005 (42)	87	Forceps (5 biopsies)	None	No range given	Overall: 75.8% ≤20 mm: 71% <30 mm: 75% >3 cm: 82.8%	None
Herth et al., 2006 (45)	54	GS Forceps	Fluoroscopy	22 ± 7 mm (14–33 mm)	Overall: 70%	PTX: 1 pt (2%)

Chung et al., 2006 (51)	113	Forceps	None	24.5 ± 8.2 mm (10–44 mm)	Overall: 78.9% <20 mm: 44.4% 20 to 30 mm:	Hemorrhage: 5 pts PTX: one pt
Yoshikawa et al., 2007 (46)	123	GS Brush/forceps	None	31.0 mm	Overall: 61.8% ≤20 mm: 29.7% >20 to ≤30: 57.9% >30 mm: 89.6%	PTX: 1 pt (0.8%)
Yamada et al., 2007 (48)	106	GS ± curette Brush/forceps	Fluoroscopy	20.8 ± 6.1 mm (9.5–30 mm)	Overall: 67% ≤15 mm: 40% >15 to ≤20: 74% >20 to ≤25: 72% >25 to ≤30: 81%	No mention
Asano et al., 2007 (52)	32	GS Forceps	Navigation with CT	21 (10–53.5 mm)	Overall: 91.2%	None
Fielding et al., 2008 (49)	140	GS Forceps	None	29 ± 12 mm (8–80 mm)	Overall: 66%	PTX: 2 pts

channel of the bronchoscope. Saline can be injected into the sheath surrounding the probe to provide a better probe-tissue interface although this is rarely necessary for peripheral lesions because of the narrow airways involved. In addition, a small amount of saline (10 cc) can be instilled into the bronchus of interest prior to probe insertion, which also promotes an improved interface and facilitates better imaging (42). The ultrasound probe rapidly rotates inside the sheath allowing a 360° field of view around the probe. This system has been used to evaluate peripheral lung lesions through the flexible bronchoscope with promising results in several case series (Table 3) (41–49).

A feasibility test in humans was published in 2002 in which EBUS-guided TBBX was compared to fluoroscopy-guided TBBX (45). The investigators failed to demonstrate a statistically significant difference in the diagnostic yield between EBUS and fluoroscopy-guided TBBX (80% vs. 76%, respectively) in 50 patients. This is perhaps attributable to the fact that all lesions were visible under fluoroscopy. EBUS technique was further refined in 2004 when Kurimoto introduced a novel technique of using EBUS with a guide sheath (EBUS-GS). The guide sheath is a hollow flexible sheath equivalent to the extended working channel (EWC) described above for ENB. The EBUS probe is passed through the guide sheath. After the EBUS probe identifies the lesion, the guide sheath is left in place while the EBUS probe is removed. Biopsy tools are then inserted through the guide sheath so that the target can be reliably reached (44,45). In Kurimoto's study, performing both brushing and TBBX, an overall diagnostic yield of 77% was achieved (69% for benign lesions and 81% for malignant lesions) (Table 3).

Diagnostic yield of EBUS-GS was not affected by the size of the lesion or fluoroscopic visualization in these studies (44,45,47). However, conflicting findings were demonstrated in another study by Yoshikawa in which there was a significantly lower diagnostic yield for lesions ≤ 20 mm compared to those > 20 mm (29.7% vs. 76%, respectively) (48). Also, addition of fluoroscopy increased the yield from 29.7% to 75.7% for those lesions ≤ 20 mm. One explanation for these contradictory findings is that Yoshikawa had a low rate of EBUS image localization at 43.2% for lesions ≤ 20 mm, compared to the previously reported rate of 66.7% for similar-sized lesions, which may have resulted in a lower diagnostic yield (47). Therefore, it is the ability to steer to a lesion and achieve localization rather than the size of the lesion that affects diagnostic yield. This was supported by data from a study by Yamada in which differences in size (≤15 mm vs. >15 mm) was significantly associated with diagnostic yield of EBUS-GS based on univariate analysis (HR 4.82, 95% CI 2.25–10.33; $p < 0.001$). However, after adjustment for the position of the probe in relation to the lung nodule on the EBUS image, lesion size was no longer significantly associated with diagnostic yield (HR 2.42, CI 0.93–6.32; $p = 0.071$) (48). This illustrates that if adequate visualization can be achieved with peripheral EBUS, then diagnostic yields are good. Diagnostic yield varies on the basis of the proximity of the probe to the lesion. When the probe is within versus adjacent versus outside, the yield is 83%, 61%, and 4%, respectively (44,48). A potentially significant weakness of the EBUS technique is the lack of navigation and steerability of the probe. It may be difficult to find the correct bronchus that will lead to the lesion of interest. Once the correct bronchus is selected, EBUS can help to verify which location is best for biopsy, but the correct bronchus may not always be found. The number of biopsies performed also seemed to have a direct correlation with the yield as well, up to a point. After five biopsies, the incremental benefit of additional biopsies was small (48).

Other factors that affect diagnostic yield include location of the lesion [left upper lobe apical posterior segment being associated with lower yield ($p = 0.003$) (45) while lingular and right middle lobe are associated with higher yield ($p < 0.03$) (46)], identification of a bronchus leading to a lesion on preprocedure CT ($p < 0.01$), solid lesions compared to mixed or pure ground glass nodules ($p = 0.05$) (46), and whether the lesion is touching the visceral pleura (74% vs. 35%, respectively) (49). Alternative methods of diagnosis should be considered for lesions anticipated to have low diagnostic yield with EBUS-GS. The guide sheath also seems to be helpful in reducing bleeding in the airways postbiopsy since it tamponades bleeding at the site of biopsy (47).

Another potentially important role of EBUS is characterizing the internal structure of the lesion to help determine the likelihood of malignancy. Kurimoto classified the internal structure of peripheral lung lesions seen with EBUS and compared them with the histologic diagnosis in 124 patients (69 patients with a surgical specimen). Classification was based on three different patterns visualized on EBUS plus vessel characteristics (53) (Table 4). Histologic comparison to the above EBUS image characteristics demonstrated that 92% of type I lesion were benign while 99% of type II and III lesions were malignant (87.5% of type II lesions being adenocarcinoma). The average time to obtain EBUS imaging was 8.38 minutes. Other image classification systems were attempted subsequently to simplify the pattern and reduce imaging time (54,55). For example, one scheme simplified and reclassified Kurimoto's original classification into three distinct patterns with elimination of vessel characteristics: "A," continuous margin; "B," absence of linear discrete air bronchograms; and "C," heterogeneity. The sensitivity and the specificity for each image pattern for malignant lesions were as follows: A, 27.64% and 93.07%; B, 91.87% and 62.38%; C, 65.04% and 90.1% (55). When all three patterns were visualized, the positive predictive value for malignancy was 100%, while the absence of all three patterns showed a negative predictive value of 93.7%. Prevalence of malignancy was 55%. Other studies have tried to simplify the scheme further and have been able to reduce mean examination time to as low as 3.49 minutes (54). At this point in time however, the optimal system for characterization of lung nodules with EBUS is not known.

Table 4 EBUS Classification for Peripheral Lung Lesion)

Types	Description
Type I	Homogeneous pattern
A	Patent vessels and patent bronchioles
B	Without vessels and bronchioles
Type II	Hyperechoic dots and linear arcs pattern
A	Without vessels
B	Patent vessels
Type III	Heterogenous pattern
A	With hyperechoic dots and short lines
B	Without hyperechoic dots and short lines

Source: From Ref. 53.

F. Multimodality Strategy

Combining different modalities may improve diagnostic yield further. For example, lack of a navigation system with EBUS can be a limiting factor since the location of the EBUS probe in relation to the lesion affects the diagnostic yield as discussed previously (44). ENB, on the other hand, can direct the biopsy forceps to the right bronchus with precision using the navigation system and the steerable probe, but cannot visually verify the lesion just prior to biopsy. This can be an issue since there is always some degree of discrepancy with target registration between the virtual CT images and real endoscopic images. Therefore, by combining EBUS and ENB, the two major obstacles of traditional diagnostic techniques can be overcome. One study that tested this hypothesis was a randomized trial that compared (*i*) ENB, (*ii*) EBUS, and (*iii*) the combination of ENB and EBUS in 118 patients (56). Patients with nondiagnostic bronchoscopy underwent subsequent surgical biopsy. The diagnostic yield for combined ENB/EBUS was significantly higher than ENB or EBUS alone, 88%, 69%, and 59%, respectively (78% prevalence for malignancy). However, for benign disease, there was no significant difference in diagnostic yield. Diagnostic yield did not vary with lesion size in this study.

IV. Conclusion

Diagnostic techniques in peripheral lung lesion have expanded dramatically in recent years with advancements in imaging technology. With multiple modalities available, it is important to select the appropriate technique on the basis of the clinical context. Each individual case should be carefully considered to determine the best technique to be used for a given clinical setting with cost-effectiveness in mind. For instance, a peripheral lesion larger than 3 cm located in the right middle lobe lateral segment would not benefit significantly from advanced techniques over plain X-ray fluoroscopy since the diagnostic yield is fairly high to begin with. The potential marginal benefit of using advanced techniques may not outweigh the cost and the time involved. In contrast, a 15-mm lesion in the right lower lobe posterior segment may require a more advanced technique, such as a combination of ENB and EBUS, as the initial procedure. Since the marginal benefit of advanced techniques is higher for smaller lesions, the higher cost may be justified. As imaging and guidance technologies continue to improve, we will need to continue to revise our diagnostic algorithms for peripheral lesions.

References

1. Cancer Facts and Figures 2008.Atlanta, GA: American Cancer Society, 2008:1–72.
2. Schreiber G, McCrory DC. Performance characteristics of different modalities for diagnosis of suspected lung cancer: summary of published evidence. Chest 2003; 123(suppl):115S–128S.
3. Wahidi MM, Govert JA, Goudar RK, et al. Evidence for the treatment of patients with pulmonary nodules: when is it lung cancer? ACCP evidence-based clinical practice guidelines 2nd ed. Chest 2007; 132(suppl): 94S–107S.
4. Baaklini WA, Reinoso MA, Gorin AB, et al. Diagnostic yield of fiberoptic bronchoscopy in evaluating solitary pulmonary nodules. Chest 2000; 117(4):1049–1054.
5. Reichenberger F, Weber J, Tamm M, et al. The value of transbronchial needle aspiration in the diagnosis of peripheral pulmonary lesions. Chest 1999; 116:704–708.

6. Haponik EF, Shure D. Underutilization of transbronchial needle aspiration: experiences of current pulmonary fellows. Chest 1997; 112:251–253.
7. Dasgupta A, Mehta AC. Transbronchial needle aspiration. An underused diagnostic technique. Clin Chest Med 1999; 20(1):39–51.
8. Yeow KM, Su IH, Tsay PK, et al. Risk factors of pneumothorax and bleeding: multivariate analysis of 660 CT-guided coaxial cutting needle lung biopsies. Chest 2004; 126:748–754.
9. Sawabata N, Ohta M, Maeda H. Fine-needle aspiration cytologic technique for lung cancer has a high potential of malignant cell spread through the tract. Chest 2000; 118:936–939.
10. Seyfer CAE, Walsh DA, Greaber CGM, et al. Chest wall implantation of lung cancer after thin-needle aspiration biopsy. Ann Thorac Surg 1989; 48:284–286.
11. Wong RS, Ketai L, Temes T, et al. Air embolus complicating transthoracic percutaneous needle biopsy. Ann Thorac Surg 1995; 59:1010–1011.
12. Aberle DR, Gamsu G, Golden JA. Fatal systemic arterial air embolism following lung needle aspiration. Radiology 1987; 165:351–353.
13. Tanaka M, Satoh M, Kawanami O, et al. A new bronchofiberscope for the study of diseases of very peripheral airways. Chest 1984; 85:590–594.
14. Tanaka M, Kawanami O, Satoh M, et al. Endoscopic observation of peripheral airway lesions. Chest 1988; 93:228–233.
15. Hasegawa S, Hiltomi S, Murakawa M, et al. Development of an ultrathin fiberscope with a built-in channel for bronchoscopy in infants. Chest 1996; 110:1543–1546.
16. Rooney CP, Wolf K, McLennan G. Ultrathin bronchoscopy as an adjunct to standard bronchoscopy in the diagnosis of peripheral lung lesions. Respiration 2002; 69:63–68.
17. Yamamoto S, Ueno K, Imamura F, et al. Usefulness of ultrathin bronchoscopy in diagnosis of lung cancer. Lung Cancer 2004; 46(1):43–48.
18. Wagner U, Walthers EM, Gelmetti W, et al. Computer-tomographically guided fiber-bronchoscopic transbronchial biopsy of small pulmonary lesions: a feasibility study. Respiration 1996; 63(3):181–186.
19. White CS, Weiner EA, Patel P, et al. Transbronchial needle aspiration: guidance with CT fluoroscopy. Chest 2000; 118:1630–1638.
20. Asano F, Matsuno Y, Komak C, et al. CT-guided transbronchial diagnosis using ultrathin bronchoscope for small peripheral pulmonary lesions. Nihon Kokyuki Gakkai Zasshi 2002; 40(1):11–16; abstract only.
21. Tsushima K, Sone S, Hanaoka T, et al. Comparison of bronchoscopic diagnosis for peripheral pulmonary nodule under fluoroscopic guidance with CT guidance. Respir Med 2006; 100:737–745.
22. Shinagawa N, Yamazaki K, Onodera Y, et al. CT-guided transbronchial biopsy using an ultrathin bronchoscope with virtual bronchoscopic navigation. Chest 2004; 125:1138–1143.
23. Shinagawa N, Yamazaki K, Onodera Y, et al. Factors related to diagnostic sensitivity using an ultrathin bronchoscope under CT guidance. Chest 2007; 131:549–553.
24. Ost D, Shah R, Anasco E, et al. A randomized trial of CT fluoroscopic guided bronchoscopy versus conventional in patients with suspected lung cancer. Chest 2008; 134(3):507–513.
25. Goldberg SN, Raptopoulos V, Boiselle PM, et al. Mediastinal lymphadenopathy: diagnostic yield of transbronchial mediastinal lymph node biopsy with CT fluoroscopic guidance—initial experience. Radiology 2000; 216:764–767.
26. Kobayashi T, Kaneko M, Kondo H, et al. CT-guided bronchoscopic barium marking for resection of a fluoroscopically invisible peripheral pulmonary lesion. Jpn J Clin Oncol 1997; 27(3):204–205.
27. Endo M, Kotani Y, Satouchi M, et al. CT fluoroscopy-guided bronchoscopic dye marking for resection of small peripheral pulmonary nodules. Chest 2004; 125:1747–1752.
28. Vining DJ, Liu K, Choplin RH, et al. Virtual bronchoscopy: relationship of virtual reality endobronchial simulations to actual bronchoscopic findings. Chest 1996; 109:549–553.

29. Hopper KD, Lucas TA, Gleeson K, et al. Transbronchial biopsy with virtual CT broncho-
     scopy and nodal highlighting. Radiology 2001; 221:531–536.
30. Tachihara M, Ishida T, Kanazawa K, et al. A virtual bronchoscopic navigation system under
     X-ray fluoroscopy for transbronchial diagnosis of small peripheral pulmonary lesions. Lung
     Cancer 2007; 57:322–327.
31. Asano F, Matsuno Y, Shinagawa N, et al. A virtual bronchoscopic navigation system for
     pulmonary peripheral lesions. Chest 2006; 130:559–566.
32. Asahina H, Yamazaki K, Onodera Y, et al.Transbronchial biopsy using endobronchial ultra-
     sonography with a guide sheath and virtual bronchoscopic navigation. Chest 2005; 128:
     1761–1765.
33. Schwarz Y, Mehta A, Ernst A, et al. Electromagnetic navigation during flexible broncho-
     scopy. Respiration 2003; 70:516–522.
34. Solomon S, White P, Acker D, et al. Real-time bronchoscope tip localization enables three-
     dimensional CT image guidance for transbronchial needle aspiration in swine. Chest 1998;
     114:1405–1410.
35. Solomon S, White P, Wiener C, et al. Three-dimensional CT-guided bronchoscopy with a
     real-time electromagnetic position sensor: a comparison of two image registration methods.
     Chest 2000; 118:1783–1787.
36. Becker HC, Herth F, Ernst A, et al. Bronchoscopic biopsy of peripheral lung lesions under
     electromagnetic guidance: a pilot study. J Brochol 2005; 12:9–13.
37. Schwarz Y, Greif J, Becker HD, et al. Real-time electromagnetic navigation bronchoscopy to
     peripheral lung lesions using overlaid CT images: the first human study. Chest 2006; 129:
     988–994.
38. Makris D, Scherpereel A, Leroy S, et al. Electromagnetic navigation diagnostic broncho-
     scopy for small peripheral lung lesions. Eur Respir J 2007; 29:1187–1192.
39. Gildea TR, Mazzone PJ, Karnak D, et al. Electromagnetic navigation diagnostic broncho-
     scopy. Am J Respir Crit Care Med 2006; 174:982–989.
40. Eberhardt R, Anantham D, Herth F, et al. Electromagnetic navigation diagnostic broncho-
     scopy in peripheral lung lesions. Chest 2007; 131:1800–1805.
41. Hurther T, Hanrath P. Endobronchial sonography: feasibility and preliminary results. Thorax
     1992; 47:565–567.
42. Paone G, Nicastri E, Lucantoni G, et al. Endobronchial ultrasound-driven biopsy in the
     diagnosis of peripheral lung lesions. Chest 2005; 128:3551–3557.
43. Herth FJ, Ernst A, Becker HD. Endobronchial ultrasound-guided transbronchial lung biopsy
     in solitary pulmonary nodules and peripheral lesions. Eur Respir J 2002; 20:972–974.
44. Kurimoto N, Miyazawa T, Okimasa S, et al. Endobronchial ultrasonography using a guide
     sheath increases the ability to diagnose peripheral pulmonary lesions endoscopically. Chest
     2004; 126:959–965.
45. Herth FJ, Eberhardt R, Becker HD, et al. Endobronchial ultrasound-guided transbronchial
     lung biopsy in fluoroscopically invisible solitary pulmonary nodules: a prospective trial.
     Chest 2006; 129:147–150.
46. Yoshikawa M, Sukoh N, Yamazaki K, et al. Diagnostic value of endobronchial ultra-
     sonography with a guide sheath for peripheral pulmonary lesions without X-ray fluoroscopy.
     Chest 2007; 131:1788–1793.
47. Kikuchi E, Yamazaki K, Sukoh N, et al. Endobronchial ultrasonography with guide-sheath
     for peripheral pulmonary lesions. Eur Respir J 2004; 24:533–537.
48. Yamada N, Yamazaki K, Kurimoto N, et al. Factors related to diagnostic yield of trans-
     bronchial biopsy using endobronchial ultrasonography with a guide sheath in small periph-
     eral pulmonary lesions. Chest 2007; 132:603–608.
49. Fielding DI, Robinson PJ, Kurimoto N. Biopsy site selection for endobronchial ultrasound
     guide-sheath transbronchial biopsy of peripheral lung lesions. Intern Med J 2008; 38:77–84.

50. Shirakawa T, Imamura F, Hamamoto J, et al. Usefulness of endobronchial ultrasonography for transbronchial lung biopsies of peripheral lung lesions. Respiration 2004; 71:260–268.
51. Chung YH, Lie CH, Chao TY, et al. Endobronchial ultrasonography with distance for peripheral pulmonary lesions. Respir Med 2007; 101:738–745.
52. Asano F, Matsuno Y, Tsuzuku A, et al. Diagnosis of peripheral pulmonary lesions using a bronchoscope insertion guidance system combined with endobronchial ultrasonography with a guide sheath. Lung Cancer 2008; 60(3):366–373 .
53. Kurimoto N, Murayama M, Yoshioka S, et al. Analysis of the internal structure of peripheral pulmonary lesions using endobronchial ultrasonography. Chest 2002; 122:1887–1984.
54. Chao TY, Lie CH, Chung YH, et al. Differentiating peripheral pulmonary lesions based on images of endobronchial ultrasonography. Chest 2006; 130:1191–1197.
55. Kuo CH, Lin SM, Chou CL, et al. Diagnosis of peripheral lung cancer with three echoic features via endobronchial ultrasound. Chest 2007; 132:922–929.
56. Eberhardt R, Anantham D, Ernst A, et al. Multimodality bronchoscopic diagnosis of peripheral lung lesions. Am J Respir Crit Care Med 2007; 176(1):36–34.

13

Bronchoscopic Treatment of Peripheral Lung Nodules

JONATHAN PUCHALSKI
Yale University School of Medicine, New Haven, Connecticut, U.S.A.

DANIEL STERMAN
University of Pennsylvania Medical Center, Philadelphia, Pennsylvania, U.S.A.

I. Introduction

The utility of the bronchoscope for diagnosing peripheral lung nodules has increased with the development of technologies to assist in accurately locating lesions beyond the operator's view. These include the use of navigational systems and ultrasound guidance for accessing peripheral lesions. Whereas surgery remains the first line of treatment for malignant lesions, other techniques are emerging for treatment when surgery is not an option. This chapter summarizes those techniques, some of which are currently present and many of which continue to develop as technology advances.

II. Background

The solitary pulmonary nodule can be defined as a single spherical lesion completely surrounded by pulmonary parenchyma, without associated adenopathy or atelectasis, <3 cm from the pleura and <3 cm in size (1). The traditional means of using transthoracic needle aspiration (TTNA) may reach a diagnostic yield of 82% to 96% but can have pneumothorax rates up to 44% (2). There are various bronchoscopic means that improve the diagnostic yield of these nodules compared with conventional fluoroscopic guidance, including electromagnetic navigation, endobronchial ultrasound, virtual bronchoscopy, and ultrathin bronchoscopy.

Electromagnetic navigation uses an electromagnetic tracking system to detect a position sensor that is guided through the bronchoscope and superimposed on previously gathered CT data (2). The reported yield of electromagnetic navigation ranges from 67% to 82%, with the highest accuracy reported for larger lesions (3). In addition to diagnostic strategies, electromagnetic navigation has been used for implanting radiofrequency monitoring devices (fiducials; RMDs) to assist with either surgical resection or radiation therapy for unresectable diseases. In one method, the electromagnetic probe is used to find the lesion and the extended working channel (EWC) is then left in place. A 19-gauge Wang needle with an inner 21-gauge needle is advanced past the EWC under fluoroscopic guidance. Once confirmed to be in the tumor, the inner 21-gauge needle is removed. The RMD is then backloaded into the sheath and advanced using a

0.66-mm guidewire. It is then placed inside or around the tumor. An alternative method employs a 5-Fr angulated Glidecath catheter into which the RMD is backloaded and deployed with a 0.66-mm guidewire (4).

Endobronchial ultrasound (EBUS) can provide cross-sectional images of the tracheobronchial wall and adjacent structures and thus can be used for mediastinal and peripheral lesions. Peripheral (radial probe) EBUS uses a very thin ultrasonic probe that is inserted through the working channel of the bronchoscope. It is passed into distal subsegments to localize parenchymal lesions. The use of endobronchial ultrasound with a guide sheath that goes through the bronchoscope, coupled with virtual bronchoscopic navigation, has been described. In this technique, an EBUS probe is inserted into the guide sheath, and the guide sheath and probe are driven to the peripheral nodule using virtual bronchoscopy. Once identified by ultrasound, the probe is removed and biopsy forceps are passed through the sheath to biopsy the lesion. The diagnostic yield was 44.4% for lesions <20 mm in size and 91.7% for lesions 20 to 30 mm in diameter using EBUS and virtual bronchoscopic navigation (5). Kurimoto et al. (6) described a diagnosis using EBUS for 76% of peripheral lesions of size <10 mm, even without the use of fluoroscopy. When combined with electromagnetic navigation, the diagnostic yield of EBUS was 88% (7). Figure 1 demonstrates images obtained by EBUS and electromagnetic navigation.

The ability to navigate the bronchoscope into peripheral subsegments is limited by the size of the bronchoscope. Several authors have described the use of an ultrathin bronchoscope for guidance further into the tracheobronchial tree. For example, the ability of an ultrathin bronchoscope with an external diameter of 3.2 mm and biopsy channel of 1.2 mm was compared with that of a 6.3-mm Olympus bronchoscope with a biopsy channel diameter of 3.2 mm under fluoroscopic guidance. Using a constant infusion of sterile saline during the procedure with the ultrathin bronchoscope, the

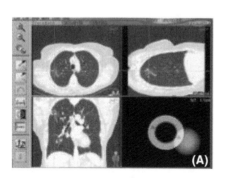
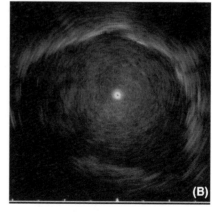

Figure 1 Two of several techniques may improve the peripheral localization of lung nodules for diagnostic and therapeutic purposes, including EMN (**A**) and peripheral EBUS (**B**). In EMN, computer-assisted technology facilitates guidance of a probe to the peripheral lesion (14). Used in conjunction with EMN or independently, peripheral EBUS allows direct confirmation that the probe is near or within the lesion. *Abbreviations*: EMN, electromagnetic navigation; EBUS, endobronchial ultrasound.

diagnostic yield was 70% for lesions <3.0 cm (8). Virtual bronchoscopy may further improve the yield of the ultrathin flexible bronchoscope. Virtual bronchoscopy can obtain a three-dimensional image of the tracheobronchial tree by using 1.0 mm sections. A virtual bronchoscopic navigational system has been described that allows for the following: animated images of bronchi that can be advanced as the bronchoscope is advanced; images that can be rotated as the bronchoscope is rotated; and a thumbnail of the images displayed as a catalog (9). Factors that improve the yield of ultrathin bronchoscopy using virtual bronchoscopic guidance include the ability to insert the ultrathin bronchoscope into the fifth or greater bronchial generation, the presence of a bronchus and pulmonary artery leading to the lesion, and the location of the lesion (10).

Although these reports describe the diagnosis of peripheral lesions, these tools can also be used to treat malignant lesions when primary modalities, such as surgery, are not feasible because of a patient's comorbid conditions, preference, or other reasons. The remainder of this chapter aims to describe techniques that can be used for the bronchoscopic treatment of peripheral lesions.

III. The Bronchoscopic Placement of Markers to Assist Resection

Several techniques are available to assist the surgeon by marking small peripheral nodules that would otherwise be difficult for the surgeon to visualize intraoperatively. These include the injection of various agents into and around nodules, such as methylene blue, radiopaque contrast, and radionuclides. Intraoperative ultrasound may be used for guidance to small lesions, as can various transthoracic approaches with fluoroscopically guided coils or CT-guided needles or hookwires (1). Davini et al. (11) described a method of radioguided surgery. Using CT guidance, they injected a solution composed of human serum albumin labeled with technetium-99 and combined with nonionic contrast. The benefits described for this solution included a longer staining duration (12 hours) compared to methylene blue (3 hours). Subsequently, CT analysis confirmed that the appropriate marking and surgical resection was then completed. They compared this method to one in which a hookwire was placed via CT-guidance into the lesion prior to resection and found comparable results. Chen and colleagues described a surgical navigational system that used computer technology similar to the electromagnetic bronchoscopy navigational systems (12). With this, a 16-gauge needle with a positioning sensor was advanced into or immediately adjacent to a lesion and methylene blue was then injected for subsequent identification by the surgeons. All lesions were successfully resected.

Whereas these radiologic techniques are valuable, bronchoscopic techniques may also be employed to mark tumors for excision and enable the surgeon to prepare for the operation ahead of time. One such method combines flexible bronchoscopy with fluoroscopic and CT guidance. Using fluoroscopic CT-guidance, the bronchoscope was used to advance a Teflon sheath through the tumor and to the visceral pleura (13). Indigo carmine (0.5 mL) was then injected with the CT used to confirm the location of the injected site. Tumors were successfully marked for excision, and it was felt that this technique caused less complication than localization via the transcutaneous approach.

Transbronchial needle injection has also been described for preoperative use in patients with non-small cell lung cancer (NSCLC). Radiolabeled technetium-99 has been injected into the visualized tumor or into the most distal subsegment visualized by bronchoscopy, successfully identifying 95% of tumors with less pneumothorax rates than transthoracic approaches. The use of this method can be accomplished at the same time as evaluation of lymph nodes for potentially upstaging cancer diagnoses (13). Needle injection under guidance of electromagnetic navigation has been described in which a 25-gauge sclerotherapy needle is placed into the EWC after the locatable guide has been removed. Indigo carmine dye (1–2 mm) is injected adjacent to the pleural surface, and an additional 0.5 mL is injected in 5-mm increments by withdrawing the catheter and needle to 5-mm proximal to the lesion (14). Surgery is expected to occur in 24 to 72 hours following this injection. Other markers placed by this technique include gold fiducials and platinum coils.

More recently, Anatham et al. (15) described a technique for electromagnetic navigation bronchoscopy–guided fiducial placement for robotic stereotactic radio-surgery. Fiducial markers were able to be deployed in 89% of patients and directly into tumors in 88% of those patients. Cyberknife planning was accomplished 7 to 10 days after placement of the markers. After this time frame, 90% of the markers were still in place, which allowed radiosurgery to proceed.

Although these modalities may help to localize lesions for surgical resection, they do not address those lesions that are not felt to be amenable to surgery. In such cases, bronchoscopic modalities may provide important therapy for peripheral malignancies.

IV. Endoluminal Techniques Employed in the Periphery

Various techniques have been used to treat central endobronchial tumors. These include, but are not limited to, direct chemotherapy injection, cryotherapy, laser, electrocautery, and transbronchial needle injection. Most of these techniques are now being considered for treatment of more peripheral-based tumors.

A. Direct Injection of Chemotherapy

The direct intratumoral injection of chemotherapeutic agents differs from intravenous chemotherapy in terms of route of delivery and mode of action. Delivered by a needle (21-gauge) catheter system, this may enable not only the precise delivery of localized chemotherapy but also higher intratumoral drug levels without toxic systemic effects (16). Endobronchial cisplatin injection has been used for tissue debulking in addition to therapy for hemoptysis and postobstructive pneumonia (17). In this technique, cisplatin (50 mg/100 mL; 4 mg/cm^2) was injected weekly up to four sessions and then monthly. A clinically satisfactory result was reported in 80% of patients. Celikiglu and colleagues (18) used up to 40 mg of cisplatin for direct injection into tumors, noting clinical improvement in 19 of 23 patients. Several other studies have examined the use of other agents for endobronchial chemotherapy, as shown in Table 1. These include intratumoral ethanol, bleomycin, methotrexate, fluorouracil, and others. It is plausible therefore, that more peripheral tumors may be injected by using transbronchial or sclerotherapy needles after localizing the lesions with the bronchoscopic techniques previously described.

Adenoviral-mediated delivery of the wild-type (or normal copy) p53 has also been investigated in patients with NSCLC and p53 gene mutation. Of 12 patients receiving monthly p53 injections, 6 had significant improvement (>25%) in airway obstruction

Table 1 Chemotherapeutic Agents Other Than Cisplatin Injected Directly into Tumors

Author	Year	Number of patients	Target lesion	Agent delivered (volume)
Fujisawa et al.	1986	13	Central airway endobronchial tumor	99.5% ethanol (0.5–0.3 mL)
Sawa et al.	1999	8	Endobronchial malignancy	99% ethanol (2 mL)
Celikoglu et al.	1997	93	Tracheobronchial malignancies	50 mg/mL 5-fluorouracil; 1 mg/mL mitomycin, 10 mg/mL bleomycin, 5 mg/mL methotrexate or 2 mg/mL mitoxantrone (1–3 mL)
Liu et al.	2000	40	Advanced bronchogenic carcinoma	Carboplatin 300 mg
Celikoglu et al.	2003	65	>50% Obstruction	50 mg/mL 5-fluorouracil (0.5–1 g)
Tursz et al.	1996	6	Endobronchial lung cancer, metastatic	Recombinant adenoviral RSV beta-gal (LacZ) (2.1 mL)
Swisher et al.	1999	5	Unresectable NSCLC	Adenoviral wt p53 cDNA (3 or 10 mL)
Schuler et al.	1998	15	IIIb or IV NSCLC	Adenoviral wt p53 cDNA (SCH 58500), 1 mL)
Nemunaitis et al.	2000	7	Endobronchial NSCLC	Adenoviral wt p53 cDNA (3 or 10 mL)
Weill et al.	2000	12	Endobronchial NSCLC	Adenoviral wt p53 cDNA (3 or 10 mL)
Schuler et al.	2001	5	Unresectable NSCLC	Adenoviral wt p53 cDNA (SCH 58500) (10 mL)
Griscelli et al.	2003	12	Unresectable NSCLC	Adenoviral TG5327 (IL-2) or RSV beta-gal (LacZ)

Although used for central lesions, it is hypothesized that new technology may enable these agents to be injected into peripheral lesions.
Source: From Ref. 13.

and 3 fulfilled criteria for partial response (19). In another study, intratumoral p53 injection (three doses) was combined with six weeks of radiotherapy (up to 60 Gy). With this combined regimen, 63% of patients had biopsy-proven nonviable tumor while only 16% had viable tumor. There was a partial or complete response in 63% of patients and stable disease in another 16%, as measured by bronchoscopic and CT evaluation (20). Again, it is plausible that this could be injected into peripheral lesions identified by bronchoscopic modalities.

B. Transbronchial Brachytherapy

Brachytherapy allows for localized tumor irradiation. Models of providing brachytherapy include the direct implantation by a tumor, implantation using an injector,

CT-guided placement, and delivery through a catheter that is inserted through the bronchoscope (21). High dose rate (HDR) transbronchial brachytherapy was developed for small peripheral lung lesions (22). A transbronchial aspiration cytology needle with the tip removed was advanced to the visceral pleura, and its precise location was verified by HRCT with 2-mm slice thickness. Barium (0.2 mL) was inserted into the peripheral bronchus to enable follow-up fluoroscopically guided placement of an applicator carrying a dummy source. Frontal and lateral X rays provided coordinates for their software, PLATO-BPS (Planning Treatment Optimization–Brachytherapy Planning System, version 13.3). Seven days later, the applicator with dummy source was reinserted, and fluoroscopy confirmed placement prior to insertion of the radioactive source (iridium-192) using an HDR afterloading system. This was performed under conscious sedation (midazolam). A radiation dose of 24 Gy at a 10 mm radius from the center of the applicator was delivered in three fractions at seven-day intervals. There was no change in the tumor size after 18 months, suggesting at least a stalling of the tumor growth. In a different patient, 15 Gy of radiation was administered in one dose with a resultant decrease in the tumor size by 75% (22). In another patient, endoluminal brachytherapy was combined with external radiation therapy by using electromagnetic navigation, endobronchial ultrasound, and CT. Electromagnetic navigation was used to localize a microsensor mounted on the tip of a dedicated catheter. The catheter was placed within the working channel of the bronchoscope, and the probe was guided to the peripheral lesion. Endobronchial ultrasound confirmed that the catheter was placed within the lesion. A 6-Fr brachytherapy catheter was then inserted and brachytherapy planned by using three-dimensional reconstruction with the catheter in place. HDR brachytherapy was performed using iridium-192 as a boost three times weekly (5 Gy for a single dose) for five days. A 12-month follow-up CT and endobronchial ultrasound showed partial remission while biopsies demonstrated complete remission (23). Intratumoral cisplatin has also been used as an adjunct to endobronchial brachytherapy for patients with stage IIIB and IV lung cancer (24).

C. Bronchoscopy-Guided Radiofrequency Ablation

Radiofrequency ablation (RFA) uses an electromagnetic wave with a frequency band similar to that of a surgical scalpel and an interchange radiofrequency electric current. Percutaneous image-guided thermal ablation of stage I to II NSCLC has been described. In this, radiofrequency or microwave ablation procedures followed by standard-fraction external-beam radiation therapy or brachytherapy were evaluated. Up to 37% of patients developed pneumothoraces and 22% required chest tube placement (25). In other studies, technical failure was encountered in 37.5% of patients receiving CT-guided RFA while 20% had "major complications," including hemothorax and bronchopleural fistula (26). The most frequent complication of RFA performed by percutaneous methods is pneumothorax, often in 10–20% of patients but reported in up to 63% of patients (27,28). Although promising for treatment, the transthoracic approach may be hindered by its significant risks (27). On the other hand, RFA may be better than conventional external-beam radiation for the treatment of the high-risk individual with NSCLC (29).

Noting success but also risks associated with the transthoracic approach, there has been effort to develop RFA that can be used through the bronchoscope. Sheep were used and a standard, noncooled RFA electrode was compared to an internally cooled RFA.

The most appropriate settings for the cooled RFA were a power output of 30 W and a flow rate of 30 to 40 mL/min. The temperature of the electrode needed to ablate the lung tissue was 50°C (30). Human applications of bronchoscopic RFA for treatment of peripheral lung lesions have not yet been reported in the medical literature.

D. Bronchoscopically Placed Markers for Real-Time Radiation Therapy

Because of complications associated with radiation, including bronchial stenosis, bronchiectasis, and significant mucosal injury, real-time radiation therapy has been improved by the use of bronchoscopically placed gold markers. The three-dimensional position of a 1.0- to 2.0-mm gold marker in or near the tumor was detected using two sets of fluoroscopies every 0.03 seconds. The radiation treatment beam would irradiate the tumor only when the marker coincided with its planned position using real-time radiation. This was feasible only for peripheral tumors and 65% of the tumors were successfully treated (31).

E. Cryotherapy

Cryotherapy is the therapeutic application of extreme cold for the local destruction of living tissue. The probe, which is typically cooled to −40°C, is applied to a lesion several times to induce several cycles of cooling and thawing (21). Wang and colleagues described over 200 cases using percutaneous cryotherapy for NSCLC using 3- and 4-mm cryoprobes. In their series, 86% of masses showed reduced or stable size (32). It is conceivable that these small probes could be used through guide sheaths directly into peripheral tumors that are found by ultrasound or electronavigational guidance.

F. Photodynamic Therapy

Photodynamic therapy (PDT) is a locoregional cancer treatment in which a systemically administered photosensitizer is activated locally by illuminating a diseased tissue with light of a suitable wavelength. Recently, the use of PDT has extended from superficial or endoluminal tumors to parenchymal tumors, such as those in the liver. It is conceivable that special catheters, fibers, and photosensitizers can be developed for interstitial PDT (33). Recently, interstitial PDT of the lung was described in rats. Zones of necrosis appeared following treatment, without damaging surrounding lung. This was accomplished via a percutaneous technique using a single fiber (34). It is possible that this technique could be expanded to include multiple fibers grouped for treatment through the bronchoscope.

V. Summary

The rapid advance of technology to aide in the diagnosis of peripheral lung lesions, coupled with the ongoing development of various treatment modalities for lung cancer, provides promise for the bronchoscopic treatment of peripheral lung tumors. Whereas electromagnetic navigation, endobronchial ultrasound, virtual bronchoscopy, and ultrathin bronchoscopy can be used to diagnose lesions, they may also facilitate the placement of markers or dye for resection or radiation. The ability to navigate beyond that which is immediately bronchoscopically visible may also assist in the direct injections of chemotherapeutic agents as well as adenoviral-mediated gene therapy, brachytherapy, cryotherapy, photodynamic therapy, or even radiofrequency ablation. As the field of interventional pulmonary continues to grow, there is no doubt that the options for bronchoscopic treatment of lung cancer will simultaneously and exponentially expand to provide additional treatment options for our patients.

References

1. Eichfeld U, Dietrich A, Ott RA. Video-assisted thoracoscopic surgery for pulmonary nodules after computed tomography-guided marking with a spiral wire. Ann Thorac Surg 2005; 79: 313–317.
2. Makris D, Scherpereel A, Leroy S, et al. Electromagnetic diagnostic bronchoscopy for small peripheral lung lesions. Eur Respir J 2007; 29:1187–1192.
3. Eberhardt R, Anatham D, Herth F, et al. Electromagnetic navigation diagnostic bronchoscopy in peripheral lung lesions. Chest 2007; 131: 1800–1805.
4. McGuire FR, Kerley JM, Ochran T, et al. Radiotherapy monitoring device implantation into peripheral lung cancers: a therapeutic utility of electromagnetic navigational bronchoscopy. J Bronchol 2007; 14:189–192.
5. Asahina H, Yamazaki K, Onodera Y, et al. Transbronchial biopsy using endobronchial ultrasonography with a guide sheath and virtual bronchoscopic navigation. Chest 2005; 128: 1761–1765.
6. Kurimoto N, Miyazawa T, Okimasa S, et al. Endobronchial ultrasound using a guide sheath increases the ability to diagnose peripheral pulmonary lesions endoscopically. Chest 2004; 126:959–965.
7. Eberhart R, Anatham D, Ernst AF-K, et al. Multimodality bronchoscopic diagnosis of peripheral lung lesions: a randomized controlled trial. Am J Respir Crit Care Med 2007; 176:36–41.
8. Rooney C, Wolf K, McLennan G. Ultrathin bronchoscopy as an adjunct to standard bronchoscopy in the diagnosis of peripheral lung lesions. Respiration 2002; 69:63–68.
9. Asano F, Matsumo Y, Shinagawa N, et al. A virtual bronchoscopic navigation system for pulmonary peripheral lesions. Chest 2006; 130:559–566.
10. Shinagawa N, Yamazaki K, Onodera Y, et al. Factors related to diagnostic sensitivity using an ultrathin bronchoscope under CT guidance. Chest 2007; 131:549–553.
11. Davini F, Gonfiotti A, Vaggelli L, et al. Thoracoscopic localization techniques for patients with solitary pulmonary nodule: radioguided surgery versus hookwire localization. J Cardiovasc Surg 2006; 47:355–359.
12. Chen W, Chen L, Yang S, et al. A novel technique for localization of small pulmonary nodules. Chest 2007; 131:1526–1531.
13. Seymour CW, Krimsky WS, Kruklitis RJ, et al. Transbronchial needle injection: a systematic review of a new diagnostic and therapeutic paradigm. Respiration, 2006; 73:78–89.
14. inReach Dye Marker Placement. Available at: http://www.superdimension.com. Accessed July 6, 2009.
15. Anantham D, Feller-Kopman D, Shanmugham L, et al. Electromagnetic navigation bronchoscopy-guided fiducial placement for robotic stereotactic radiosurgery of lung tumors: a feasibility study. Chest 2007; 132:930–935.
16. Celikoglu F, Celikoglu SI, Goldberg EP. Bronchoscopic intratumoral chemotherapy of lung cancer. Lung Cancer 2008; 61:1–12.
17. Jabbardarjani H, Kharabian S, Reza Masjedi M. Endobronchial chemotherapy in malignant airway lesions of the lung. J Bronchol 2007; 14:242–245.
18. Celikoglu F, Celikoglu SI, York AM, et al. Intratumoral administration of cisplatin through a bronchoscope followed by irradiation for treatment of inoperable non-small cell obstructive lung cancer. Lung Cancer 2006; 51:225–236.

19. Weill MD, Mack MM, Roth MJ, et al. Adenoviral-mediated p53 gene transfer to non-small cell lung cancer through endobronchial injection. Chest 2000; 118:966–970.

20. Swisher SG, Roth JA, Komaki R, et al. Induction of p53-regulated genes and tumor regression in lung cancer patients after intratumoral delivery of adenoviral p53 (INGN 201) and radiation therapy. Clin Cancer Res 2003; 9:93–101.

21. Bollinger C, Mathur P. ERS/ATS statement on interventional pulmonology. Eur Respir J 2002; 19:356–373.

22. Kobayashi T, Kaneko M, Sumi M, et al. CT-assisted transbronchial brachytherapy for small peripheral lung cancer. Jap J Clin Oncol 2006; 30(2):109–112.

23. Harms W, Krempien R, Grehn C, et al. Electromagnetically navigated brachytherapy as a new treatment option for peripheral pulmonary tumors. Strahlenther Onkol 2006; 182(2): 108–111.

24. Nader DA. Intratumoral chemotherapy as an adjunct to endobronchial brachytherapy. Chest 2007; 132:459S.

25. Grieco CA, Simon CJ, Mayo-Smith WW, et al. Percutaneous image-guide thermal ablation and radiation therapy: outcomes of combined treatment for 41 patients with inoperable stage I/II non-small-cell lung cancer. J Vasc Interv Radiol 2006; 17(7):1117–1124.

26. Jin GY, Han YM, Lee YS, et al. Radiofrequency ablation using a monopolar wet electrode for the treatment of inoperable non-small cell lung cancer: a preliminary report. Korean J Radiol 2008; 9:140–147.

27. Haasbeek CJ, Senan S, Smit EF, et al. Critical review of nonsurgical treatment options for stage I non-small cell lung cancer. Oncologist 2008; 13:303–319.

28. Hiraki THG, Iishi T, Sano Y, et al. Percutaneous radiofrequency ablation for clinical stage I non-small cell lung cancer: results in 20 nonsurgical candidates. J Thorac Cardiovasc Surg 2007; 134(5):1306–1312.

29. Fernando H. Radiofrequency ablation to treat non-small cell lung cancer and pulmonary metastases. Ann Thorac Surg 2008; 85:S780–S784.

30. Sushima K, Koizumi T, Tanabe T, et al. Bronchoscopic guided radiofrequency ablation as a potential novel therapeutic tool. Eur Respir J 2007; 29:1193–1200.

31. Harada T, Shirato H, Ogura S, et al. Real-time tumor-tracking radiation therapy for lung carcinoma by the aid of insertion of a gold marker using bronchofiberscopy. Cancer 2002; 95:1720–1727.

32. Wang H, Littrup P, Duan Y, et al. Thoracic masses treated with percutaneous cryotherapy: initial experience with more than 200 procedures. Radiology 2005; 235:289–298.

33. Vogl T, Eichler K, Mack M, et al. Interstitial photodynamic laser therapy in interventional oncology. Oncology 2004; 14:1063–1073.

34. Fielding D, Buonaccorsi GM, Hanby A, et al. Fine-needle interstitial photodynamic therapy of the lung parenchyma. Chest 1999; 115:502–510.

14

Percutaneous Dilational Tracheostomy

CARLA LAMB
Lahey Clinic Medical Center, Burlington, Massachusetts, U.S.A.

I. Introduction

Tracheostomy as an open surgical procedure in the operating room setting has spanned over a hundred years and has been the classic standard approach to the airway. Percutaneous dilational tracheostomy (PDT) performed at the patient bedside has gained wide acceptance over the past 15 years (1–5). The actual technique continues to be modified, but has been based on the Seldinger technique with percutaneous serial dilations over a guidewire. Ciaglia described the initial percutaneous technique in 1985. This was further modified with the Ciaglia Blue Rhino technique using a single dilation technique. Other methods of performing PDT have been described (1–5). Most recently, a balloon dilation technique has been introduced to establish the tracheostomy tract. The advantages of PDT include the ability to avoid transport of a critically ill patient to an operating room setting, reduction in the time between decision to perform tracheostomy and actual procedure, avoiding the need for general anesthesia, as well as cost savings by avoiding the need for operative room and its personnel. There has also been more interest in performing bedside open surgical tracheostomy (OST) to provide similar benefits. PDT is a natural extension of OST but is a less invasive technique that can be performed by otolaryngologists, general surgeons, interventional pulmonologists, and intensivists. PDT has proven to be safe and effective, with complication rates comparable to OST. In many centers patient evaluation and PDT occur the same day (6–16). While the debate over patient selection, timing to tracheostomy, as well as technique continues, the need for proper procedural training along with development of a complimentary team is universally agreed upon by all specialties performing this procedure (17–20). Tracheostomy has become a relatively common procedure, provided in both the surgical and medical critical care settings for those patients requiring prolonged mechanical ventilator support because of a wide range of diseases such as extensive burns, trauma, significant cardiopulmonary disease, and neuromuscular or neurologic disease. As the general population ages, the severity of critical illness increases along with the likelihood of prolonged respiratory failure. The transition from translaryngeal intubation to tracheostomy is expected to optimize pulmonary toilet and patient comfort, to reduce the need for sedation, and to potentially improve the process of weaning from mechanical ventilator. The ability to identify specific patient parameters upon initial presentation with acute respiratory failure, which indicate those most likely to require mechanical ventilator support for greater than seven days, may allow for more timely transition to tracheostomy. Presently, there is increasing clinical data on the benefits of early tracheostomy in specific medical patient populations as well as in the trauma and surgical arena (17–28). Animal and clinical models have been developed to assess the impact of early versus late tracheostomy on the airway. Mucosal damage to the proximal airways and vocal cords can occur within three to seven days of endotracheal tube placement. Despite these data there is no universal agreement on timing to tracheostomy. There is a growing trend to advise early tracheostomy when mechanical ventilator support is anticipated for greater than 10 days. This chapter will focus on PDT with a review of the airway anatomy and procedural technique, patient selection, indications with special population considerations, contraindications, distinguishing early versus late complications, and timing of tracheostomy.

II. Overview of Anatomy

Knowledge of basic airway anatomy, along with surrounding structures of the neck, is required when approaching the patient for PDT (Figs. 1 and 2). The tracheal length is 10 to 13 cm, including 18 to 22 cartilaginous rings with an anterior-posterior diameter of 1.8 cm and lateral diameter of 2 cm. The trachea begins approximately 1.5 cm below the vocal cords. It is important to consider possible variation in this anatomy and a number of factors that may alter the usual landmarks. For example, the presence of tracheal

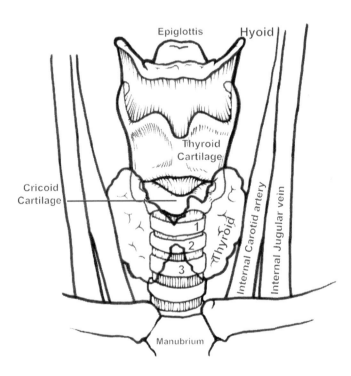

Figure 1   Important anatomic structures and landmarks (Vinald Francis medical artist).

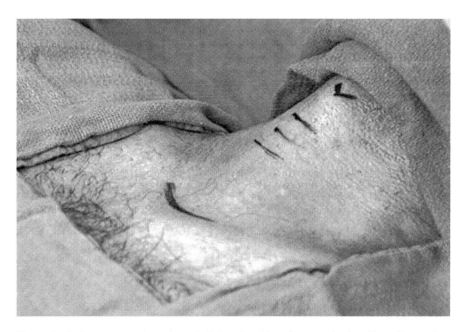

Figure 2 Patient anatomy (superior to inferior: thyroid cartilage notch, thyroid cartilage, crico-thyroid membrane, cricoid cartilage, tracheal rings, and sternal notch).

deviation, a goiter, kyphoscoliosis or obesity (BMI > 30) may impact the decision in terms of procedural approach. Ultrasound is an additional tool that may extend evaluation beyond visual inspection and palpation of standard landmarks. Ultrasound may help to avoid vascular structures such as the inferior thyroid vein, an aberrant anterior jugular vein, a high brachiocephalic vein, or even a high-riding innominate artery that might not otherwise be recognized. External visual anatomic cues and bronchoscopic tracheal anatomy must be understood and reliably recognized by the person performing the tracheostomy as well the assisting bronchoscopist. The endoscopic anatomy and entry position for the tracheostomy are the key in establishing the most optimal location for placement. This is between tracheal intercartilagenous spaces one and two or two and three. Correct placement reduces the likelihood of malposition and the incidence of tracheal stenosis (Fig. 3). Proper patient positioning is a key step in identifying these anatomic landmarks. The neck is kept somewhat hyperextended with an infrascapular towel roll and the head is maintained in a midline position. Custom tracheostomy tubes should be available for patients who are obese or morbidly obese (BMI > 30) with a deep trachea or a significantly large neck diameter. The tubes should be able to accommodate either the length from neck to trachea entry and/or the length of the distal component of the tracheostomy as a poor-fitting tube can have a significant impact on the ability to maintain adequate ventilation on the ventilator. Using the serial dilator kit, these custom tracheostomy tubes can be loaded onto the dilator and be passed during the initial PDT procedure. Additionally, patients with severe kyphoscoliosis or pectus excavatum may have anatomic distortion such that standard tracheostomy tubes may rest

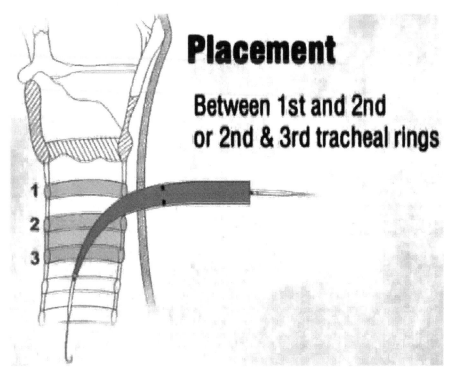

Placement

Between 1st and 2nd or 2nd & 3rd tracheal rings

Figure 3 Dilator placement demonstrating recommended entry position between tracheal cartilages. *Source*: courtesy of Cook Medical.

aberrantly in the airway and thus require special consideration in terms of tracheostomy tube placement and positioning.

III.   Patient Selection and Timing of Tracheostomy

Patient selection criteria for tracheostomy by PDT or OST are basically the same; however, there are some instances where surgical tracheostomy is superior to PDT. Patients with a large tumor or goiter obscuring palpable landmarks would be better served with a surgical approach. A patient whose thyroid cartilage and sternal notch are in such proximity that the tracheal cartilages cannot be palpated, as seen with severe kyphoscoliosis, should also be considered for OST. General indications for tracheostomy include (Table 1) an anticipated need for prolonged mechanical ventilation, improved management of respiratory secretions, relieving of upper airway obstruction, facilitating weaning from mechanical ventilation, reducing potential endotracheal tube associated laryngeal injury, improving patient comfort, reducing sedation requirements, improving mobility, allowing oral feeding, and enhancing communication and vocalization. Tracheostomy also minimizes extubation risk, and may be required before transfer to a long-term acute care facility. Contraindications to PDT can be divided

Table 1 Indications for PDT Indications (and Potential Benefits)

Prolonged mechanical ventilation: anticipated >7 days
Improved management of respiratory secretions
Relief of airway obstruction
Enhance patient comfort while weaning from mechanical ventilation (reduction of sedation
    requirements, increased mobility, enhanced communication)
Reduction of extubation risk in a known difficult airway
Failed extubation
Obviates need for transfer of a critically ill patient to the operating room for surgical tracheostomy
    (PDT and bedside surgical tracheostomies are comparable)

Table 2 Contraindications for PDT

Relative contraindications
    Unstable cervical spine
    Prior neck surgery or radiation to site
    Extensive burns to the neck
    Morbid obesity (BMI > 40)
    $FiO_2\% \geq 60\%$
    $PEEP \geq 15$
    Surgical wounds near planned site
    Large thyroid goiter or local malignancy at planned site
        Anatomic variations include severe tracheal deviation and superficial vasculature at planned
            site (ultrasound can assist to avoid these)
    Severe tracheomalacia
Absolute contraindications
    Infants
    Clinical instability
    Uncorrectable coagulopathy
    Significant infection at the anticipated site
    Emergency airway access
    Patient unlikely to survive >48 hr
    Unable to define/palpate tracheal anatomy after proper patient positioning
    Absence of informed consent
    Lack of appropriate operator training

Note that some of the traditional relative and absolute contraindications are now being reevaluated (see
section on single-center and multicenter experience).

into absolute and relative (Table 2), but as will be discussed later, some of these are
being challenged. The procedurist should evaluate each patient case by case. Operator
experience and expertise may also influence procedure selection (Tables 1 and 2).
Proper procedural training is necessary. Published guidelines from the American College of Chest Physicians (ACCP) and The American Thoracic Society/European
Respiratory Society have recommended a minimum of 20 supervised procedures to be
performed (29–30).

A designated procedural team and preprocedure planning are important. It is
helpful to have a standard checklist when evaluating the patient for PDT (Table 3). The

Table 3 Procedure Team and Preprocedure Checklist

Team members

  Procedurist (with or without assistant): Guides steps of procedure and assures safety of patient and communication of all team members

  Bronchoscopist: Inspects airway, collects any bronchoscopic samples, familiar with endoscopic landmarks to confirm puncture site and maintains control of the airway

  Bronchoscopy technician: Provides all necessary bronchoscopic equipment for procedure and specimen handling

  Bronchoscopy nurse: assists bronchoscopist in management of endotracheal tube repositioning throughout the procedure

  Respiratory therapist: confirms patient ventilator settings and provides 100% FiO_2 while reports oxygen saturation during the procedure

  ICU nurse: provides continuous assessment of the patient and provides sedation, analgesia and paralytic agents as requested

Preprocedure checklist

  Consent signed

  All coagulopathies with lab and medication list review have been addressed

  Identifies the anticipated difficult airway and has necessary reintubation equipment available

  Proper patient positioning and verifies key anatomic landmarks

  Verifies ventilator setting and oxygenation

  Initiates universal protocol and timeout

  Coordinates and communicates stepwise throughout the procedure

---

decision to perform PDT requires awareness of the so-called big picture of the clinical status of the patient and an anticipation of the potential need for the intervention. PDT can be considered as early as on day one of mechanical ventilation when anticipation for prolonged mechanical ventilation is expected. Early tracheostomy can generally be defined as between two and seven days of mechanical ventilation. Another rule of thumb is to consider tracheostomy when there is anticipation that the patient will likely require greater than 14 days of ventilator support.

IV. Technique of PDT

The technique of PDT can be described as a Seldinger method with dilations occurring over a guidewire and stylet. This section will review the most widely accepted technique and briefly review some of the variations (31–34). A stepwise approach using a pre-procedure checklist with a procedural team is ideal (Table 3). The Patient is positioned with a towel roll between the scapula, resulting in extension of the neck and improved definition of neck anatomy. Maintaining the neck and head in a midline position throughout the procedure prevents inadvertent anatomic distortion that might impact on tube placement. Universal Protocol compliance assures that all necessary staff and personnel are present and agree. It is most important to anticipate the presence of a difficult airway in the event of accidental extubation and to confirm that intubation equipment is readily available. As the majority of these patients are receiving mechanical ventilation, the technique assumes the presence of an endotracheal tube. However, a laryngeal mask airway can be safely used in selected patients. This approach might be appropriate for an outpatient with progressive neuromuscular disease requiring long-term airway management with tracheostomy. The patient should be evaluated for coagulation abnormalities and the presence of uremia. PDT can be performed if the prothrombin time/international normalized ratio (INR) is ≤1.5 times control and the platelet count is ≥50,000. If uremia is present, intravenous 1-desamino-8-D-arginine vasopressin at 0.3 μg/kg can be administered one hour prior to the procedure and again after the procedure to reduce the associated bleeding risk. Appropriate holding of anticoagulant agents and antiplatelet agents is also recommended.

Prior to sterile prep and drape, the vital landmarks are marked to maintain orientation throughout the procedure (Fig. 2). Topical anesthetic with 1% lidocaine with epinephrine within the subcutaneous tissue and pretracheal fascia is administered. The liberal use of intravenous narcotics and benzodiazepines or propofol followed by a paralytic agent prevents unnecessary movement, such as coughing because of tracheal stimulation. The patient is preoxygenated on 100% oxygen and the ventilator is placed on a set rate, pressure, or volume. Although PDT can be performed without the use of bronchoscopy, it is felt that bronchoscopy enhances optimal placement of the needle and guidewire. Direct visualization allows for immediate confirmation of tracheal entry in between 10 o'clock and 2 o'clock positions. In addition, bronchoscopy confirms entry between the first and second or second and third tracheal cartilage rings. It is important that the bronchoscopist is familiar with the endoscopic appearance of the first tracheal ring in order to position the bronchoscope well within the endotracheal tube to avoid inadvertent puncture of the bronchoscope by the introducer needle. Bronchoscopic visualization is not required during the entire procedure. Limiting bronchoscopy time avoids progressive hypercapnea or hypoxemia because of obstruction of the endotracheal tube/ventilator circuit by the scope. Bronchoscopy is best utilized during initial entry, for confirming that the direction of the guidewire is distal in the trachea, and that there is no inadvertent false tract entry during the actual tracheostomy placement. Lastly, it allows suctioning of any periprocedural bleeding or clots, and confirms final positioning of the tracheostomy in the airway. As the operators gain additional experience, the reduced time of the procedure also significantly reduces bronchoscopy time in the airway and reduces the risk of significant hypercapnea.

PDT establishes a stoma to the trachea by means of the modified Seldinger technique. This most widely used approach uses a single-dilator method, which is described below. After sterile prep and drape, topical anesthetic, intravenous sedation and analgesia, and a muscle relaxant, a 1 to 1.5-cm skin incision is made guided by the previously identified landmarks (Fig. 4). This incision may be made vertically or horizontally, and is situated over the area between the first and fourth tracheal cartilaginous rings. Often a blunt dissecting clamp can be used to gently spread the pretracheal planes of subcutaneous tissue to allow for deep palpation of the tracheal rings. This clamp can also be used to apply pressure on the anterior tracheal wall to confirm the anticipated point of entry with the bronchoscopist. The introducer needle is passed through the incision and between the tracheal rings. Airway entry is confirmed with the appearance of easily aspirated air bubbles into the saline-filled syringe attached to the introducer needle. The bronchoscopist confirms to the point of entry. Without bronchoscopic visualization, an entry into the lateral wall of the trachea might also demonstrate the air

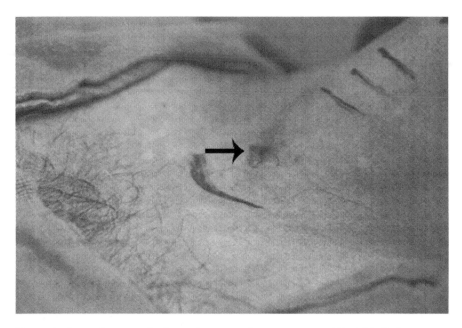

Figure 4 Anatomic entry point for tracheostomy. *Source*: courtesy of Cook Medical.

bubbles in the syringe. In this case the guidewire might feed through the lateral wall, thus creating a false tract. A guidewire is then passed into the trachea via the introducer needle, which should pass freely without resistance. The introducer needle is then removed. A punch dilator is passed over the guidewire, creating the initial tract for subsequent dilations. A small catheter is then placed over the guidewire to prevent kinking of the guidewire as the large dilator or serial dilators are inserted into the trachea, creating the stoma (Fig. 5). The tracheostomy tube is preloaded onto a dilator/ loader and passed over the guidewire and catheter into the newly established tract (Fig. 6). A balloon dilation technique as an alternative approach has been recently introduced with the idea that it may create less tissue trauma while establishing an acceptable tract; however, this new technique requires further evaluation and comparison of patient characteristics with the standard technique (Fig. 7).

V. Complications of PDT (Early Versus Late)

The complications associated with PDT are generally the same as that of surgical tracheostomy; however, those specific to PDT will be highlighted. Table 4 provides a general overview. PDT is a less invasive procedure with infrequent to rare, significant or life-threatening complications. Although complications rates of 5% to 30% have been reported, these are often not separated between self-limited complications and those requiring significant intervention (35–37). Complications most commonly reported are bleeding, infection, malposition, and stenosis. Death has been reported in 0.3% to 1.6% of cases (35–38). Case reports of lethal complications include aortic arch laceration,

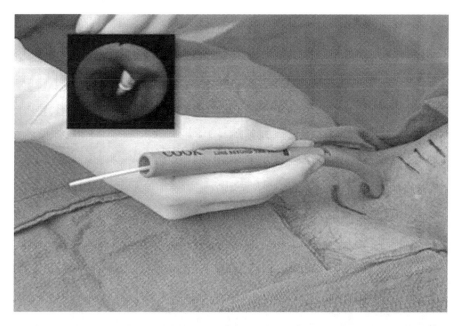

Figure 5 Dilating catheter and stylet with guidewire introduced into trachea with endoscopic view.

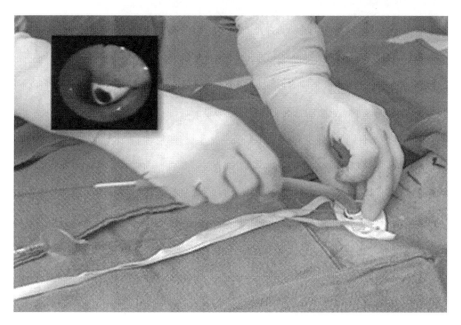

Figure 6 Tracheostomy tube over loading device with stylet and guidewire into trachea with endoscopic view. *Source*: courtesy of Cook Medical.

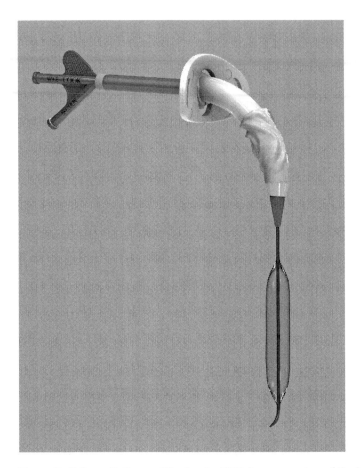

Figure 7 Balloon dilation modification for PDT. *Source*: courtesy of Cook Medical.

hemorrhage, and multifactorial hypoxemia (39–40). Other complications cited include arrhythmias, bronchospasm, transient hypoxemia or hypotension, pneumothorax, tracheal granulation tissue, subcutaneous emphysema, loss of guidewire, paratracheal insertion via a false tract, premature decannulation or extubation, tracheomalacia, fistulae of the esophagus, obstruction of the tracheostomy because of posterior tracheal wall edema, and persistent stoma. Complications should also be categorized as early or late. Often early is defined as within the first 48 hours of the procedure, whereas late and long-term complications are seen within weeks of the procedure. Many of the complications in the literature are often self-limited and require little to no intervention and therefore should be categorized as minor. Those requiring significant medical or surgical intervention would be considered as major complications. It is important to have well-established surgical backup in the event of some of these complications to insure patient safety and timely intervention.

Table 4 Complications of PDT

Early minor complications (occurring within 48 hr of procedure and requiring little to no intervention)
  Bleeding
  Hypoxemia
  Hypercapnea
  Hypotension or arrhythmia
  Bronchospasm
Early major complications
  Bleeding requiring transfusion or surgical repair
  Posterior tracheal wall puncture or tear
  Bronchoscope needle puncture during introduction of needle into trachea
  False tract or paratracheal insertion
  Pneumothorax
  Fracture of tracheal cartilage resulting in tracheal tube balloon puncture at time of procedure
    (requiring immediate replacement and repeat procedure because of immature tract)
  Obstruction of the tracheostomy tube (because of blood clot/secretions obstructing the tube or
    improper sizing of the tube or because of obstruction by the posterior tracheal wall)
  Decannulation and loss of airway
  Death
Delayed complications
  Tracheostomy tube occlusion
  Decannulation (unanticipated)
  Tracheomalacia
  Tracheoesophageal fistula
  Tracheal granulation tissue at entry site (may lead to proximal airway obstruction)
  Tracheal stenosis
  Vocal cord dysfunction
  Persistent stoma
  Aspiration and swallowing dysfunction
  Tracheoinnominate artery fistula

VI. Special Consideration in Specific Patient Populations and Extended Indications for PDT

Some conditions that were initially considered contraindications to this procedure have been reclassified because of less complications and improved patient outcomes than had been expected. It should be noted that tracheostomy is generally an elective procedure and safety guidelines should be enforced routinely. The decision to perform PDT should be individualized, and operator experience and skill will directly impact this. Some of the patient populations include obese patients, coagulopathic patients, neurosurgical patients, patients with limited cervical spine mobility, cardiothoracic patients, and burn patients. The literature suggests that in these specific populations PDT may still be performed safely without significant differences in complication rates when compared with the general population undergoing PDT (41–46). In patients where patient positioning was limited or landmark anatomy was difficult (obesity or c-spine limitations) to palpate, use of ultrasound may offer a means to perform PDT safely. Also in these patients if the thyroid cartilage can be palpated, then PDT can be safely performed.

In the cardiothoracic group there was no increased risk of mediastinitis after PDT. In burn patients, the incidence of pulmonary sepsis or local infection from PDT compared with OST was lower. In refractory coagulopathic patients, as seen in liver disease, PDT was performed safely despite an INR >1.5 and platelet counts <50,000 both on the day of the procedure and 72 hours following PDT (45). The study protocol provided blood products prior to the procedure to establish a normal INR and platelet counts greater than 50,000. Although this goal could not be uniformly achieved, when compared with those with no coagulopathy or mild coagulopathy, there were no deaths reported as a direct consequence of PDT. One of the refractory coagulopathic patients required a moderate amount of blood product support in the periprocedure period because of PDT-related bleeding; however, no surgical intervention was required. Extended indications may also include the role of PDT in emergent airway access by the skilled operator.

VII.   Review of Large Single-Center and Multicenter PDT Experiences

There are several published single-center or multicenter series of PDT experience that include both retrospective chart reviews as well as prospective database collection. One single-center report of 824 patients undergoing PDT noted that the average duration of intubation before PDT was 10 days and the mean procedure time was 15 minutes (37). The intraoperative complication rate was 6% and premature extubation was cited as the most common complication. The procedure-related death rate was 0.6%. The most common postprocedural complication was bleeding in 5%. The mean follow-up of greater than one year reported a tracheal stenosis rate of 1.6%. It was noted that that patients who did get tracheal stenosis had prolonged translaryngeal intubation prior to actual tracheostomy. The authors concluded that early time to tracheostomy may reduce the long-term potential complication of tracheal stenosis. The authors also concluded that PDT is both a safe and effective alternative to OST in those intubated patients requiring elective tracheostomy. Another group reported a multicenter prospective study of 326 patients undergoing PDT (36) and highlighted both early results and long-term outcome. The Ciaglia method was utilized. One hundred and six patients were ultimately decannulated and evaluated by plain tracheal radiography. There were two procedure-related deaths because of 0.6% and 9.5% perioperative and postoperative complications, respectively. Only one of the 106 patients who were decannulated had clinically sig-nificant tracheal stenosis at six months from initial PDT. Of patients who demonstrated some element of tracheal stenosis, 43.4% defined at least 10% reduction in the tracheal cross-sectional area. Most stenoses were felt not to be clinically significant. At our institution a retrospective database was established to specifically review early com-plications of PDT in the higher risk patient populations (47). We included those patients requiring high PEEP or who had morbid obesity, prior tracheostomy, a short neck, cervical spine traction, or coagulopathy As a result of this effort, a preprocedure checklist was created and used in each patient being evaluated for PDT. A prospective database is currently ongoing. Among our 550 patients, 40% had short neck, and 45 patients had undergone prior tracheostomy or had prior surgery at the site. There was a high rate of obesity, with 51% having a BMI of >30. Complications in the first 48 hours occurred in 4.9%. The most common complications were transient hypoxemia and bleeding; all were self-limited and minor. Of patients who had excessive bleeding, five had documented use of clopidigrel or were uremic during the hospital stay. No complication resulted in a procedure-related death. No statistically significant difference in complication rates was observed with any of the risk factors including obesity, use of anticoagulants during the same hospital stay, $FiO_2 > 50\%$, INR over 1.5 platelets less than 50,000, cervical spine traction, or PEEP > 10. However, in patients who had the combination of thrombocytopenia, uremia, and a history clopidigrel use, there was a higher incidence of bleeding complications. We found no significant difference in complication rates in patients with high-risk neck factors such as a short neck, prior neck radiation, or prior tracheostomy as long as the tracheal anatomic landmarks could be palpated. We concluded that some of the relative contraindications to PDT should be reevaluated and further studies in these patient populations regarding early and late complications should be performed to determine whether modification of current guidelines should occur.

VIII. Conclusion

PDT is both a safe and efficient procedure now widely used in the intensive care unit setting. Since its initial introduction, there have been modifications and simplification of the technique of PDT. Proper patient selection, more standardized preprocedural planning, and an experienced PDT team enhance overall success of the procedure. This procedure is comparable to the standard of OST but has a number of advantages as cited in this chapter. Further evidence-based studies will be helpful in comparing the new balloon dilation approach with the well-established Ciaglia Blue Rhino method. It will also be helpful to better define the particular characteristics of those ICU patients who will require more than seven days of mechanical ventilator support to offer them PDT in a more timely manner. Additionally, follow-up studies are needed to define the relationship between length of intubation prior to PDT and the incidence of long-term tracheal complications.

References

1. Rovner MS. Percutaneous dilatational tracheotomy. Clin Pulm Med 2001; 8(2):78–87.
2. Wahid MM, Feller-Kopman D, Ernst A. Deciding when to use percutaneous dilatational tracheostomy. J Respir Dis 2003; 24(5):195–199.
3. Cobean R, Beals M, Moss C, et al. Percutaneous dilatational tracheostomy: a safe, cost-effective bedside procedure. Arch Surg 1996; 131:265–271.
4. Polderman KH, Spijkstra JJ, de Bree R, et al. Percutaneous dilatational tracheostomy in the ICU. Chest 2003; 123:1595–1602.
5. Al-Ansari MA, Hijazi MH. Clinical review: percutaneous dilatational tracheostomy. Crit Care 2006; 10(202):1–9.
6. Paran H, Butnaru G, Hass I, et al. Evaluation of a modified percutaneous tracheostomy technique without bronchoscopic guidance. Chest 2004; 126:868–871.
7. Raghuraman G, Rajan S, Marzouk JK, et al. Is tracheal stenosis caused by percutaneous tracheostomy different from that by surgical tracheostomy? Chest 2005; 127:879–885.
8. Antonelli M, Michetti V, Di Palma A, et al. Percutaneous translaryngeal versus surgical tracheostomy: a randomized trial with 1-yr double-blind follow-up. Crit Care Med 2005; 33(5):1015–1020.
9. Freeman BD, Isabella K, Lin N, et al. A meta-analysis of prospective trials comparing percutaneous and surgical tracheostomy in critically Ill patients. Chest 2000; 118:1412–1418.

10. Grover A, Robbins J, Bendick P, et al. Open versus percutaneous dilatational tracheostomy: efficacy and cost analysis. Am Surg 2001; 67:297–302.

11. Bacchetta MD, Girardi LN, Southard EJ. Comparison of open versus bedside percutaneous dilatational tracheostomy in the cardiothoracic surgical patient: outcomes and financial analysis. Ann Thorac Surg 2005; 79:1879–1885.

12. Johnson JL, Cheatham NL, Sagraves SG. Percutaneous dilational tracheostomy: a comparison of single-versus multiple –dilator techniques. Crit Care Med 2001; 29(6):1251–1254.

13. Silvester W, Goldsmith D, Uchina S, et al. Percutaneous versus surgical tracheostomy: a randomized controlled study with long-term follow-up. Crit Care Med 2006; 34(8): 2145–2152.

14. Angel L, Simpson CB. Comparison of surgical and percutaneous dilational tracheostomy. Clin Chest Med 2003; 24:423–429.

15. Delaney A, Bagshaw SM, Nalos M. Percutaneous dilatational tracheostomy versus surgical tracheostomy in critically ill patients: a systematic review and meta-analysis. Crit Care 2006; 10:1–13.

16. Higgins K, Punthakee X. Meta-analysis comparison of open versus percutaneous tracheostomy. Laryngoscope 2007; 117:447–454.

17. Goettler CE, Fugo JR, Bard MR, et al. Predicting the need for early tracheostomy: a multifactorial analysis of 992 intubated trauma patients. J Trauma 2006; 60:991–996.

18. Clum SR, Anderson WM, Rumbak M. The timing of tracheotomy in patients requiring prolonged mechanical ventilation. J Bronchol 2008; 15(4):247–259.

19. Rumbak M, Newton M, Truncale T, et al. A prospective, randomized study comparing early percutaneous dilational tracheotomy to prolonged translaryngeal intubation (delayed tracheotomy) in critically ill medical patients. Crit Care Med 2004; 32(8):1689–1694.

20. Moller MG, Slaikeu JD, Bonelli P, et al. Early tracheostomy versus late tracheostomy in the surgical intensive care unit. Am J Surg 2005; 189:293–296.

21. Blot F, Melot C. Indications, timing, and techniques of tracheostomy in 152 french ICUs. Chest 2005; 127:1347–1352.

22. Durbin C. Indications for and timing of tracheostomy. Respir Care 2005; 50(4):483–487.

23. Shirawi N, Arabi Y. Bench to bedside review: early tracheostomy in critically ill trauma patients. Crit Care 2006; 10:1–12.

24. Maziak D, Meade MO, Todd TR. The timing of tracheotomy: a systematic review. Chest 1998; 114:605–609.

25. Hsu CL, Chen KY, Chang CH, et al. Timing of tracheostomy as a determinant of weaning success in critically ill patients: a retrospective study. Crit Care 2005; 9:46–52.

26. Arabi Y, Haddad S, Shirawi N, et al. Early Tracheostomy in intensive care trauma patients improves resource utilization: a cohort study and literature review. Crit Care 2004; 8:347–352.

27. Crofts SL, Alzeer A, McGuire GP. A comparison of percutaneous and operative tracheostomies in intensive care patients. Can J Anesth 1995; 42:775–779.

28. Chintamani JK, Singh JP, Kulshreshtha P, et al. Early tracheostomy in closed head injuries: experience at a tertiary center in a developing country—a prospective study. BMC Emerg Med 2005; 5:1–8.

29. Ernst A, Silvestri GA, Johnstone D. Interventional pulmonary procedures: guidelines from the american college of chest physicians. Chest 2003; 123(5):1693–1717.

30. Bolliger CT, Mathur PN, Beamis JF, et al. ERS/ATS statement on interventional pulmonology european respiratory society and american thoracic society. Eur Respir J 2002; 19(2):356–373.

31. Durbin CG. Techniques for performing tracheostomy. Respir Care 2005; 50(4):488–496.

32. Brambrink A. Percutaneous dilatation tracheostomy: which technique is the best for the critically ill patient, and how can we gather further scientific evidence? Crit Care 2004; 8:319–321.

33. Groves D, Durbin CG. Tracheostomy in the critically ill: indications, timing and techniques. Curr Opin Crit Care 2007; 13:90–97.

34. deBoisblanc BP. Percutaneous dilational tracheostomy techniques. Clin Chest Med 2003; 24:399–407.

35. Pandit RA, Jacques TC. Audit of over 500 percutaneous dilational tracheostomies. Crit Care Resusc 2006; 8(2):146–150.

36. Walz MK, Peitgen K, Thurauf N, et al. Percutaneous dilatational tracheostomy-early results and long-term outcome of 326 critically ill patients. Intensive Care Med 1998; 24:685–690.

37. Kearney PA, Griffen MM, Ochoa JB, et al. A single-center 8-year experience with percutaneous dilational tracheostomy. Ann Surg 2000; 231(5):701–709.

38. Beiderlinden M, Walz MK, Sander A, et al. Complications of bronchoscopically guided percutaneous dilational tracheostomy: beyond the learning curve. Intensive Care Med 2002; 28:59–62.

39. Ayoub OM, Griffiths MV. Aortic arch laceration: a lethal complication after percutaneous tracheostomy. Laryngoscope 2007; 117:176–178.

40. Shlugman D, Satya-Krishna R, Loh L. Acute fatal haemorrhage during percutaneous dilatational tracheostomy. Br J Anaesth 2003; 90:517–520.

41. Browd SR, MacDonald JD. Percutaneous dilational tracheostomy in neurosurgical patients. Neurocrit Care 2005; 2:268–273.

42. Gravvanis AI, Tsoutsos DA, Iconomou TG, et al. Percutaneous versus conventional tracheostomy in burned patients with inhalation injury. World J Surg 2005; 29:1571–1575.

43. Hubner N, Rees W, Seufert K, et al. Percutaneous dilatational tracheostomy done early after cardiac surgery- outcome and incidence of mediastinitis. Thorac Cardiovasc Surg 1998; 46:89–92.

44. Sustic A, Krstulovic B, Eskinja N, et al. Surgical tracheostomy versus percutaneous dilational tracheostomy in patients with anterior cervical spine fixation: preliminary report. Spine 2002; 17:1942–1945.

45. Auzinger G, O'Callaghan GP, Bernal W, et al. Percutaneous tracheostomy in patients with severe liver disease and a high incidence of refractory coagulopathy: a prospective trial. Crit Care 2007; 11:110–119.

46. Stamenkovic SA, Morgan IS, Pontefract DR, et al. Is early tracheostomy safe in cardiac patients with median sternotomy incisions? Ann Thorac Surg 2000; 69:1152–1154.

47. Lamb CR, Gonzalez A, Collins T, et al. A review of percutaneous dilational tracheostomy in a single center of 550 patients: reevaluation of the contraindications. Abstract/Poster 15th World Congress for Bronchology, Tokyo, Japan, March 30–April 2, 2008.

15

Training in Interventional Pulmonology

JESSICA S. WANG and GERARD A. SILVESTRI
Medical University of South Carolina, Charleston, South Carolina, U.S.A.

I. Introduction

"See one, do one, teach one" is an ever-present adage in medicine in reference to learning and teaching procedures. Essentially, this phrase implies that the physician-in-training should be proficient to perform a procedure after just one observation and to teach after just one performance. Obviously, this adage does not work in clinical practice, especially for more complicated procedures such as bronchoscopy.

With advancements in technology over the last several decades, a broad range of procedures have become available to the interventional pulmonologist. They are broadly defined as diagnostic or therapeutic procedures with applications in the pulmonary and critical care setting, as well as the otolaryngology, surgical, and anesthesia fields. With the explosion of new technologies, the field has grown to include a multitude of interventions, and with this growth has come the question of education, proficiency, and the determination of competency in this field.

II. Definition of Interventional Bronchoscopy

Interventional bronchoscopy encompasses procedures using bronchoscopic and pleuroscopic techniques to diagnose and treat a spectrum of thoracic disorders. The European Respiratory Society with the American Thoracic Society (ERS/ATS) defines interventional bronchoscopy as "the art and science of medicine as related to the performance of diagnostic and invasive therapeutic procedures that require additional training and expertise beyond that required in a standard pulmonary medicine training programme" (1). Table 1 lists the interventional pulmonology procedures described by the American College of Chest Physicians (ACCP) and the ERS/ATS (1,2).

Interventional procedures can be performed with rigid and/or flexible bronchoscopy with each having their own distinct advantage (3). Rigid bronchoscopy is used in the management of massive hemoptysis, tracheobronchial stenosis, foreign body removal, tumor resection, deeper biopsy, obstructing lesions with coring and dilation of strictures, debridement and clot removal, as well as for ventilation during bronchoscopy. Most other biopsy procedures can be performed with a flexible fiberoptic bronchoscope, but some may require specific devices such as ultrasound. TBNA is considered a "blind" biopsy of mediastinal and hilar lymph nodes, but endobronchial ultrasound with fine-needle aspiration (EBUS/FNA) allows for direct visualization of those nodes and can evaluate the depth of tumor invasion (4–12). Autofluorescence

Table 1   Interventional Procedures

Rigid bronchoscopy
Diagnostic procedures
    TBNA
    Autofluorescence
    EBUS
Treatment procedures
    Laser therapy
    Electrocautery and argon plasma coagulation
    Cryotherapy
    Brachytherapy
    Photodynamic
    Stents
Pleuroscopic procedures
    Transthoracic needle aspiration/biopsy
    Tube thoracostomy
    Pleuroscopy
    Percutaneous pleural biopsy
Oxygen therapies
    Percutaneous dilatational tracheotomy
    Tracheal oxygen therapy

bronchoscopy is used to visualize and biopsy endoluminal abnormalities that may indicate premalignant or malignant lesions (1,2).

Airway compression can be managed via flexible or rigid bronchoscopy. Neodymium:yttrium-aluminum-garnet (Nd:YAG) for laser therapy has good penetration and fair precision but has risk of endobronchial fire if the patient is on a high concentration of supplemental oxygen. Endobronchial cryotherapy does not work well on paucicellular tissue and cannot offer rapid symptomatic relief (1–3,13). Brachytherapy is effective for central airway lesions and is typically used with laser therapy or external radiation. Photodynamic therapy works by injecting the target lesion with a photosensitizing agent, but follow-up bronchoscopy is often necessary to debride the necrotic tissue (1–3,13). Silicone or plastic tracheobronchial stents are placed with rigid bronchoscopy, and expandable metallic stents can be placed with flexible bronchoscopy.

The diagnosis and management of pleural diseases and creation of artificial airways also fall under the realm of interventional bronchoscopy. Pleuroscopy is less invasive than video-assisted thoracoscopic surgery, is performed with local anesthesia and conscious sedation, and is used for evaluation of undiagnosed effusion and for pleural or lung biopsy (2,3). Pleural biopsy can also be performed percutaneously. Recurrent malignant pleural effusions causing dyspnea can be managed with tube thoracotomy using large- or small-bore, tunneled catheters (i.e., Pleurex catheters) (13). Percutaneous dilatational tracheostomy placement creates a tracheal stoma through sequential dilation, and tracheostomy tubes can be inserted with bronchoscopic guidance. Transtracheal oxygen therapy procedure used for oxygen delivery is similar to tracheostomy placement except that the stoma created is smaller (1,2,13).

Interventional bronchoscopy is wide ranging and consists of many procedures that overlap in their purpose.

III.   Current Status of Bronchoscopy Training

Bronchoscopy training has evolved over time. Stories from established pulmonologists who learned bronchoscopy less than 15 years ago often refer to their first bronchoscopy as a terrifying experience (14). Their initial introduction to a bronchoscope often occurred only moments before inserting the scope into a patient and consisted of little instruction with perhaps a few minutes of practice on a model. Current bronchoscopy training across the fields of medicine, surgery, and anesthesia has evolved in an effort to improve the safety and quality of the procedure and to give the novice bronchoscopist experience in handling the bronchoscope. There are several methods of endoscopy training that include cadaveric or animal models, nonanatomical training models, and endoscopic simulators.

The use of animal and/or human cadaver models has been studied for the teaching of bronchoscopy (15,16). Ram et al. developed a series of exercises using a pig model (16). They concluded that these exercises would not only help trainees learn and practice the basic psychomotor skills necessary to perform bronchoscopy, but also could assist a trained specialist in the maintenance of their skills. In 2006, Hatton et al. used embalmed donated cadavers to give anesthesiology residents experience with percutaneous cricothyrotomy, retrograde intubation, and fiberoptic intubation, which are invasive procedures used in the management of the difficult airway (15). Prior to this study, most of the participants did not feel comfortable at all with the first two procedures, but some had previous experience with bronchoscopy. After the study, the residents felt more comfortable performing all three procedures correctly although the difference was not significant for fiberoptic intubation because of their prior experience with bronchoscopy. The authors did agree that the use of cadavers is limited by the "inability to reproduce hemorrhage, muscle spasm, or hematoma ... [and] decreased joint and tissue mobility."

Another method that has been studied used nonanatomical models to aid in dexterity training (17). The two models studied were the "choose the hole" model and the Dexter model. The former consists of three wooden panels with labeled holes through which the bronchoscope is guided. The Dexter is a system that consists of a model that can be changed, a training manual, an image chart, and a map. The trainees practiced on the models, then performed five bronchoscopies on the other study participants. They were graded by time to visualization of various bronchial locations and by a previously validated Global Rating Scale. Participants who used the Dexter system performed better, but they had also spent more time with the models prior to performing the live bronchoscopy. Interestingly, this study did not include a control group that did not undergo model training because such a control group was considered unethical. The majority of those who learn bronchoscopy have never used any model prior to performing an initial procedure.

Simulators have garnered more notice and have been recommended for training in basic bronchoscopy. They have the advantage of not needing to use animals or human cadavers and of being able to simulate patient responses (i.e., cough, hemorrhage). While the cost of this technology is high, the hope is that it will decrease over time, making the technology available at most teaching institutions (18). The use of simulators in the aviation, aeronautics, and nuclear industries has been cited as examples of the benefit of virtual reality training. Colt et al. studied five novice fellows who underwent an eight-hour course on bronchoscopy (four hours of group instruction, followed by four hours of individual simulator practice) and compared them with four skilled physicians who had performed over 200 bronchoscopies each (19). They were evaluated on the bronchoscopy simulator and on an inanimate bronchoscopy model. Scores were based on dexterity (graded by bronchial wall collisions avoided), accuracy (defined by the number of bronchial segments entered), and speed. They found no difference in the two groups after the novices completed their training session. Another study by Blum in the cardiothoracic surgery literature showed that only an hour of training with a bronchoscopy simulator was necessary for novice PGY1 bronchoscopists to be nearly as competent as experienced residents (20). The use of simulators can also give the trainee more comfort and confidence with using the bronchoscope (21). While simulators can improve the dexterity of the bronchoscopist, other aspects of the procedure such as understanding the appropriate indications, contraindications, risks, and benefits of the procedure must be mastered.

IV. Interventional Pulmonology Training

Currently, advanced training in interventional bronchoscopy outside of a traditional pulmonary fellowship program consists of four possible pathways: (*i*) exposure and teaching during a traditional pulmonary and critical care fellowship, (*ii*) short courses of several days duration of instruction with some hands-on experience usually in an animal lab, (*iii*) mini-sabbaticals consisting of several months of more intensive training, and (*iv*) subspecialty fellowship year(s) in designated interventional pulmonology programs much like interventional cardiology. There is debate as to whether some of these methods are sufficient to gain adequate understanding and proficiency in these procedures. In an editorial in *Chest* in 1978, Dr. W. Faber, a thoracic surgeon, stated that he did not believe it was appropriate to train the occasional endoscopist and that physicians should be required to "define what they hope to accomplish in their endoscopic practice" (22). He could not have imagined the increase in the number and complexity of procedures, leading to a call for advanced training in interventional pulmonology.

The short courses that teach a specific procedure (i.e., EBUS) are ideal for those who have finished formal training and hope to incorporate new technologies into their practices. The courses typically have a didactic portion followed with some hands-on experience with simulators or animal models. A short course of simulator training for flexible bronchoscopy has been shown to be successful in teaching the technical skills needed, and perhaps this type of education could be translated into other procedures (19). The biggest drawback of these programs is the lack of real experience performing the procedure on a patient under direct supervision of an experienced interventionalist. With current guidelines, these courses cannot offer the repetition needed to become competent in these procedures.

Alternately, mini-sabbaticals are longer in duration and allow the trainee to focus solely on the procedure(s) to be learned. These several-month training courses can offer the experience needed to become "competent" in the procedures in an environment where they are performed on a regular basis. However, the drawback is that the trainee has to be in a situation to be able to take several months away from their practice, which can be expensive and impractical. In addition, institutions throughout the United States and Europe have increased the restrictions placed upon visiting trainees, making this type of instruction difficult to find.

Currently, additional subspecialty fellowship training is not mandatory for interventional pulmonology, and, where appropriate, such training can be incorporated into a traditional three-year fellowship program if the patient population is sufficient.

The initiation of dedicated year of subspecialty training in interventional pulmonology is the topic of debate based on both the expertise that can be gained and the volume that most pulmonologists will encounter. Similar fellowships exist in both cardiology and gastroenterology. They both call for an additional year of training beyond the traditional generic track with an examination required for certification. On one side of the debate is the general belief that an additional fellowship will allow the trainee to perform enough procedures to be competent, and the greater number of procedures performed translates into decreased morbidity and mortality. One survey by Haponik of 59 representative pulmonary fellows showed a wide variation in procedural exposure and in methods of training across pulmonary fellowship programs (23). Pastis et al. reviewed fellows' attitudes toward training (24). In their survey, they found that general pulmonary fellows do not feel well trained in more complex interventional procedures and that 52.7% would be interested in advanced training with 93.5% feeling that it is reasonable to require minimal numbers of supervised procedures for certification. Another survey of pulmonary fellowship directors found that the procedures to which fellows were exposed varied considerably (25). It demonstrated that some programs with a dedicated interventional pulmonologist had an increased likelihood of training in some but not all advanced procedures. But having an interventional pulmonologist did not correlate with achieving an adequate number of procedures suggested to attain competency. Thus, a dedicated interventional fellowship will allow a trainee to obtain competency, but not for every procedure. Others advantages of a dedicated interventional training program include improved scope and quality of research, better-defined standards of practice, and creation of a larger pool of interventional pulmonologists to teach within academic centers, thus advancing the field (26).

Conversely, most pulmonologists in practice do not perform advanced procedures beyond fellowship training. Most community or non-"megaclinic" institutions lack the infrastructure to support a physician performing these procedures (27), and they do not have a referral base for these interventions, which decreases the opportunity to perform them on a regular basis. Additionally, no standard of care or clear data exists to quantify or qualify competence in these advanced procedures (such as board examinations).

V. Defining Competence

The most important question for training of anything is "What defines competence?" This is a simple question without a simple answer, especially when patient safety is an issue. In school, written and oral examinations are used to assess understanding. But procedural competence not only requires the demonstration of the technical skills to complete the task, but also includes an understanding of the indications, risks, and possible complications, as well as the need for repeated performance and possibly testing of the ability to perform the procedure.

A quick and simplistic method to determine competence is to use numbers of procedures performed as an indication of acquired ability. Dull attempted to analyze proficiency in flexible fiberoptic bronchoscopy on the basis of diagnostic accuracy (28). In his study, he concluded that 100 bronchoscopies are sufficient to reach competencies. In 1982, the ACCP released their *Guidelines for Competency and Training in Fiberoptic Bronchoscopy*, stating that the "minimum number of procedures to allow one to be able to anticipate problems and complications is 50 diagnostic bronchoscopies" under supervision (29). Others have written editorials stating their opinions on adequate numbers (30). But one thoracic surgeon aptly concluded that numbers may not be sufficient to ensure competence and that the "performance of the procedure on a regular basis" is more important (31).

For interventional bronchoscopy, the ERS/ATS published their "ERS/ATS Statement on Interventional Pulmonology" in 2002, which defined the procedures, recommended the equipment and personnel necessary, described the techniques and complications, and listed the numbers of procedures performed needed to achieve and maintain competence (1). The ACCP followed in 2003 with their guidelines, which also based competence on the number of procedures performed (2) (Table 2).

Using number criteria to judge competence is based on the thought that "practice makes perfect," but repetitive practice may not fully allow the trainee to completely understand the procedure itself or the complications and management of the possible risks involved. A novice pianist may practice a song repeatedly to perfection at home, but when that pianist is playing that same song in a recital on a stage with bright lights and a crowd, the situation can complicate the musician's ability to perform well. In the same way, the ability to perform a diagnostic bronchoscopy and being able to deal with the complications that can occur during that procedure differ.

One hundred flexible bronchoscopies are recommended by the ACCP to be deemed competent in this procedure (2). It is still unclear if numbers of procedures performed can solely be used to assess the skills necessary to be considered competent. In a recent study by Crawford, only three of six trainees who had performed more than 200 flexible bronchoscopies were able to locate, identify, and enter all required bronchial segments (32). None of the trainees who had performed less than that were able to do the same. Alternately, in another study, nine novice bronchoscopists who were initially trained with a simulator were compared to nine experienced bronchoscopist who had each performed between 200 and 1000 bronchoscopies (33). The difference between them in the number of segments studied and the economy of performance disappeared after merely the second bronchoscopy, and the difference in the number of wall collisions disappeared after only five attempts. Neither study states that the ability to enter certain segments or other endpoints defines proficiency, but both used those criteria to grade the study participants.

VI. Aviation Training as a Model

As noted above, simulators in bronchoscopy have been studied as a tool to provide novice trainees an introduction to the procedures to make their initial patient contact safer. But perhaps the bronchoscopy community should take more from the aviation industry than simply the use of simulators.

In 2003, the FAA began developing the FAA Industry Training Standards (FITS) program plan that comprises various methods of training pilots. This program is

Table 2 ACCP and ERS/ATS Guidelines for Competence in Interventional Pulmonology
Procedures

	ACCP		ERS/ATS	
Procedures	Number needed for competence	Number of years to maintain competence	Number needed for competence	Number of years to maintain competence
Rigid bronchoscopy	20	10	20	10–15
TBNA	25	10	25*	
Autofluorescence	20	10	Proven expertise	
EBUS	50	20	40	25
Laser	15	10	≥20	10–15
Electrocautery and argon plasma coagulation	15	10	≥10	5–10
Cryotherapy	10	5	≥10	5–10
Brachytherapy	5	5	≥5	5–10
Photodynamic	10	5	≥10	5–10
Stents	20	10	≥10	5–10
Transthoracic needle aspiration/biopsy	10	10	≥10	5–10
Tube thoracostomy	10	5		
Pleuroscopy	20	10		
Percutaneous pleural biopsy	5	5		
Percutaneous dilatational tracheotomy	20	10	5–10	10
Tracheal oxygen therapy	10	5	≥5	≥5

* Obtain 10 positive specimens with cytology needles prior to attempting to use histology needles.

multitiered with the ultimate goal of keeping pilots up-to-date and producing training
standards. These programs include Safer Skies, which is an attempt to determine root
causes and how to break the chain of events that occur, as well as scenario-based
training (SBT) with learner-centered grading, which may be applicable to the bronchoscopy community.

In the development of SBT instruction, the FAA focused on the learning theory of
E. L. Thorndike who developed the law of readiness (basic knowledge and skills), law of
exercise (repetition and practice), and law of effect (emotional reaction of student to
stimulus as negative versus positive reinforcement) (34). Three additional laws were
used: law of primacy (learn the correct procedures at first application), law of intensity
(learning as immediate and dramatic as the real situation), and the law of recency
(training close to actual practice). Additionally, the FAA implemented several rules for
their instructors that can be applied to all training: First, the student conducts a

preprocedural plan. Second, avoid overloading the student with too many new tasks or information at one time. Third, avoid teaching very complex or important items during a time when there are other distractions. Fourth, use varying cues for teaching such as verbal, visual, and tactile. Fifth, relate new knowledge to previous understanding. And sixth, give the trainee time to process before moving onto next teaching item.

The SBT is aimed at first instructing students in the traditional didactic manner to give them basic knowledge. Then that knowledge is put into practice in simulated scenarios that are based on the learning objective. Finally, the learners would be continually evaluating themselves with learner-centered grading that consists of more than just a self-assessment of their abilities. In the FITS manual, the trainee should describe the physical characteristics and cognitive elements of the scenario, explain the concepts and procedures, plan and execute the procedure in an actual situation, and perform the procedure after gathering all the pertinent information and assessing the risks (34,35).

In the bronchoscopy community, this more comprehensive method of training can be used as an example in an effort to standardize training and introduce the trainee to a variety of situations. For example, a curriculum can be devised to teach the basic knowledge of bronchoscopy or other advanced procedures including the indications, risk, and complications. One course has been developed and is currently available online called Bronchoscopy International (www.bronchoscopy.org). It contains a four-part curriculum that takes the novice bronchoscopist through the knowledge and skills needed to learn bronchoscopy: Essential Bronchoscopist, Flexible Bronchoscopy Step by Step, the Art of Bronchoscopy, and BronchAtlas. Through self-learning and question-answer modules, the Essential Bronchoscopist section teaches the basic knowledge of bronchoscopy including anatomy and abnormalities, instrumentation, cleaning, safety, and complications. Flexible Bronchoscopy Step by Step consists of exercises for performing bronchoscopy that incorporates instructor evaluation and learner self-assessment of skill. The trainees are evaluated on the ability to traverse through the various segments of the bronchial tree and identify those segments. And in the end, the trainees do a self-evaluation of their comfort with the procedure. The Art of Bronchoscopy emphasizes the "philosophy" of bronchoscopy and the principles of the procedure, such as staying in the midline and slowing down to think before acting. In the BronchAtlas section, clinical cases are presented to teach recognition of anatomy and abnormalities, description of those abnormalities, and how to communicate. And finally, Bronchoscopy International allows bronchoscopists throughout the world to share their images and cases in the BronchAtlas. This curriculum does bring the novice through many good components to teach bronchoscopy, but simulation can add to this training course.

A bronchoscopy simulator gives the trainee practice with manual dexterity skills before performing an actual bronchoscopy on a patient. The simulator is able to make some assessments as to wall collisions, segments entered, and length of procedure, giving feedback on the correct performance (18). The simulator sessions can be designed to teach the basic procedure and offer opportunities to practice that procedure. But as one becomes more comfortable with basic bronchoscopy, other more complex scenarios can be created in a stepwise fashion to teach the student how to handle more complicated situations, such as hemorrhage or lung collapse. When the basic skills needed to perform a procedure have been obtained, the learner should be evaluated by an instructor for readiness to perform an actual bronchoscopy. The trainees should be able to assess the patient and explain to the instructor the indications and plan for the procedure before

Table 3 Components of Training

Components	Definition	Methods of obtaining
Knowledge	Understanding reasons for procedure	Web-based curriculum
	Understanding risks, benefits and complications	Textbooks
		Monographs
		Scientific publications
Anatomy	Identifying all structures germane to the procedure	Use of simulators, inanimate models, animal labs, cadavers, humans
	Identifying abnormalities	
Technical skills	Understanding equipment	Use of simulators, inanimate models, animal labs, cadavers, humans
	Knowing the procedural steps and protocols	
Practice	Mastering of procedures	Supervised and mentored performance with patients
Testing	Assessing abilities and skills	Feedback from simulator
		Written tests
		Supervised evaluation of performance

starting the procedure. They should also be able to assess any of the possible risks in a particular patient. After the procedure, both should then review the procedure together to address any issues or questions as well as to assess the execution of the procedure. This curriculum can be used for any procedure and for the novice as well as for the practicing bronchoscopists who are learning new or honing their skills. With this situation, all courses of basic and more advanced procedural training can be taught with the hope of improving procedural quality and performance (Table 3) (23).

VII. Conclusion

In summary the techniques within the field of interventional pulmonology continue to increase in number and complexity as technology advances. This heightens our awareness of the gaps that currently exist in educating clinicians to perform complex procedures. Closing this gap can be accomplished with the caveat that a "one size fits all" solution is not currently available. There are components to the mastery of any procedure that are common: a structured educational curriculum, practice on an inanimate model or simulator, supervision of cases by an experienced practitioner, and repetition. Since interventional pulmonology is a new field, drawing from the expertise of others (e.g., the aviation industry) can provide an educational framework from which to learn and teach. Programs like Bronchoscopy International that can provide the basics have already made a foray into this type of instruction. As procedures become more advanced, new modules will need to be developed. The question of competence is a constant concern for novice and seasoned bronchoscopists learning new techniques. It is overly simplistic to rely only on competency numbers for certification to perform these procedures as those criteria do not verify that the practitioner is aware of or prepared for any complications. English biologist and writer Thomas Henry Huxley once wrote, "Perhaps the most valuable result of all education is the ability to make yourself do the thing you have to do, when it ought to be done, whether you like it or not; it is the first lesson that ought to be learned; and however early a man's training begins, it is probably the last lesson that he learns thoroughly."

References

1. Bolliger CT, Mathur PN, Beamis JF, et al. ERS/ATS statement on interventional pulmonology. European Respiratory Society/American Thoracic Society. Eur Respir J 2002; 19(2): 356–373.
2. Ernst A, Silvestri GA, Johnstone D. Interventional pulmonary procedures: Guidelines from the American College of Chest Physicians. Chest 2003; 123(5):1693–1717.
3. Seijo LM, Sterman DH. Interventional pulmonology. N Engl J Med 2001; 344(10):740–749.
4. Herth F, Becker HD, Ernst A. Conventional vs endobronchial ultrasound-guided transbronchial needle aspiration: a randomized trial. Chest 2004; 125(1):322–325.
5. Herth F, Ernst A, Schulz M, et al. Endobronchial ultrasound reliably differentiates between airway infiltration and compression by tumor. Chest 2003; 123(2):458–462.
6. Herth FJ, Becker HD, Ernst A. Ultrasound-guided transbronchial needle aspiration: an experience in 242 patients. Chest 2003; 123(2):604–607.
7. Herth FJ, Rabe KF, Gasparini S, et al. Transbronchial and transoesophageal (ultrasound-guided) needle aspirations for the analysis of mediastinal lesions. Eur Respir J 2006; 28(6): 1264–1275.
8. Hurter T, Hanrath P. Endobronchial sonography: feasibility and preliminary results. Thorax 1992; 47(7):565—567.
9. Kurimoto N, Murayama M, Yoshioka S, et al. Analysis of the internal structure of peripheral pulmonary lesions using endobronchial ultrasonography. Chest 2002; 122(6):1887–1894.
10. Kurimoto N, Murayama M, Yoshioka S, et al. Assessment of usefulness of endobronchial ultrasonography in determination of depth of tracheobronchial tumor invasion. Chest 1999; 115(6):1500–1506.
11. Yasufuku K, Chiyo M, Sekine Y, et al. Real-time endobronchial ultrasound-guided transbronchial needle aspiration of mediastinal and hilar lymph nodes. Chest 2004; 126(1): 122–128.
12. Yasufuku K, Nakajima T, Chiyo M, et al. Endobronchial ultrasonography: current status and future directions. J Thorac Oncol 2007; 2(10):970–979.
13. Wahidi MM, Herth FJ, Ernst A. State of the art: interventional pulmonology. Chest 2007; 131 (1):261–274.
14. Silvestri GA. The evolution of bronchoscopy training. Respiration 2008; 76(1):19–20.
15. Hatton KW, Price S, Craig L, et al. Educating anesthesiology residents to perform percutaneous cricothyrotomy, retrograde intubation, and fiberoptic bronchoscopy using preserved cadavers. Anesth Analg 2006; 103(5):1205–1258.
16. Ram B, Oluwole M, Blair RL, et al. Surgical simulation: an animal tissue model for training in therapeutic and diagnostic bronchoscopy. J Laryngol Otol 1999; 113(2):149–151.
17. Martin KM, Larsen PD, Segal R, et al. Effective nonanatomical endoscopy training produces clinical airway endoscopy proficiency. Anesth Analg 2004; 99(3):938–944, table of contents.
18. Kvale PA, Mehta AC. Training bronchoscopists for the new era. Clin Chest Med 2001; 22(2): 365–372, ix.
19. Colt HG, Crawford SW, Galbraith O, III. Virtual reality bronchoscopy simulation: a revolution in procedural training. Chest 2001; 120(4):1333–1339.

20. Blum MG, Powers TW, Sundaresan S. Bronchoscopy simulator effectively prepares junior residents to competently perform basic clinical bronchoscopy. Ann Thorac Surg 2004; 78(1): 287–291; discussion 287–291.

21. Chen JS, Hsu HH, Lai IR, et al Validation of a computer-based bronchoscopy simulator developed in Taiwan. J Formos Med Assoc 2006; 105(7):569–576.

22. Faber LP. Bronchoscopy training. Chest 1978; 73(5 suppl):776–778.

23. Haponik EF, Russell GB, Beamis JF Jr., et al. Bronchoscopy training: current fellows' experiences and some concerns for the future. Chest 2000; 118(3):625–630.

24. Pastis NJ, Nietert PJ, Silvestri GA. Fellows' perspective of their training in interventional pulmonary procedures. J Bronchol 2005; 12:88–95.

25. Pastis NJ, Nietert PJ, Silvestri GA. Variation in training for interventional pulmonary procedures among US pulmonary/critical care fellowships: a survey of fellowship directors. Chest 2005; 127(5):1614–1621.

26. Feller-Kopman D. Is a dedicated 12-month training program required in interventional pulmonology? Pro: dedicated training. J Bronchol 2004; 11(1):62–64.

27. Gildea TR. Is a dedicated 12-month training program required in interventional Pulmonology? Con: Dedicated training. J Bronchol 2004; 11(1):65–66.

28. Dull WL. Flexible fiberoptic bronchoscopy. An analysis of proficiency. Chest 1980; 77(1): 65–67.

29. Guidelines for competency and training in fiberoptic bronchoscopy. Section on Bronchoscopy, American College of Chest Physicians. Chest 1982; 81(6):739.

30. Torrington KG. Bronchoscopy training and competency: how many are enough? Chest 2000; 118(3):572–573.

31. Rocco G, Rizzi A, Robustellini M, et al. Training and competence in bronchoscopy. The thoracic surgeon's viewpoint. Chest 1993; 103(4):1305–1306.

32. Crawford SW, Colt HG. Virtual reality and written assessments are of potential value to determine knowledge and skill in flexible bronchoscopy. Respiration 2004; 71(3):269–275.

33. Moorthy K, Smith S, Brown T, et al. Evaluation of virtual reality bronchoscopy as a learning and assessment tool. Respiration 2003; 70(2):195–199.

34. FAA Industry Training Standards (FITS). Scenario Based Training: Course Developers Guide, 2005; 1. Available at : http://www.faa.gov/training_testing/training/fits.

35. FAA-Industry Training Standards (FITS). Program Plan, 2003; 2.3.

16
Role of Bronchoscopy in Transplant Patients

CHRISTOPHE VON GARNIER
Bern University Hospital, Bern, Switzerland

PRASHANT CHHAJED
Department of Pulmonology and Centre for Sleep Studies, Fortis Hiranandani Hospital, Vashi, Navi Mumbai, India

I. Introduction

The number of patients with lung, other solid organ, and hematopoietic stem cell transplantation (HSCT) is steadily increasing in many countries. Overall prognosis has improved with evolving immunosuppressive regimens, surveillance protocols, as well as diagnosis and treatment of pulmonary complications. Bronchoscopy remains a key investigation to diagnose infectious and noninfectious transplantation-related conditions and treat complications in the lung graft.

II. Flexible Bronchoscopy—Technical Review

Flexible bronchoscopy (FB) is routinely performed under moderate sedation and local anesthetic to perform an inspection, bronchoalveolar lavage (BAL), mucosal biopsy, transbronchial biopsy (TBB), and/or transbronchial needle aspiration.

A. Premedication and Sedation

In most centers, premedication for FB is usually limited to inhalation with short-acting bronchodilators in patients with obstructive pulmonary disease (1). Preinterventional administration of atropine is not routinely recommended because of nonsignificant differences in bronchodilation, secretions, use of normal saline, bleeding, desaturation, and arrhythmias (2,3). In general, the aims of an appropriate sedation are to maintain adequate patient comfort while safely performing bronchoscopy. Patient acceptance of bronchoscopy is directly related to the appropriateness of the sedation—if insufficient, 60% of patients find it unpleasant and 25% refuse to have a repeat investigation (3–5). An emerging modern concept for endoscopy is the continuum of sedation, in which patients shift between different sedation levels as required, from minimal sedation/anxiolysis, to moderate sedation/analgesia (formerly referred to as conscious sedation), and to deep sedation/analgesia (6). For bronchoscopy, the most appropriate level of sedation is moderate sedation/analgesia, defined as a medication-induced depression of consciousness during which the patient purposefully responds to verbal commands, no specific interventions are required to maintain a patent airway, spontaneous ventilation is appropriately maintained, and cardiovascular function is stable (6). Generally, a benzodiazepine (e.g., midazolam) combined with an opiate (e.g., fentanyl) to induce sedation and analgesia/cough suppression, respectively, is titrated to achieve the desired depth of sedation/analgesia. There is an increased requirement for drugs in patients with cystic fibrosis, lung transplantation, or HSCT (7,8). In such patients, propofol may be a drug of choice to obtain adequate sedation for bronchoscopy (7). Patients with HIV and drug abuse may also need higher doses of sedation during bronchoscopy (7).

B. Monitoring During Bronchoscopy

During bronchoscopy, patients are continuously monitored with pulse oximetry to assess oxygen requirements. Lung transplant recipients are at particular risk for desaturation events during FB for several reasons: sedation-related central respiratory depression, allograft dysfunction, and upper or central airway obstruction (9). Patients with severe heart disease or significant hypoxia should also be monitored with an ECG to detect arrhythmias. Though transcutaneous carbon dioxide monitoring during bronchoscopy is feasible, patient groups that benefit from this measurement still need to be clearly defined (10). As patients with lung, other solid organ, or HSCT may present with significant pulmonary impairment that require a diagnostic FB, cautious monitoring is essential during the procedure to guarantee maximal safety.

C. Bronchoalveolar Lavage

Performing BAL allows obtaining a microbiological sample and the cellular composition of the alveolar space in a specific lobe or segment of interest. Typically, in lung transplant recipients, a lavage sample is sent routinely for cytology, aerobic culture, and fungal studies at every bronchoscopy. During the procedure, the bronchoscope is wedged in a segmental or subsegmental bronchus, followed by the instillation of total of 100 mL of prewarmed normal saline, in 20 mL aliquots that is subsequently aspirated for further examination. The technique for performing BAL is identical in patients with lung, other organ, or HSCT. Most guidelines recommend that patients at increased risk for bleeding (uremia, immunosuppression, liver disease, coagulation disorders, or thrombocytopenia) have their platelet count and coagulation capacity (prothrombin time, partial thromboplastin time, and INR) measured prior to the intervention (11). Baseline examination of BAL fluid generally includes bacterial stain (gram, acid-fast bacilli) and immunostains for the detection of specific organisms (e.g., PCP, cytomegalovirus). A cell count is not routinely performed in transplant patients. Furthermore, staining with specific fluorochrome-labeled antibodies allows performing flow cytometric analysis for more in-depth analysis of cellular profiles (e.g., CD4+:CD8+ ratio). More recently, some centers have used BAL in IFN-γ release assays for the diagnosis of tuberculosis and the measurement of specific compounds, such as myeloperoxidase, eosinophilic cationic protein, and IL-8 in the surveillance of the lung allograft posttransplant (12,13).

D. Transbronchial Lung Biopsy

Transbronchial lung biopsy is usually performed under fluoroscopic guidance, with or without maintaining a wedge position during the entire procedure (14,15). Under uniplanar or biplanar fluoroscopic guidance, 1.8- to 2.4-mm fenestrated ellipsoid or crocodile biopsy forceps are advanced into the lung periphery to obtain parenchymal specimen from the left (usually lower lobe and lingular segments) and right (usually lower and middle lobes), or from focal radiological abnormalities (16–19). When performing TBB with the wedge technique, the bronchoscope is advanced as far as possible into a segmental/subsegmental bronchus, and the forceps extruded and guided under fluoroscopy to the periphery until a resistance is felt, retracted 1 to 2 cm, opened, and biopsy taken during expiration. When performing the wedge technique, the bronchoscope is maintained at its localization during the entire procedure, whereas without wedging during TBB the forceps is advanced under visual control into the segment of interest. In lung allograft 10 or more biopsies are recommended to minimize sampling error and enhance the diagnostic yield, whereas for other transplant patients less biopsies may be required, depending on the clinical situation (16–19). Specimens may be placed in normal saline for microbiology, but are mostly fixed in formaldehyde solution, embedded, serially cut, and stained, for example, with hematoxylin, specific immunostains (e.g., CMV and PCP), or PCR (e.g., tuberculosis) (20).

E. Balloon Dilatation and Bronchoplasty

Dilatation of strictures with a balloon may be performed either through a rigid or a flexible bronchoscope. The technique consists of advancing the balloon through the stricture and inflating it under visual or fluoroscopic control at increasing diameters in a stepwise manner. The choice of the balloon diameter is determined by the bronchoscopic inspection of the stenosis and its morphological features in CT radiographs. Different balloons and corresponding inflation devices are presently marketed—usually controlled application of 6 to 12 atm results in diameters ranging from 4 to 20 mm on predetermined balloon lengths of 40 to 80 mm. The balloon is inserted through the working channel, optimally placed within the stenosis and inflated at increasing pressures, each step being held up to one minute with cautious monitoring of blood pressure, heart rhythm, and oxygen saturation. The balloon may be inflated either with normal saline or with a radiopaque solution if fluoroscopic guidance is utilized. If required, this procedure may be repeated at several occasions until the desired result is achieved (21,22). Though rare, reported complications include pain, airway laceration, and recurrent stenosis (23).

F. Airway Stenting

Stents are tubular devices deployed in an airway to maintain its patency in conditions was extrinsic or intrinsic compression, or when both exist. A variety of stents exist on the market, though none will offer only advantages without the potential drawbacks, such as mucus plugging, migration, fracture, bacterial colonization, hemoptysis, erosion, and affordability. However, from the range of stents currently available, a suited one may be chosen that will be most appropriate for a particular situation. Broadly, these devices are categorized into silicone, metal, and hybrid stents, each with their own advantages and disadvantages (23). Metallic and hybrid stents are manufactured from nitinol, a nickel titanium alloy endowed with advantageous mechanical properties, excellent biocompatibility, and good tissue tolerance. Metallic stents can be inserted with a rigid or flexible bronchoscope, whereas placing a silicone stent always requires a rigid bronchoscope. The general procedure consists localizing and measuring the length of the stenosis and then predilatating either with a balloon or with the rigid bronchoscope. The stent is then deployed with the help of an introducer (silicone stents) or inserted with a wire-guided stent delivery system and deployed under visual or fluoroscopic control (metallic and hybrid stents).

III. Procedure-Related Complications and Management
A. Hypoxia

FB may cause hypoxia, partly because of drug-related central hypoventilation and upper airway obstruction. Additional factors causing hypoxia are airway obstruction by the FB (shunt effect), large amounts of fluid in the airways (e.g., BAL fluid and local anesthetic), and excessive suctioning. The British Thoracic Guidelines recommend maintaining oxygen saturation more than 90% to prevent cardiac arrhythmias by routine oxygen supplementation during the procedure (11). The simple insertion of a nasopharyngeal tube and transient withdrawal of the bronchoscope during procedures reversed 88% of the hypoxic events, as these are mostly related to upper airway obstruction (9). Patients who did not respond to this effective measure received pharmacological reversal of their sedation or manual bag ventilation, and rarely endotracheal intubation with ventilation (9). Though optional, the availability of an anesthetist, propofol, back-up rigid bronchoscopy, and fluoroscopy is desirable when performing bronchoscopy (24,25). Patient's desaturation events during and prior to FB are successfully treatable with preventive insertion of a nasopharyngeal tube prior to any subsequent bronchoscopic procedure (9). The risk factors associated with hypoxia during the procedure were male gender, obstructive sleep apnea, and increased BMI.

B. Pneumothorax

Pneumothorax following FB with TBB is reported to occur in 1% to 6% of cases and up to 14% in mechanically ventilated patients (26–33). Though fluoroscopic guidance for TBB did not decrease pneumothorax rates, it is recommended for the biopsy of localized lung lesions (11,34–36). About half of the patients with post-TBB pneumothorax required drainage with a chest tube (32,37). Most bronchoscopists will perform a routine CXR one hour after the procedure to exclude a pneumothorax, as suggested by the BTS guidelines (11). This approach has recently been challenged by a study that analyzed 350 post-TBB, showing that the CXR confirmed a pneumothorax requiring drainage only in symptomatic patients (32). The authors suggested that only symptomatic patients require a post-TBB CXR, as pneumothoraces in asymptomatic patients were small and did not lead to chest tube placement.

C. Bleeding

Major bleeding during FB is a rare complication, reported in less than 1% of the bronchoscopies (38–40). Clinically relevant hemorrhage was more common with transbronchial than with endobronchial biopsies, especially when performed in the presence of diffuse lung disease (1.6–4.4%) (39,41,42). The risk of bleeding is higher in ventilated patients, but seems unrelated to the type of biopsy forceps utilized (33,43). Conditions commonly associated with increased risk of bleeding are uremia, pulmonary hypertension, thrombocytopenia, coagulation disorders, liver disease, and immunosuppression (44,45). Of the inhibitors for platelet aggregation, aspirin did not lead to increased bleeding complications during TBB, but clopidogrel and the combination of the two drugs were significantly associated with hemorrhages (40,46).

Most bronchscopists will employ one of three approaches, or a combination, when confronted with bleeding: (1) maintaining a wedge position in a segmental or subsegmental bronchus to tamponade the bleeding; (2) instilling ice-cold normal saline, diluted adrenaline, or glypressin (vasopressin derivative) intrabronchially via the working channel of the bronchoscope (47); (3) back-and-forth suctioning to maintain a clear vision; or (4) utilizing an endobronchial balloon (14,15,39). Furthermore, compared to the topical administration, intravenous vasopressin was equally effective but led to increased diastolic blood pressure (47). Rarely, bronchial arterial embolization or surgical procedures have to be adopted.

IV. Value of Bronchoscopy in Management of Transplant Recipients

In transplant recipients other than lung transplant, FB is generally indicated in the workup of radiographic changes under immunosuppression. In lung transplant patients, however, there are several indications for FB: (*i*) early posttransplantation; (*ii*) surveillance, diagnostic, and follow-up TBB; (*iii*) therapeutic interventions: suture removal, dilatation, laser photocoagulation, diathermy and argon plasma electrocoagulation, and stent placement; (4) research protocols.

A. Inspection in Lung Transplantation

Most centers will perform FB on day 1 to 2, day 7, and day 14 post transplant and/or prior to discharge. Visualization of the bronchial anastomoses is an essential part of any FB performed post lung transplant to detect dehiscence, defects, or signs of inflammation. As bronchial arteries are not anastomosed to the systemic arterial blood supply, posttransplant viability of the graft tracheobronchial tree relies on blood supply from the pulmonary circulation. Therefore, some degree of ischemia in the perianastomotic region extending into lobar bronchi is usually present, especially early after transplantation. Caution should apply while performing a bronchoscopy to minimize additional trauma through vigorous suction, as this may worsen mucosal ischemia. Any excess secretions should be gently cleared with saline flushes. The TEGLA scale, a classification to report ischemic injury, has been proposed, consisting of a visual grading of the following parameters: (*i*) thickness, (*ii*) extent of injury, (*iii*) granulation tissue, (*iv*) loose sutures, and (*v*) anastomotic/airway complications (48).

B. Bronchoalveolar Lavage

BAL fluid examination is a key investigation in the workup of lung radiographic changes in immunosuppressed hosts with solid organ and HSCT. BAL facilitates detection of infectious complications (bacterial, viral, fungal, protozoan) through a combination of microbiological cultures, cytological morphology, immunohistochemical stains, and molecular biology approaches such as PCR. Bacterial infections lead to a neutrophilic alveolitis with an increase in total cell counts. A differential diagnosis to be considered in the presence of neutrophilia in lung transplant (LT) recipients is rejection and bronchilitis obliterans. Lymphocytic alveolitis is the hallmark of a viral infection that usually decreases the ratio of CD4+ to CD8+ T cells because of a relative increase in CD8+ cytotoxic/suppressor T cells (49). BAL eosinophilia is usually found with fungal infection, but may also be associated with rejection, asthma, or acute eosinophilic pneumonia (50,51). BAL is sensitive for the diagnosis of *Pseudomonas aeruginosa* infections, frequently found in cystic fibrosis LT recipients and in broncholitis obliterans syndrome (52). Immunosuppression increases the risk for opportunistic infections such as *Pneumocystis jiroveci* pneumonia (formerly PCP), cytomegalovirus (CMV) pneumonitis, and invasive pulmonary aspergillosis (IPA). The prophylactic administration of trimethoprim-sulfamethoxazole (TMP-SMX) in immunosuppressed transplant recipients effectively prevents PCP infections (52–54). CMV pneumonitis is a diagnosis made on the basis of the donor/recipient organ status, serology, culture, cytomorphology, antigen detection, and PCR amplification. Serologic criteria compatible with an active CMV infection are a fourfold rise in CMV-specific IgG or newly detected IgM antibodies. Antibody tests to detect CMV antigen in cells are a rapid method to detect early CMV infection (55). PCR-based assay for the detection of CMV DNA is an additional test available in the armamentarium for CMV diagnosis, but this technique still requires standardization and validation in larger studies (56,57). *Aspergillus* colonization of the airways in the immunosuppressed host is a risk factor to develop invasive pulmonary aspergillosis, but BAL in LT patients is neither specific nor sensitive enough to be clinically useful (49). Though colonization with *Aspergillus* is common in LT patients, invasive growth occurs infrequently but causes high mortality rates (58–60). Therefore, most lung transplant centers will initiate antifungal treatment when *Aspergillus* colonization is documented in sputum, bronchial secretions, or BAL.

In patients with HSCT, the reported diagnostic yield of bronchoscopy is up to 74%, influencing therapeutic decisions in 41% of the patients (61–65). In this patient group, the reported diagnostic yield of TBB (with unrevealing BAL) is low (5–12%) and complication rates of TBB are higher (4–9%) (61,62,66–68). To our knowledge, no prospective randomized controlled trial exists to date in which the effect of routine bronchoscopy on prolonged survival of HSCT patients has been investigated, and it is questionable whether such a study will be performed in the future because of ethical issues. Most clinicians will balance empiric treatment, diagnostic uncertainty, and potentially life-threatening adverse events against the risks, moderate diagnostic yield, and low impact on treatment decisions of bronchoscopy.

C. Transbronchial Lung Biopsy

Obtaining histological samples from the lung with TBB remains a method of choice to investigate infiltrates in immunocompromized transplant patients. In particular for LT patients, TBB allows assessing the pulmonary graft for rejection and/or infection, either as a routinely performed surveillance or as a diagnostic procedure in the presence of unexplained lung functional decline (>10% reduction in FEV1), radiographic changes (infiltrates, masses, nodules), or respiratory symptoms (17,69).

The Lung Rejection Study Group (LRSG) provided a classification and grading of pulmonary allograft rejection, reporting the degree of acute rejection as the extent of perivascular mononuclear infiltrate (A descriptor), the degree of airway inflammation (B descriptor), and presence or absence of bronchiolitis obliterans, as well as chronic vascular rejection (69). Importantly, the LRSG has also recommended that at least five TBB specimen should be taken during each procedure for optimal diagnostic yield (69). Up to 20% of the biopsy specimen may be unsatisfactory because of insufficient lung parenchyma, mechanical distortion, blood clot formation, and sampling of airways only

(70,71). Most centers will routinely obtain more than 10 samples to maximize quality and minimize sampling error.

The necessity, frequency, and timing of routine surveillance TBB in LT to diagnose early rejection and CMV infection still generate controversy. In their single-center study on 81 LT recipients, Valentine et al. found no difference between a group that had received 0 to 1 TBB/BAL and those that had more than 1 TBB/BAL performed during three-year follow-up (72). Another study did not detect significant differences in BOS prior to and after ceasing routine surveillance TBB (73). On the other hand, in a large study evaluating 1235 TBB in LT recipients, the diagnostic yield for surveillance TBB in clinically stable patients was 28% in the first three months, and only 11% in the 4- to 12-month interval (17). These data are similar to a 26% diagnostic yield reported by Baz et al. in 157 surveillance TBB (74). On the basis of these observations, the risk-to-benefit ratio of surveillance TBB six months post transplant is questionable. It has recently been shown that patients who develop multiple A1 rejections develop an earlier onset of bronchiolitis obliterans and may warrant alternative immunosuppressive strategies (75).

V. Role of Interventional Bronchoscopy in Lung Transplantation

Complications in the lung allograft are still seen in 7% to 14% of LT recipients despite improved operative techniques and optimized immunosuppressive protocols (76–80). Perianastomotic ischemia leads to airway stenosis and malacia, the two most frequent complications. Operative techniques such as omental wrap, direct revascularization, forced telescoping, and discontinued steroid therapy do not alter the frequency of anastomotic problems (80). The indications for a therapeutic FB are airway stenosis, tracheobronchomalacia, obstructing granulation tissue, anastomotic dehiscence, and mucus plugging (48). Interventions performed during FB include suture removal, balloon dilatation, ablation of granulation tissue (electrocautery, laser photocoagulation), and metallic stent placement (76,81). Balloon dilation is indicated in stenotic lesions occluding more than 50% of the airway lumen that cause dypsnea, decreased lung function, and inability to clear secretions distally to the stenosis (76). Performing this procedure during FB is safe and can be repeated as required, avoiding subsequent stent insertion in up to a quarter of the patients (76). Stent placement is indicated when stenotic lesions do not respond to a couple of balloon dilation attempts, significant bronchomalacia exists, or if anastomotic dehiscence occurs. In an analysis of stent placement for 11 post-LT anastomosis complications (2 anastomosis dehiscence, 5 tracheobronchomalacia, 4 bronchial stenoses), Saad et al. reported immediate resolution of symptoms in nine patients (82%) (82). Stent-related complications, mostly minor in nature, in this series included infection (36%) and granuloma formation (27%), but only one migration and one hemoptysis. Subsequently, Mughal et al. analyzed seven patients with post-LT dehiscence successfully treated with uncovered self-expanding metallic stents (SEMS) (83). Stent insertion resulted in complete healing of the dehiscent anastomosis. Complications included three stent stenoses and one stent migration, and two patients requiring repeat stent insertion because of bronchomalacia after stent removal. Therefore, temporary utilization of SEMS in life-threatening bronchial dehiscence provides a safe and minimal invasive treatment option.

VI. Role of Bronchoscopy in Fundamental Research

FB may provide access to different anatomical compartments of the respiratory tract and allows obtaining both tissue and cells samples from these regions for research purposes. Potentially, mucosal biopsies and bronchial brushings provide samples from the main conducting airways, whereas TBB and BALF reflect the more peripheral parenchymal compartment and alveolar space. Obliterative bronchiolitis limits post-LT survival; therefore, active research in this area is of utmost importance. One in vitro method to study the biology of fibroblasts and their response to immunosuppressive drugs consists of obtaining fibroblast cultures from TBB in LT recipients (84,85). BAL fluid may be utilized to assess the composition of immune cells in the alveolar space and measure levels of cytokines, chemokines, and growth factors. Nicod et al. showed that alveolar macrophages in lung allograft displayed upregulated CD80, CD83, and CD86 during early or late rejection (86). Elevated levels of IL-6, IL-8, TGFβ, and PDGF in BAL fluid were associated with BOS (87,88). Taken together, FB provides an invaluable research tool in transplanted patients to assess the effect of immunosuppression on the respiratory tract and also provide insight into post-LT changes that affect lung allograft survival.

References

1. Stolz D, Pollak V, Chhajed PN, et al. A randomized, placebo-controlled trial of bronchodilators for bronchoscopy in patients with COPD. Chest 2007; 131(3):765–772.
2. Cowl CT, Prakash UB, Kruger BR. The role of anticholinergics in bronchoscopy. A randomized clinical trial. Chest 2000; 118(1):188–192.
3. Williams T, Brooks T, Ward C. The role of atropine premedication in fiberoptic bronchoscopy using intravenous midazolam sedation. Chest 1998; 113(5):1394–1398.
4. Macfarlane JT, Storr A, Wart MJ, et al. Safety, usefulness and acceptability of fibreoptic bronchoscopy in the elderly. Age Ageing 1981; 10(2):127–131.
5. Rees PJ, Hay JG, Webb JR. Premedication for fibreoptic bronchoscopy. Thorax 1983; 38(8): 624–627.
6. Rex DK. Review article: moderate sedation for endoscopy: sedation regimens for non-anaesthesiologists. Aliment Pharmacol Ther 2006; 24(2):163–171.
7. Chhajed PN, Wallner J, Stolz D, et al. Sedative drug requirements during flexible bronchoscopy. Respiration 2005; 72(6):617–621.
8. Chhajed PN, Aboyoun C, Chhajed TP, et al. Sedative drug requirements during bronchoscopy are higher in cystic fibrosis after lung transplantation. Transplantation 2005; 80(8): 1081–1085.
9. Chhajed PN, Aboyoun C, Malouf MA, et al. Management of acute hypoxemia during flexible bronchoscopy with insertion of a nasopharyngeal tube in lung transplant recipients. Chest 2002; 121(4):1350–1354.
10. Chhajed PN, Rajasekaran R, Kaegi B, et al. Measurement of combined oximetry and cutaneous capnography during flexible bronchoscopy. Eur Respir J 2006; 28(2):386–390.
11. British Thoracic Society guidelines on diagnostic flexible bronchoscopy. Thorax 2001; 56(suppl 1):i1–i21.
12. Glanville AR. The role of bronchoscopic surveillance monitoring in the care of lung transplant recipients. Semin Respir Crit Care Med 2006; 27(5):480–491.
13. Strassburg A, Jafari C, Ernst M, et al. Rapid diagnosis of pulmonary TB by BAL enzyme-linked immunospot assay in an immunocompromised host. Eur Respir J 2008; 31(5):1132–1135.
14. Zavala DC. Pulmonary hemorrhage in fiberoptic transbronchial biopsy. Chest 1976; 70(5): 584–588.

15. Chhajed PN, Aboyoun C, Malouf MA, et al. Risk factors and management of bleeding associated with transbronchial lung biopsy in lung transplant recipients. J Heart Lung Transplant 2003; 22(2):195–197.
16. Higenbottam T, Stewart S, Penketh A, et al. Transbronchial lung biopsy for the diagnosis of rejection in heart-lung transplant patients. Transplantation 1988; 46(4):532–539.
17. Hopkins PM, Aboyoun CL, Chhajed PN, et al. Prospective analysis of 1,235 transbronchial lung biopsies in lung transplant recipients. J Heart Lung Transplant 2002; 21(10):1062–1067.
18. Scott JP, Fradet G, Smyth RL, et al. Prospective study of transbronchial biopsies in the management of heart-lung and single lung transplant patients. J Heart Lung Transplant 1991; 10(5 pt 1):626–636; discussion 636–637.
19. Scott JP, Smyth RL, Higenbottam T, et al. Transbronchial biopsy after lung transplantation. J Thorac Cardiovasc Surg 1991; 101(5):935–937.
20. Park DY, Kim JY, Choi KU, et al. Comparison of polymerase chain reaction with histopathologic features for diagnosis of tuberculosis in formalin-fixed, paraffin-embedded histologic specimens. Arch Pathol Lab Med 2003; 127(3):326–330.
21. Chhajed PN, Malouf MA, Glanville AR. Bronchoscopic dilatation in the management of benign (non-transplant) tracheobronchial stenosis. Intern Med J 2001; 31(9):512–516.
22. Sheski FD, Mathur PN. Long-term results of fiberoptic bronchoscopic balloon dilation in the management of benign tracheobronchial stenosis. Chest 1998; 114(3):796–800.
23. Folch E, Mehta AC. Airway interventions in the tracheobronchial tree. Semin Respir Crit Care Med 2008; 29(4):441–452.
24. Chhajed PN, Glanville AR. Management of hypoxemia during flexible bronchoscopy. Clin Chest Med 2003; 24(3):511–516.
25. Chhajed PN, Aboyoun C, Malouf MA, et al. Prophylactic nasopharyngeal tube insertion prevents acute hypoxaemia due to upper-airway obstruction during flexible bronchoscopy. Intern Med J 2003; 33(7):317–318.
26. Hernandez Blasco L, Sanchez Hernandez IM, Villena Garrido V, et al. Safety of the transbronchial biopsy in outpatients. Chest 1991; 99(3):562–565.
27. Broaddus C, Dake MD, Stulbarg MS, et al. Bronchoalveolar lavage and transbronchial biopsy for the diagnosis of pulmonary infections in the acquired immunodeficiency syndrome. Ann Intern Med 1985; 102(6):747–752.
28. Milam MG, Evins AE, Sahn SA. Immediate chest roentgenography following fiberoptic bronchoscopy. Chest 1989; 96(3):477–479.
29. Frazier WD, Pope TL Jr., Findley LJ. Pneumothorax following transbronchial biopsy. Low diagnostic yield with routine chest roentgenograms. Chest 1990; 97(3):539–540.
30. Reissig A, Kroegel C. Accuracy of transthoracic sonography in excluding post-interventional pneumothorax and hydropneumothorax. Comparison to chest radiography. Eur J Radiol 2005; 53(3):463–470.
31. Ahmad M, Livingston DR, Golish JA, et al. The safety of outpatient transbronchial biopsy. Chest 1986; 90(3):403–405.
32. Izbicki G, Shitrit D, Yarmolovsky A, et al. Is routine chest radiography after transbronchial biopsy necessary?: A prospective study of 350 cases. Chest 2006; 129(6):1561–1564.
33. O'Brien JD, Ettinger NA, Shevlin D, et al. Safety and yield of transbronchial biopsy in mechanically ventilated patients. Crit Care Med 1997; 25(3):440–446.
34. Joyner LR, Scheinhorn DJ. Transbronchial forceps lung biopsy through the fiberoptic bronchoscope. Diagnosis of diffuse pulmonary disease. Chest 1975; 67(5):532–535.
35. de Fenoyl O, Capron F, Lebeau B, et al. Transbronchial biopsy without fluoroscopy: a five year experience in outpatients. Thorax 1989; 44(11):956–959.
36. Puar HS, Young RC Jr., Armstrong EM. Bronchial and transbronchial lung biopsy without fluoroscopy in sarcoidosis. Chest 1985; 87(3):303–306.

37. Pue CA, Pacht ER. Complications of fiberoptic bronchoscopy at a university hospital. Chest 1995; 107(2):430–432.
38. Pereira W Jr., Kovnat DM, Snider GL. A prospective cooperative study of complications following flexible fiberoptic bronchoscopy. Chest 1978; 73(6):813–816.
39. Cordasco EM Jr., Mehta AC, Ahmad M. Bronchoscopically induced bleeding. A summary of nine years' Cleveland clinic experience and review of the literature. Chest 1991; 100(4): 1141–1147.
40. Herth FJ, Becker HD, Ernst A. Aspirin does not increase bleeding complications after transbronchial biopsy. Chest 2002; 122(4):1461–1464.
41. Mitchell DM, Emerson CJ, Collins JV, et al. Transbronchial lung biopsy with the fibreoptic bronchoscope: analysis of results in 433 patients. Br J Dis Chest 1981; 75(3):258–262.
42. Hue SH. Complications in transbronchial lung biopsy. Korean J Intern Med 1987; 2(2): 209–213.
43. Loube DI, Johnson JE, Wiener D, et al. The effect of forceps size on the adequacy of specimens obtained by transbronchial biopsy. Am Rev Respir Dis 1993; 148(5):1411–1413.
44. Borchers SD, Beamis JF Jr. Flexible bronchoscopy. Chest Surg Clin N Am 1996; 6(2):169–192.
45. Papin TA, Lynch JP III, Weg JG. Transbronchial biopsy in the thrombocytopenic patient. Chest 1985; 88(4):549–552.
46. Ernst A, Eberhardt R, Wahidi M, et al. Effect of routine clopidogrel use on bleeding complications after transbronchial biopsy in humans. Chest 2006; 129(3):734–737.
47. Breuer HW, Charchut S, Worth H, et al. Endobronchial versus intravenous application of the vasopressin derivative glypressin during diagnostic bronchoscopy. Eur Respir J 1989; 2(3): 225–228.
48. Chhajed PN, Tamm M, Glanville AR. Role of flexible bronchoscopy in lung transplantation. Semin Respir Crit Care Med 2004; 25(4):413–423.
49. Tiroke AH, Bewig B, Haverich A. Bronchoalveolar lavage in lung transplantation. State of the art. Clin Transplant 1999; 13(2):131–157.
50. Bewig B, Stewart S, Bottcher H, et al. Eosinophilic alveolitis in BAL after lung transplantation. Transpl Int 1999; 12(4):266–272.
51. Yousem SA. Graft eosinophilia in lung transplantation. Hum Pathol 1992; 23(10):1172–1177.
52. Nunley DR, Grgurich W, Iacono AT, et al. Allograft colonization and infections with pseudomonas in cystic fibrosis lung transplant recipients. Chest 1998; 113(5):1235–1243.
53. Kramer MR, Stoehr C, Lewiston NJ, et al. Trimethoprim-sulfamethoxazole prophylaxis for Pneumocystis carinii infections in heart-lung and lung transplantation—how effective and for how long? Transplantation 1992; 53(3):586–589.
54. Green H, Paul M, Vidal L, et al. Prophylaxis for Pneumocystis pneumonia (PCP) in non-HIV immunocompromised patients. Cochrane Database Syst Rev 2007; (3):CD005590.
55. Egan JJ, Barber L, Lomax J, et al. Detection of human cytomegalovirus antigenaemia: a rapid diagnostic technique for predicting cytomegalovirus infection/pneumonitis in lung and heart transplant recipients. Thorax 1995; 50(1):9–13.
56. Barber L, Egan JJ, Lomax J, et al. A prospective study of a quantitative PCR ELISA assay for the diagnosis of CMV pneumonia in lung and heart-transplant recipients. J Heart Lung Transplant 2000; 19(8):771–780.
57. Bhorade SM, Sandesara C, Garrity ER, et al. Quantification of cytomegalovirus (CMV) viral load by the hybrid capture assay allows for early detection of CMV disease in lung transplant recipients. J Heart Lung Transplant 2001; 20(9):928–934.
58. Cahill BC, Hibbs JR, Savik K, et al. Aspergillus airway colonization and invasive disease after lung transplantation. Chest 1997; 112(5):1160–1164.
59. Nunley DR, Ohori P, Grgurich WF, et al. Pulmonary aspergillosis in cystic fibrosis lung transplant recipients. Chest 1998; 114(5):1321–1329.

60. Helmi M, Love RB, Welter D, et al. *Aspergillus* infection in lung transplant recipients with cystic fibrosis: risk factors and outcomes comparison to other types of transplant recipients. Chest 2003; 123(3):800–808.

61. Patel NR, Lee PS, Kim JH, et al. The influence of diagnostic bronchoscopy on clinical outcomes comparing adult autologous and allogeneic bone marrow transplant patients. Chest 2005; 127(4):1388–1396.

62. White P, Bonacum JT, Miller CB. Utility of fiberoptic bronchoscopy in bone marrow transplant patients. Bone Marrow Transplant 1997; 20(8):681–687.

63. Dunagan DP, Baker AM, Hurd DD, et al. Bronchoscopic evaluation of pulmonary infiltrates following bone marrow transplantation. Chest 1997; 111(1):135–141.

64. Feinstein MB, Mokhtari M, Ferreiro R, et al. Fiberoptic bronchoscopy in allogeneic bone marrow transplantation: findings in the era of serum cytomegalovirus antigen surveillance. Chest 2001; 120(4):1094–1100.

65. Glazer M, Breuer R, Berkman N, et al. Use of fiberoptic bronchoscopy in bone marrow transplant recipients. Acta Haematol 1998; 99(1):22–26.

66. Hofmeister CC, Czerlanis C, Forsythe S, et al. Retrospective utility of bronchoscopy after hematopoietic stem cell transplant. Bone Marrow Transplant 2006; 38(10):693–698.

67. Huaringa AJ, Leyva FJ, Giralt SA, et al. Outcome of bone marrow transplantation patients requiring mechanical ventilation. Crit Care Med 2000; 28(4):1014–1017.

68. Huaringa AJ, Leyva FJ, Signes-Costa J, et al. Bronchoalveolar lavage in the diagnosis of pulmonary complications of bone marrow transplant patients. Bone Marrow Transplant 2000; 25(9):975–979.

69. Yousem SA, Berry GJ, Cagle PT, et al. Revision of the 1990 working formulation for the classification of pulmonary allograft rejection: Lung Rejection Study Group. J Heart Lung Transplant 1996; 15(1 pt 1):1–15.

70. Husain AN, Siddiqui MT, Montoya A, et al. Post-lung transplant biopsies: an 8-year Loyola experience. Mod Pathol 1996; 9(2):126–132.

71. Pomerance A, Madden B, Burke MM, et al. Transbronchial biopsy in heart and lung transplantation: clinicopathologic correlations. J Heart Lung Transplant 1995; 14(4):761–773.

72. Valentine VG, Taylor DE, Dhillon GS, et al. Success of lung transplantation without surveillance bronchoscopy. J Heart Lung Transplant 2002; 21(3):319–326.

73. Tamm M, Sharples LD, Higenbottam TW, et al. Bronchiolitis obliterans syndrome in heart-lung transplantation: surveillance biopsies. Am J Respir Crit Care Med 1997; 155(5): 1705–1710.

74. Baz MA, Layish DT, Govert JA, et al. Diagnostic yield of bronchoscopies after isolated lung transplantation. Chest 1996; 110(1):84–88.

75. Hopkins PM, Aboyoun CL, Chhajed PN, et al. Association of minimal rejection in lung transplant recipients with obliterative bronchiolitis. Am J Respir Crit Care Med 2004; 170(9): 1022–1026.

76. Chhajed PN, Malouf MA, Tamm M, et al. Interventional bronchoscopy for the management of airway complications following lung transplantation. Chest 2001; 120(6):1894–1899.

77. Shennib H, Massard G. Airway complications in lung transplantation. Ann Thorac Surg 1994; 57(2):506–511.

78. Griffith BP, Hardesty RL, Armitage JM, et al. A decade of lung transplantation. Ann Surg 1993; 218(3):310–318; discussion 318–320.

79. Schafers HJ, Haydock DA, Cooper JD. The prevalence and management of bronchial anastomotic complications in lung transplantation. J Thorac Cardiovasc Surg 1991; 101(6): 1044–1052.

80. Schmid RA, Boehler A, Speich R, et al. Bronchial anastomotic complications following lung transplantation: still a major cause of morbidity? Eur Respir J 1997; 10(12):2872–2875.

81. Chhajed PN, Malouf MA, Tamm M, et al. Ultraflex stents for the management of airway complications in lung transplant recipients. Respirology 2003; 8(1):59–64.

82. Saad CP, Ghamande SA, Minai OA, et al. The role of self-expandable metallic stents for the treatment of airway complications after lung transplantation. Transplantation 2003; 75(9): 1532–1538.

83. Mughal MM, Gildea TR, Murthy S, et al. Short-term deployment of self-expanding metallic stents facilitates healing of bronchial dehiscence. Am J Respir Crit Care Med 2005; 172(6): 768–771.

84. Tamm M, Roth M, Malouf M, et al. Primary fibroblast cell cultures from transbronchial biopsies of lung transplant recipients. Transplantation 2001; 71(2):337–339.

85. Azzola A, Havryk A, Chhajed P, et al. Everolimus and mycophenolate mofetil are potent inhibitors of fibroblast proliferation after lung transplantation. Transplantation 2004; 77(2): 275–280.

86. Nicod LP, Joudrier S, Isler P, et al. Upregulation of CD40, CD80, CD83 or CD86 on alveolar macrophages after lung transplantation. J Heart Lung Transplant 2005; 24(8):1067–1075.

87. Scholma J, Slebos DJ, Boezen HM, et al. Eosinophilic granulocytes and interleukin-6 level in bronchoalveolar lavage fluid are associated with the development of obliterative bronchiolitis after lung transplantation. Am J Respir Crit Care Med 2000; 162(6):2221–2225.

88. Bergmann M, Tiroke A, Schafer H, et al. Gene expression of profibrotic mediators in bronchiolitis obliterans syndrome after lung transplantation. Scand Cardiovasc J 1998; 32(2): 97–103.

Index

ACCP. *See* American College of Chest Physicians (ACCP)

Acute respiratory distress syndrome (ARDS), 111

AIR trial. *See* Asthma Intervention Research (AIR) trial

Airway anatomy
overview, 210–212

Airway anesthesia
superior laryngeal nerve block, 174–175
transtracheal/translaryngeal injection, 175–176

Airway passages
blockade of
EBV. *See* Endobronchial valve (EBV)
endobronchial coils, 148
endobronchial occluders, mechanical, 143–148
endobronchial spigots, 143
silicone balloons, 143

Airway smooth muscle (ASM), 152
asthma and, 152–153
contraction, physiologic basis for, 153

Airway stenting, 237–238

Airway stents
choice of, 56–57
indications for, 46–47
insertion techniques, 57
overview, 45–46
types of, 47–55

5-ALA. *See* 5-aminolevulinic acid (5-ALA)

Alair® Bronchial Thermoplasty System, 152, 155

Alair catheter, 156, 157

Alair controller, 155, 156

Alfentanil, 181

α-2A. *See* Alpha-2A (α-2A)

Alpha-2A (α-2A), 179

Alveolus stent, 56

American College of Chest Physicians (ACCP), 213, 224
guidelines for competence in interventional pulmonology, 230

American Society of Anesthesiologists (ASA), 161
physical status classification, 170

American Thoracic Society (ATS), 224

American Thoracic Society/European Respiratory Society, 213

5-Aminolevulinic acid (5-ALA), 35

Analgesia
procedural sedation and, 168–169

Anesthesia
complications under, 21–22, 159–160, 169
airway, superior laryngeal nerve block, 174–175
field block, 174
local, 172–174

Angiogenic squamous dysplasia (ASD), 68

Anticoagulation, 137

Aortic allografts
tracheal transplantation with, 58

APC. *See* Argon plasma coagulation (APC)

AQLQ. *See* Asthma Quality of Life Questionnaire (AQLQ)

ARDS. *See* Acute respiratory distress syndrome (ARDS)

Argon plasma coagulation (APC), 10, 15, 16–18

ASA. *See* American Society of Anesthesiologists (ASA)

ASD. *See* Angiogenic squamous dysplasia (ASD)

ASM. *See* Airway smooth muscle (ASM)
Aspergillus, 240
Asthma
  bronchoconstriction in, 153
  pathophysiology of, ASM and, 152–153
Asthma Intervention Research (AIR)
    trial, 162
Asthma Quality of Life Questionnaire
    (AQLQ)
  responses to, 164, 165
ATS. *See* American Thoracic Society
    (ATS)
Autofluorescence bronchoscopy
  limitations of, 64–65
  literature review, 63–64
  overview, 61–63
Aviation training, 229–232

BAL. *See* Bronchoalveolar lavage (BAL)
Balloon dilatation, 237, 241
Balloon dilation
  technique, 216
Balloon-expandable stents, 52
Benign tumors
  treatment with curative intent, 11
Benzodiazepines (BZD), 173, 176–178
Biologic agents
  LVR using, 149
Biosense®, 190
Bleeding
  during FB, 238–239
  TPC insertion and, 137
Blind biopsy, 224
Brachytherapy. *See* Endobronchial
    brachytherapy (EBT)
British Thoracic Society, 173
Bronchial thermoplasty, 152–166
  histopatholology, 154
  overview of, 152–153
  patient management
    feasibility study, 162–166
    postprocedure care, 161–162
    preparation and premedication, 159
    sedation, 160–161
    topical anesthesia, 159–160
  patient selection, 158

[Bronchial thermoplasty]
  physiologic basis, 153
  preclinical studies of, 153–154
  procedure of
    equipment, 155
    overview, 155
    technique, 155–158
Bronchoalveolar lavage (BAL), 186, 236,
    239–240
Bronchogenic carcinoma, 122
Bronchoscopic lung volume reduction
    (BLVR)
  airway passages, blockade of. *See* Airway
    passages
  in COPD, 141–150
  extra-anatomical pathways, opening of,
    148–149
  techniques of, 142
Bronchoscopic thermal vapor ablation
    (BTVA), 149–150
Bronchoscopy, 1
  considerations on day of, 160
  CT fluoroscopic guidance for, 188–189
  electromagnetic navigation and guidance
    for, 190
  FB. *See* Flexible bronchoscopy (FB)
  flexible, 187
  interventional. *See* Interventional
    bronchoscopy
  placement of markers, 202–203
  RFA, 205–206
  rigid, 224
  role of, in fundamental research, 242
  simulators in, 229–232
  techniques
    peripheral pulmonary lesions and,
      diagnosis of, 186–196
    training, current status of, 226–227
    transbronchial, 204–205
    treatment of peripheral lung nodules,
      200–206
    overview, 200–202
  ultrathin, 188
  virtual, 189, 202
Bronchus Technologies Inc., 148
Bryan-Dumon Series II rigid
    bronchoscope, 5

BTVA. *See* Bronchoscopic thermal vapor ablation (BTVA)
Bupivacaine, 174
BZD. *See* Benzodiazepines (BZD)

Cancer
lung. *See* Lung cancer
CAO. *See* Central airway obstruction (CAO)
Carcinoma in situ (CIS), 63
Cardiovascular system
effects, opioids and, 181
toxicity and, 173
Catheter
blockage, 136
insertion technique, 124–131
placement of, 124
removal technique, 131
Cellulitis, 136
Cellvizio, 76
Central airway obstruction (CAO), 9
treatment of, 10
types of, 10
Central nervous system (CNS)
effects, opioids and, 180
toxicity and, 173
Chemotherapeutic agents
direct intratumoral injection of, 203–204
Chest tube pleurodesis, 133
Chronic obstructive pulmonary disease (COPD)
bronchoscopic lung volume reduction in, 141–150
Chylothorax, 135
Ciaglia Blue Rhino technique, 209
Cirrhosis, 178
CMV pneumonitis. *See* Cytomegalovirus (CMV) pneumonitis
CNS. *See* Central nervous system (CNS)
Colon cancer
Raman spectroscopy (RS), 71
Competence, 228–229
Convex probe EBUS (CP-EBUS), 87
equipment for, 88–90
procedure for, 90–92

[Convex probe EBUS (CP-EBUS)]
results for, 92–93
tip of, 89
Convulsions, 173
COPD. *See* Chronic obstructive pulmonary disease (COPD)
CP-EBUS. *See* Convex probe EBUS (CP-EBUS)
Cryoprobe, 26
Cryotherapy, 206. *See also* Endobronchial cryotherapy (ECT)
Curative intent, treatment with
benign tumors, 11
malignant tumors, 11–12
Cyberknife, 203
Cyclops forceps, 7
CYP enzymes. *See* Cytochrome P450 (CYP) enzymes
Cytochrome P450 (CYP) enzymes, 176
Cytomegalovirus (CMV) pneumonitis, 240

DAFE, 63
Deep sedation, 169
Desmethyldiazepam, 177
DEX. *See* Dexmedetomidine (DEX)
Dexmedetomidine (DEX), 179–180
Dexter system, 226
Diazepam, 177
Dilator
placement of, 212
Diode lasers
for photosensitizers, 35
Drug-induced sedation-analgesia, 169
Dumon bronchoscope, 22
Dumon stent, 48–51
comparison of, 50
placement of, 57
Dumon Y stent, 51
Dynamic stent, 51–52

EBRT. *See* External beam radiation therapy (EBRT)
EBT. *See* Endobronchial brachytherapy (EBT)

EBUS. *See* Endobronchial ultrasound (EBUS)

EBUS-GS. *See* EBUS with a guide sheath (EBUS-GS)

EBUS with a guide sheath (EBUS-GS), 194

ECT. *See* Endobronchial cryotherapy (ECT)

Electrocautery, 16–18
  clinical experience, 18
  equipment for, 16–18
  logistics for, 18
  use of, 21

Electromagnetic navigation bronchoscopy, 190, 191, 200

Emphasys Inc., 143

Emphasys one-way valve, 143

Emphysema, 141, 148

Empyema, 136

Endobronchial brachytherapy (EBT)
  complications for, 33–34
  history of, 30
  indications for, 32–33
  radiographs of, 31
  scientific basis of, 30
  technical aspects, 30–32

Endobronchial cisplatin injection, 203

Endobronchial coils, 148

Endobronchial cryotherapy (ECT)
  characteristics of, 28
  complications for, 29–30
  during flexible bronchoscopy, 28
  history of, 25
  indications for, 28–29
  for lung cancer, 28
  for removal of granulation tissue, 29
  scientific basis, 26
  technical aspects, 26–28

Endobronchial occluders
  EBV. *See* Endobronchial valve (EBV)
  endobronchial coils, 148
  endobronchial spigots, 143
  silicone balloons, 143

Endobronchial spigots, 143

Endobronchial therapy
  equipment used for, 27

Endobronchial ultrasound (EBUS), 9, 190, 192–195, 201, 205

[Endobronchial ultrasound (EBUS)]
  classification for peripheral lung lesion, 195
  types of, 86

Endobronchial valve (EBV), 143–148
  Zephyr, 143–144

Endoscopic ultrasound-guided fine-needle aspiration (EUS-FNA), 93–94
  in lymph node, 94

Endotracheal (ET) tube, 11

ERS. *See* European Respiratory Society (ERS)

ERS/ATS. *See* European Respiratory Society with the American Thoracic Society (ERS/ATS)

ET. *See* Endotracheal (ET) tube

Euphorigenic mood alteration, 178

European Respiratory Society (ERS), 224

European Respiratory Society with the American Thoracic Society (ERS/ATS), 224
  guidelines for competence in interventional pulmonology, 230

EUS-FNA. *See* Endoscopic ultrasound-guided fine-needle aspiration (EUS-FNA)

EWC. *See* Extended working channel (EWC)

Exhale Emphysema Treatment System, 148

Extended working channel (EWC), 190, 194, 200

External beam radiation therapy (EBRT), 32

Extra-anatomical pathways
  opening of, 148–149

FAA Industry Training Standards (FITS), 229

FB. *See* Flexible bronchoscopy (FB)

FCFM. *See* Fibered confocal microscopy (FCFM)

FDA. *See* Food and Drug Administration (FDA)

FDG-PET. *See* Fluoro-deoxy-glucose positron emission tomography (FDG-PET) scan

FEAT. *See* Fluorescein-enhanced autofluorescence thoracoscopy (FEAT)
Fentanyl, 161, 181–182
FEV$_1$. *See* Forced expiratory volume in one
  second (FEV$_1$)
Fibered confocal microscopy (FCFM)
  in bronchoscopy, 77
  history of, 76
  limitations of, 77–78
  literature review, 76–77
  medical system, 76
  overview, 76
Field block anesthesia, 174
FITS. *See* FAA Industry Training Standards
  (FITS)
Flexible bronchoscope
  design of, 3
  procedures performed under
    anesthesia, 22
  use of, 21
Flexible bronchoscopy (FB)
  airway stenting, 237–238
  BAL, 236
  balloon dilatation and bronchoplasty, 237
  bleeding during, 238–239
  hypoxia, 238
  monitoring during, 236
  overview, 61
  pneumothorax, 238
  premedication for, 235–236
  sedation, 235–236
  transbronchial lung biopsy, 236–237
  transplant recipients, bronchoscopy in
    management of
    BAL, 239–240
    lung transplantation, inspection in, 239
    transbronchial lung biopsy, 240–241
Flumazenil, 177
Fluorescein-enhanced autofluorescence
  thoracoscopy (FEAT), 107
Fluoro-deoxy-glucose positron emission
  tomography (FDG-PET) scan, 12
Fluoroscopy
  real-time CT, 188–189
Food and Drug Administration (FDA), 179
Forced expiratory volume in one second
  (FEV$_1$), 148

Fospropofol disodium, 179
Freeze-thaw cycles
  in ECT, 26

GABA. *See* Gamma-aminobutyric acid
  (GABA)
Gamma-aminobutyric acid (GABA), 176
Global Rating Scale, 226
Glycopyrrolate, 159

HDR. *See* High dose rate (HDR)
  brachytherapy
HDR, transbronchial brachytherapy.
  See High dose rate (HDR),
  transbronchial brachytherapy
Hematopoietic stem cell transplantation
  (HSCT), 235
Hematoporphyrin derivative, 34
Hemer bronchoscope, 6
High dose rate (HDR)
  brachytherapy, 30
  transbronchial brachytherapy, 205
High-magnification bronchovideoscopy
  (HMB), 68
Histopatholology
  bronchial thermoplasty, 154
HMB. *See* High-magnification
  bronchovideoscopy (HMB)
Hood stent, 51
HPV. *See* Hypoxic pulmonary
  vasoconstriction (HPV)
HSCT. *See* Hematopoietic stem cell
  transplantation (HSCT)
Hyoid bone, 172
Hypoproteinemia, 173
Hypoxia, 238
Hypoxic pulmonary vasoconstriction
  (HPV), 172

IBV. *See* Intrabronchial valve (IBV)
Ideal stents
  characteristics of, 46
Ikeda, Shigeto, 61
IM. *See* Intramuscular (IM) administration

Immunosuppression, 240
Infections
    as risk of TPC, 135–136
INR. *See* International normalized ratio
    (INR)
Interleukin-8, 112
International normalized ratio (INR),
    214
Interventional bronchoscopy
    advanced training in, 227–228
    competence, 228–229
    defined, 224–225
    procedures, 225
    role of, in LB, 241
Interventional pulmonology, 168
    anesthesia techniques
        local, 172–174
    equipment and personnel, 170–171
    N₂O sedation, 182–183
    patient evaluation and preparation,
        169–170
    PCS, 182
    physiology, 171
        lateral decubitus position, 171–172
    procedural sedation and analgesia,
        168–169
        BZD, 176–178
        DEX, 179–180
        ketamine, 180
        neuromuscular blockade, 183
        opioids. *See* Opioids
        pharmacology, 176–183
        propofol, 178–179
Intrabronchial valve (IBV)
    Spiration Umbrella, 144
Intraluminal bronchoscopic treatment
    with early cancer, 10
Intramuscular (IM) administration, 159
Intravenous (IV) administration, 159
Invasive pulmonary aspergillosis (IPA),
    240
IPA. *See* Invasive pulmonary aspergillosis
    (IPA)
Ir-192. *See* Iridium-192 (Ir-192)
Iridium-192 (Ir-192), 30
IV. *See* Intravenous (IV) administration

Jabbing method
    for TBNA, 86
Jackson, Chevalier, 2
Jet ventilation, 5

Ketamine, 180
Killian, Gustav, 1

LABA. *See* Long-acting β-agonists (LABA)
Laser. *See* Light amplification of stimulated
    emission of radiation (Laser)
Laser resection
    argon plasma coagulation, 15
    equipment for bronchoscopic
        applications, 14
    indications for, 15
    of recurrent endoluminal growth of
        thymoma, 13
Lateral decubitus position, 171–172
Lidocaine, 173–174
LIFE device, 63
LIFE lung system, 68
Light amplification of stimulated emission
    of radiation (Laser), 12
    equipment for bronchoscopic
        applications, 14
Liquid nitrogen, 26
Local anesthetics, 172–174
Long-acting β-agonists (LABA), 162
Lorazepam, 176
LRSG. *See* Lung Rejection Study Group
    (LRSG)
LT recipients. *See* Lung transplant (LT)
    recipients
Lung cancer
    early stage, defined, 33
    patients with
        palliative treatment, 10–11
        treatment with curative intent, 11–12
    Raman spectroscopy (RS), 71
Lung parenchyma
    biopsy technique, 110
Lung Rejection Study Group (LRSG),
    240

Lungs
  cancer, MPE and, 122
  transplantation, inspection in, 239
  trapped, 133–134
Lung transplant (LT), 239, 240
  role of interventional bronchoscopy in, 241
Lung volume reduction (LVR), 141
  using biologic agents, 149
  using thermal ablation, 149–150
Lung volume reduction surgery (LVRS), 141
LVR. *See* Lung volume reduction (LVR)
LVRS. *See* Lung volume reduction surgery (LVRS)

Malignant pleural effusion (MPE), 98, 102–104
  carcinoma metastatic to pleura, 102–104
  chylothorax and, 135
  lung cancer and, 122
  management of, 122
    pleurodesis, 123
    TPC for. *See* Tunneled pleural catheter (TPC)
  mesothelioma, 104, 134
  outpatient drainage of, 123
    costs associated with, 133
    hospitalization, 133
    insertion technique, 124–131
    patient selection, 124
    removal technique, 131
    spontaneous pleurodesis, 132–133
    symptom control, 132
  overview, 122
Malignant tumors
  treatment with curative intent, 11–12
Mallampati airway classification, 169
Markers
  placement of, bronchoscopic, 202–203
    for real-time radiation therapy, 206
Mauna Kea Technologies, 76
Medical thoracoscopy
  complications of, 111
  contradictions in, 111

[Medical thoracoscopy]
  diagnostic limitations of, 108
  in differentiating benign from malignant causes of pleural effusions, 106–107
  indications for, 98–99
  malignant pleural effusions, 102–104
  for mesothelioma, 98
  parenchymal lung disease, 107–108
  pleural biopsy technique, 108–109
  of pleural effusions of unknown etiology, 99–102
  of pleural thickening, 107
  of recurrent pneumothorax, 107
  therapeutic uses of, 111–116
  thoracoscopes, 110
  of tuberculous pleural effusions, 104–105
Meperidine, 181
Mepivacaine, 174
Mesothelioma, 134
Metallic stents
  alveolus stent, 56
  Palmaz stent, 52–53
  self-expanding stents, 53–54
  Strecker stents, 52–53
  types of, 50
  Ultraflex stents, 53–54
Microdebrider
  clinical experience, 20
  equipment for, 18–20
  rotating tip tracheal, 19
Midazolam, 161, 177
Mild exacerbations
  rate of, 162, 163
Minimal sedation, 169
Minsky, Marvin, 76
Minute ventilation, 181
Moderate sedation, 169
Monaldi–Brompton technique, 141
Mono-L-aspartyl chlorin e6 (NPe6), 36
Montgomery T-tube, 48
Morphine, 181
MPE. *See* Malignant pleural effusion (MPE)
Mycobacterium tuberculosis, 105

Naloxone, 182
Narrow-band imaging (NBI)
  color videobronchoscopes with, 67
  limitations of, 68
  literature review, 67–68
  overview, 66
  rationale, 66–67
National Cancer Center Hospital, Tokyo, 2
NBI. *See* Narrow-band imaging (NBI)
Nd:YAG. *See* Neodymium:yttrium-
    aluminum-garnet (Nd:YAG)
Nd-YAG laser, 17
Neck
  anatomic structure, 210
Neodymium:yttrium-aluminum-garnet
    (Nd:YAG), 225
Neuromuscular blockade, 183
Nitrous oxide (N$_2$O), 26
  sedation, 182–183
NMDA receptors. *See* N-methyl-D-
    aspartate (NMDA) receptors
N-methyl-D-aspartate (NMDA) receptors,
    180
Non–small cell lung cancer (NSCLC), 25,
    84, 202
Noppen stent, 51
Normeperidine, 180
N$_2$O sedation. *See* Nitrous oxide (N$_2$O)
    sedation
Nothing per os (NPO), 170
NPe6. *See* Mono-L-aspartyl chlorin e6
    (NPe6)
NPO. *See* Nothing per os (NPO)
NSCLC. *See* Non-small cell lung cancer
    (NSCLC)

OCT. *See* Optical Coherence Tomography
    (OCT)
OCT optical interferometer, 73
Olympus CF-100L colonoscope, 77
Olympus EVIS EXERA II models, 67
ONCOLIFE, 63
  in FCFM, 63
Open surgical tracheostomy (OST), 209
Opioids
  antagonism, 182

[Opioids]
  cardiovascular effects, 181
  CNS effects, 180
  fentanyl, 181–182
  naloxone, 182
  respiratory effects, 181
Optical biopsy forceps, 109
Optical coherence tomography (OCT)
  in carcinoma, 75
  in vivo study, 74
  history of, 72–73
  literature review, 73–74
  overview, 72
  in tracheobronchial disease, 73
Optical forceps, 7
OST. *See* Open surgical tracheostomy (OST)

Palliative treatment
  lung cancer, patients with, 10–11
Palmaz stent, 52–53
  placement of, 57
PaO$_2$. *See* Partial pressure of oxygen (PaO$_2$)
Papanicolaou staining, 91
Parenchymal lung disease, 107–108
Parietal pleura
  biopsy of, 108–109
Partial pressure of oxygen (PaO$_2$), 172
Patient-controlled sedation (PCS), 182
PCS. *See* Patient-controlled sedation (PCS)
PDT. *See* Photodynamic therapy (PDT)
Pentax Safe-3000, 63
Peripheral lung lesion
  EBUS classification for, 195
Peripheral lung nodules
  bronchoscopic treatment of, 200–206
    bronchoscopic placement of markers,
      202–203
    cryotherapy, 206
    direct injection of chemotherapy,
      203–204
    overview, 200–202
    PDT, 206
    radiofrequency ablation,
      bronchoscopy-guided, 205–206
    real-time radiation therapy, 206
    transbronchial brachytherapy, 204–205

Peripheral pulmonary lesions
  diagnosis of
    bronchoscopic approaches, 186, 187
    bronchoscopic techniques for, 186–196
    CT fluoroscopic guidance for
      bronchoscopy, 188–189
    electromagnetic navigation, 190, 191
    endobronchial ultrasound, 190,
      192–195
    percutaneous approach, 187
    ultrathin bronchoscopy, 188
    virtual bronchoscopy, 189
Photodynamic therapy (PDT), 12, 25, 206,
    209–221, 225
  airway anatomy, 210–212
  balloon dilation modification for, 218
  complications in, 37–38, 216, 218–219
  contraindications for, 213
  experiences
    multicenter series of, 220–221
    single-center series of, 220–221
  extended indications for, 219–220
  history of, 34
  indications for, 36–37, 213
  laser system and cylindrical diffusing tip
    used for, 35
  preprocedure checklist, 214
  procedure team, 214
  scientific basis, 34
  technical aspects of, 35–36
  technique, 214–216
  tracheostomy. *See* Tracheostomy
Photofrin II, 18
Piggyback method, 86
  for TBNA, 86
Planning Treatment Optimization–
    Brachytherapy Planning System
    (PLATO-BPS), 205
PLATO-BPS. *See* Planning Treatment
    Optimization-Brachytherapy
    Planning System (PLATO-BPS)
Pleural biopsy, 225
Pleural effusions, 99–102
  bronchoscopy, 99
  in differentiating benign from malignant
    causes of, 106–107
  studies for, 99–100

Pleural porosity, 107
Pleural thickening
  diagnosis of, 107
Pleurodesis, 111–116, 123, 134
  chest tube, 133
  spontaneous, 132–133
Pleuroscopy, 98, 225
PleurX®, 124
Pneumocystis jiroveci, 240
Pneumothorax, 136, 238
Polyethylene catheter, 30
Polyflex stent, 51
  placement of, 57
Primary spontaneous pneumothoraces
    (PSP), 107
Propofol, 178–179
Prothrombin time, 214
Pseudomonas aeruginosa, 240
PSP. *See* Primary spontaneous
    pneumothoraces (PSP)

Radial probe EBUS (RP-EBUS), 86–87
  equipment for, 87–88
  indications for, 88
  procedure for, 88
Radiofrequency ablation (RFA), 205–206
Radiofrequency monitoring devices
    (RMD), 200
Radiofrequency (RF), 152
  controller, Alair, 155
Raman effect, 69
Raman spectroscopy (RS)
  in colon cancer, 70
  history of, 69
  limitations of, 71–72
  literature review, 70–71
  in lung cancer, 71
  overview, 69
  rationale for, 69–70
Real-time radiation therapy
  markers for, bronchoscopically placed,
    206
Recurrent pneumothorax
  diagnosis of, 107
Research in Severe Asthma (RISA) trial,
    163–165

Respiratory system
  effects, opioids and, 181
RF. *See* Radiofrequency (RF)
RFA. *See* Radiofrequency ablation (RFA)
Rigid bronchoscope
  Bryan-Dumon series II, 5
Rigid bronchoscopy, 224
  design of, 3
  history of, 1–3
  new innovations in, 3–7
  overview, 1
RISA trial. *See* Research in Severe Asthma
      (RISA) trial
RMD. *See* Radiofrequency monitoring
      devices (RMD)
RP-EBUS. *See* Radial probe EBUS
      (RP-EBUS)
RS. *See* Raman spectroscopy (RS)

Safer Skies, 230
SBT. *See* Scenario-based training (SBT)
Scenario-based training (SBT), 230
Sedation, 160–161
  α-2A receptor, 179
  continuum and physiologic function, 169
  deep, 169
  minimal, 169
  moderate, 169
  N₂O, 182–183
  PCS, 182
  procedural, and analgesia, 168–169
    BZD, 176–178
    DEX, 179–180
    ketamine, 180
    neuromuscular blockade, 183
    opioids. *See* Opioids
    pharmacology, 176–183
    propofol, 178–179
    recovery after, 183–184
Self-expanding metallic stents (SEMS), 241
Self-expanding stents, 53–54
Silicone balloons, 143
Simulators
  in bronchoscopy, 229–232
Solitary pulmonary nodule (SPN), 187
Spiration®, 143
Spiration Umbrella IBV, 144

SPN. *See* Solitary pulmonary nodule (SPN)
Spontaneous pleurodesis, 132–133
Sputum cytology, 65
Staphylococcus aureus, 136
Stent, Charles, 45
Stent alert card, 57
Stent placement, 241
Storz D-Light, 63
Strecker stents, 52–53
  placement of, 57
Superior laryngeal nerve
  block, anesthesia and, 174–175
Suspension laryngoscopy, 19

Tanno, Naohiro, 72
TBB. *See* Transbronchial biopsy (TBB)
TBBX. *See* Transbronchial biopsy (TBBX)
TBNA. *See* Transbronchial needle aspirate
      (TBNA); Transbronchial needle
      aspiration (TBNA)
Texas R.I.B. bronchoscope, 6–7
Thermal energy, 21
Thoracoscopes, 110
  rigid, 110
  semi-rigid, 110
Thoracoscopic talc pleurodesis (TTP), 111
  indication for, 112
  patient selection for, 116
  side effects and complications
      of, 114–115
  techniques of, 112–113
  vs. bedside pleurodesis, 113–114
Thoracoscopy, 106, 133
TMP-SMX. *See* Trimethoprim-
      sulfamethoxazole (TMP-SMX)
Toxicity
  manifestations of lidocaine, 173
TPC. *See* Tunneled pleural catheter (TPC)
Tracheal transplantation
  with aortic allografts, 58
Tracheoscope, 4
Tracheostomy, 209
  airway anatomy, 210–212
  anatomic entry point for, 216
  patient selection criteria for, 212–214
  timing of, 212–214
Transbronchial biopsy (TBB), 235

Transbronchial biopsy (TBBX), 186
Transbronchial brachytherapy, 204–205
Transbronchial lung biopsy, 236–237,
 240–241
Transbronchial needle aspirate (TBNA),
 148
Transbronchial needle aspiration (TBNA),
 186
 bronchoscopic view of, 85
 complications for, 86
 diagnostic yield of, 86
 equipment for, 85
 penetrating techniques for, 86
 jabbing method, 86
 piggyback method, 86
 procedure for, 85–86
Transthoracic needle aspiration (TTNA),
 200
Transtracheal lidocaine injection, 175–176
Trimethoprim-sulfamethoxazole
 (TMP-SMX), 240
TTNA. *See* Transthoracic needle aspiration
 (TTNA)
TTP. *See* Thoracoscopic talc pleurodesis
 (TTP)
Tube stents
 characteristics of, 47
 dumon stent, 48–51
 dynamic stent, 51–52
 hood stent, 51
 major advantages of, 48
 montgomery T-tube, 48
 noppen stent, 51
 placement, 57
 polyflex stent, 51
Tumor seeding, 136
Tunneled pleural catheter (TPC), 122–136
 chylothorax and, 135
 mesothelioma and, 134
 for nonmalignant disease, 135
 pleural effusions, outpatient drainage of,
 123
 costs associated with, 133
 hospitalization, 133
 insertion technique, 124–131
 patient selection, 124
 removal technique, 131

[Tunneled pleural catheter (TPC)
 pleural effusions, outpatient drainage of]
 spontaneous pleurodesis, 132–133
 symptom control, 132
 risks of
 anticoagulation, difficulties
 reinitiating, 137
 bleeding, 137
 catheter blockage, 136
 infection, 135–136
 loculation of fluid, 136
 pneumothorax, 136
 tumor seeding, 136

Ultraflex stents, 53–54
 covered and uncovered, 55
 placement of, 57
Ultrasound, 211
Ultrathin bronchoscopy, 188
Universal Protocol, 214

VacLok syringe, 91
Vasoconstrictors, 172–173
VATS. *See* Video-assisted thoracic surgery
 (VATS)
Ventilation-perfusion relationship *(V/Q),*
 172
Video-assisted thoracic surgery (VATS), 99
Virtual bronchoscopy, 189, 202
Visceral pleura
 biopsy technique, 110
V/Q. See Ventilation-perfusion relationship
 (V/Q)

Wallstent, 53–54
 covered and uncovered, 54
Wolf Company, 6

Xenon lamp, 66

Zephyr®, 143
Zephyr EBV, 143–144